T0349417

DEATH OF A RACEHORSE

AN AMERICAN STORY

KATIE BO LILLIS

SIMON & SCHUSTER

NEW YORK AMSTERDAM/ANTWERP LONDON TORONTO SYDNEY/MELBOURNE NEW DELHI

Simon & Schuster
1230 Avenue of the Americas
New York, NY 10020

For more than 100 years, Simon & Schuster has championed authors and the stories they create. By respecting the copyright of an author's intellectual property, you enable Simon & Schuster and the author to continue publishing exceptional books for years to come. We thank you for supporting the author's copyright by purchasing an authorized edition of this book.

No amount of this book may be reproduced or stored in any format, nor may it be uploaded to any website, database, language-learning model, or other repository, retrieval, or artificial intelligence system without express permission. All rights reserved. Inquiries may be directed to Simon & Schuster, 1230 Avenue of the Americas, New York, NY 10020 or permissions@simonandschuster.com.

Copyright © 2025 by KBL Books LLC

All rights reserved, including the right to reproduce this book or portions thereof in any form whatsoever. For information, address Simon & Schuster Subsidiary Rights Department, 1230 Avenue of the Americas, New York, NY 10020.

First Simon & Schuster hardcover edition May 2025

SIMON & SCHUSTER and colophon are registered trademarks of Simon & Schuster, LLC

Simon & Schuster strongly believes in freedom of expression and stands against censorship in all its forms. For more information, visit BooksBelong.com.

For information about special discounts for bulk purchases, please contact Simon & Schuster Special Sales at 1-866-506-1949 or business@simonandschuster.com.

The Simon & Schuster Speakers Bureau can bring authors to your live event. For more information or to book an event, contact the Simon & Schuster Speakers Bureau at 1-866-248-3049 or visit our website at www.simonspeakers.com.

Interior design by Kyle Kabel

Manufactured in the United States of America

1   3   5   7   9   10   8   6   4   2

Library of Congress Cataloging-in-Publication Data is available.

ISBN 978-1-6680-1701-2
ISBN 978-1-6680-1703-6 (ebook)

For my mother, Robin Traywick Williams,
who taught me to love the Thoroughbred

Though some may think, and I'll agree,
That only God can make a tree,
Before God thought of trees, it's said,
His mind was on the Thoroughbred.

—Paul Mellon,
  "Thoroughbreds," 1975

This book draws its title from a 1949 column by W. C. Heinz, perhaps the finest turf writer who ever lived, documenting the fatal breakdown of Air Lift, the full brother to Assault, in his first start as a two-year-old at the old Jamaica racecourse in Queens, New York.

CONTENTS

CHARACTER LIST

Listed with their title at the time of the events recounted in the book

1/ST: Racing company owned by the Stronach family and operating Santa Anita, Gulfstream, and Pimlico

Andrew Adams: Prosecutor, Department of Justice

Aqueduct Racetrack: Racetrack, New York

Rick Arthur: Equine medical director, California Horse Racing Commission

Bob Baffert: Trainer, California

Vince Baker: Baffert's longtime veterinarian, California

John Bassett: Quarter horse trainer and friend of Bob Baffert

Clark Brewster: Lawyer for Bob Baffert

Belmont Park: Racetrack, New York

Geoff Berman: US attorney, Southern District of New York

Chad Brown: Trainer, New York

P. J. Campo: Vice president of racing, Santa Anita

Bill Carstanjen: CEO, Churchill Downs Inc.

Churchill Downs: Racetrack and home of the Kentucky Derby

Coolmore: Breeding and racing business operating in Ireland, the United States, and elsewhere

Brice Cote: Track investigator, Meadowlands

Rick Dane Jr.: Harness trainer, New Jersey

Joe Drape: Reporter, *New York Times*

Rick Dutrow: Trainer, New York

Tony Dutrow: Trainer, New York

Equestology: Drug manufacturing and distribution company owned by Seth Fishman

Fasig-Tipton: Bloodstock sales company, Kentucky

Seth Fishman: Veterinarian, Florida

Lisa Giannelli: Sales representative, Equestology

Randal Gindi: Racehorse owner, New York

Gulfstream Park: Racetrack, Florida

Jeffrey Gural: Owner of the Meadowlands, New Jersey

Adrienne Hall: Harness trainer, Ohio and Florida

Arthur Hancock: Breeder, Kentucky

Seth Hancock: Breeder, Kentucky

Robert Hanratty: Special Agent, FBI

Tim Harrington: Investigator, 5 Stones Intelligence

Dr. Alexander Harthill: Veterinarian, Kentucky; deceased

Stuart S. Janney III: Chairman, Jockey Club

Jockey Club: Thoroughbred breed registry, New York

Keeneland Association: Racetrack and bloodstock sales company, Kentucky

D. Wayne Lukas: Trainer, United States

Mitch McConnell: Majority leader, US Senate (R-KY)

Claude R. "Shug" McGaughey: Trainer, New York

Sheikh Mohammed bin Rashid al Maktoum: Ruler of Dubai, founder and owner of Godolphin racing and breeding operation

Mike Marlow: Assistant trainer for Bob Baffert, California

George Maylin: Director, New York Equine Drug Testing Programs

Meadowlands: Harness racetrack, New Jersey

Sarah Mortazavi: Prosecutor, US Department of Justice

Karen Murphy: Lawyer, New York

Jorge Navarro: Trainer, Florida

New York Racing Association: Not-for-profit corporation operating Belmont Park, Saratoga, and Aqueduct

Chris Oakes: Harness trainer

Mike Pegram: Racehorse owner and friend of Bob Baffert

Ogden "Dinny" Phipps: Former chairman, Jockey Club

Pimlico: Racetrack, Maryland

Todd Pletcher: Trainer, New York

Kristian Rhein: Veterinarian, New York

Gail Rice: Breeder of Medina Spirit, Florida

Shaun Richards: Special agent, FBI

Tim Ritvo: CEO, Santa Anita

Craig Robertson: Lawyer for Bob Baffert

Rick Sams: Former lab director, HFL Sports Science, Kentucky
Robert Sangster: Racehorse breeder and owner
Santa Anita Park: Racetrack, California
Saratoga Race Course: Racetrack, New York
Mary Scollay: Director, Racing Medication and Testing Consortium
Jason Servis: Trainer, New Jersey and New York
Belinda Stronach: Chairman, CEO and president, 1/ST
Nick Surick: Harness trainer, New Jersey
Mike Tannuzzo: Trainer, New York
David Tinsley: Founder and chairman, 5 Stones Intelligence
Bruce Turpin: Special agent, FBI
Mary Kay Vyskocil: Judge, US Southern District of New York
Tim Yakteen: Trainer and former assistant trainer to Bob Baffert, California
Marcus Zulueta: Trainer, Florida

PROLOGUE

On a quiet morning near Pasadena, California, in the December offseason of 2021, that year's Kentucky Derby winner, Medina Spirit, was on the racetrack for a routine morning workout.

Something had gone horribly wrong.

It wasn't a terribly fast effort for Medina Spirit, a dark brown horse with just the tiniest white star, like a freckle in the middle of his forehead. He covered five-eighths of a mile in precisely one minute and one and two-fifths of a second under his regular exercise rider, Juan Ochoa. An official track clocker marked the time to disseminate to gamblers across the country, so they could keep track of how the horse was training, mining the workout for clues about how well he might run in his next race, later that month.[1] But there was little urgency this time of year. Racing's year-end championships, the Breeders' Cup, were over—Medina Spirit had finished second—and his next race was considered only a warm-up run for a $20 million race in Saudi Arabia in late February. With all the controversy about his Derby win and the status of his trainer still a matter of regulatory adjudication, it wasn't at all clear what races he might even be entered into after that. Medina Spirit had failed a drug test after winning the Derby, and his sixty-eight-year-old trainer, Bob Baffert, was now facing suspensions at some of the country's most important racetracks.

Baffert sat in his usual seat in the open-air grandstand at Santa Anita Park, watching. The workout had been rescheduled from the day before, when a dense fog had rolled into Los Angeles and made exercising horses impossible. The fog had cleared and business as usual had resumed. A handheld radio that was connected to a receiver in Ochoa's ear rested on the seat next to Baffert, unused.

In fact, Baffert was feeling the early tug of impending vindication that morning. He had just gotten some good news that he hoped would clear both his name and Medina Spirit's, laboratory testing he thought should prove that the positive test was the result of an innocent mistake. It had been an emotionally trying year for Baffert, a year that had left him feeling bewildered and betrayed by the sport he had dedicated his life to for the past forty years. Surely now his fortunes were turning. Fate was—once again—coming home to roost in his barn.

Medina Spirit and Ochoa galloped easily around the oval. Palm trees quivered in the chill morning breeze. The San Gabriel Mountains stood like sentinels in the distance, the unencumbered view along the backstretch of the track making them appear looming.

As they came to the end of the workout, finish line in sight, something in the horse changed beneath Ochoa's hands, beneath the toe of his boots perched in the irons. Baffert saw it instantly. He knew this horse—every flick of his ears and ripple of muscle was a language that he could understand. The rhythm of the horse's stride had changed. Medina Spirit was laboring.

Medina Spirit should not have been struggling. He was in peak physical condition and the workout had not been overly hard. Moreover, the horse was a trier. He had what horsemen speak of in hushed and reverent tones: heart.

No one had expected Medina Spirit to make anything of himself on the racetrack. His mother failed to produce milk in time for his birth, and Medina Spirit had to be bottle-fed in the beginning. He had an obscure pedigree, the first foal of a mare with no accomplishments and a stallion that no one had ever heard of. He was sold as a one-year-old, known as a "yearling," for just $1,000—an age at which the top prospects sell for $1 million or more.[2]

But Medina Spirit had also been the biggest of the foals born at his farm, even though he was the youngest. He was pushy in the paddock with his friends, a scrapper. He played hard.[3] The next year, at a sale for unraced two-year-olds, Medina Spirit caught the eye of a buyer for one of Baffert's wealthy clients.

Baffert was America's most successful and recognizable horse trainer. With a shock of lanky white hair and a pair of blue-tinted sunglasses, he stood out even in the spectacle of gaudy hats and too-loud suits on the TV broadcasts of the Kentucky Derby. Reporters loved him, and he loved reporters. He was always good for a colorful quote and he usually had the best horse in the race. By the time he trained Medina Spirit, he had won the Derby a record-tying six times and the Triple Crown twice—racing's most elusive and sought-after prize, in which a single horse wins the Kentucky Derby, the Preakness Stakes, and the Belmont Stakes. Before Baffert, no one had won the Triple Crown since 1978. Most of the horses in his barn were blue bloods worth millions of dollars, their pedigrees a cashmere map of generations of prized Thoroughbreds.

But Medina Spirit had a quality that Baffert recognized. At two, he was tall, if a bit lean and weedy. His body had the easy balance of an athlete. Later, Baffert would remember some of the pieces of his anatomy that suggested his potential as a racehorse: A good, sturdy hind leg to provide power. A good shoulder, the scapula laid back at an open angle to allow the horse to reach forward and pull the ground under him. He was a beautiful mover, deceptively fast with an almost liquid stride.

Thanks to his junk pedigree, Medina Spirit would command only $35,000, a tiny sum in the rarefied market for top-level racehorses. But he quickly established himself in Baffert's barn. The horse, Baffert recalled later, had no bottom. You couldn't tire him out. In workouts, Baffert would pick up his two-way radio and tell the exercise rider to keep going on him, keep pushing him past the wire. He could work a mile and a quarter or more—something few other trainers in America ask of their horses—and not be blowing when he came back to the barn.

Still, Medina Spirit spent most of his two- and three-year-old years overshadowed by other, flashier-pedigreed horses in Baffert's stable. Even after he had gained entry to racing's most important race, the Kentucky Derby, bettors sent him to the post at 12-1—a long shot.

With the regally bred Mandaloun glued to his shoulder in the final stretch, Medina Spirit won by only a half a length. He had to fight for it. Two other horses, late closers who had conserved energy during the early stages of the race, were flying up the tails of the two lead horses. But the plain brown horse from nowhere refused to yield. The racecaller's voice swelled to a crescendo as he crossed the finish line: *Bob Baffert does it again! Medina Spirit has won the Kentucky Derby!*

So Baffert knew something wasn't right that December morning when he saw the horse suddenly begin to struggle in a routine workout. It wasn't just that the horse was tiring, it was the way he was moving. That liquid stride had morphed into something jerky and painful. His tail flagged into the air unnaturally. Baffert reached for his radio to tell Ochoa to stop, thinking that something had gone wrong in the horse's hind end. Ochoa was already standing up in the stirrup irons to signal the horse to slow. Medina Spirit took a few peg-legged strides, his front legs stiff and unbending against the ground.

Then he collapsed.

Somewhere behind Baffert, someone said, "Oh my God, no."

Medina Spirit was dead by the time the racetrack vet got to him. He was only three years old. Most horses live into their twenties, sometimes into their thirties.

Watching from the rail, other trainers instantly knew what had happened. The stiff-legged strides, the grotesque fall—both were telltale signs of a heart attack.

They knew something else too: This wasn't the first time one of Bob Baffert's horses had dropped dead of a heart attack. It wasn't even the second, or the third. A decade before, seven horses in Baffert's stable had died abruptly of suspected cardiac-related causes in less than two years—nine times the rate of other trainers stabled in the state of California.

More to the point, Medina Spirit wasn't just any horse in Baffert's barn. Blood and urine samples drawn from Medina Spirit in the hours after his miraculous win in the Kentucky Derby seven months before had revealed the presence of an anti-inflammatory corticosteroid called betamethasone, which is illegal to have in a horse's bloodstream on race day. Baffert's team had insisted that the overage was infinitesimal and came from a topical cream used for a skin rash—but the racetrack and the regulatory body in charge of overseeing horse racing in the state of Kentucky argued that distinction was irrelevant. The drug was banned on race day for a reason: it has the potential to mask pain that a horse could run through and injure himself. Two months after Medina Spirit's death, he would be officially stripped of his victory in the Derby.

Then there was the fact that Baffert had received four other medication positives in the year leading up to the race, including one in late 2020 for the same drug that had been found in Medina Spirit.

Baffert had operated under a cloud of suspicion for his entire career. For decades, rumors swirled around the backstretch of every racetrack from California to New York that the most dominant trainer in the country was giving his horses a little chemical help. Some people believed there was no way he was that good without doping his horses. Others believed he was exactly that good, and chalked up the rumors to racetrack gossip and jealousy.

Medina Spirit's positive in the Kentucky Derby had thrust every quiet whisper, every rumor ever traded behind the stable gates, into the glare of the public spotlight. It swallowed the Baffert barn. Baffert went on a blitz of media appearances, trying to explain the overage. In the early hours following the news of the positive, he gave a press conference in which he insisted the horse had never received betamethasone. He was widely mocked for rambling, speculative explanations that at times bordered on the absurd. (He told Fox News that he was being "canceled.")[4] By week's end, *Saturday Night Live* was in on the action, devoting three minutes of its "Weekend Update" segment to mocking Baffert's protestations that he had not doped the horse to win the Derby.

Meanwhile, the commercial power centers of horse racing, long dominated by old and blue-blooded East Coast institutions, moved swiftly to eject the sport's most famous and controversial face. Churchill Downs, the home of the Kentucky Derby, banned Baffert-trained horses for two years. The top racetracks in New York also sought to suspend Baffert for two years. *Enough was enough*.

Behind the scenes, the sport of Thoroughbred horse racing was in a moment of profound peril. The year before Medina Spirit's victory, the Justice Department had indicted twenty-seven trainers, veterinarians, drug suppliers, and distributors in a sprawling doping scheme that drew widespread media interest. The year before that, in 2019, cable news networks across the country had feverishly covered a cluster of what the racing industry calls "catastrophic breakdowns"—a horse that breaks one of the myriad fragile bones in its legs and must be euthanized—at Santa Anita, California's premier racetrack. More than forty horses died at Santa Anita that year. (None of Baffert's horses were among them.) Pundits attributed the parade of deaths to rampant drugging of horses. The Los Angeles County district attorney launched an investigation that threatened to impose legal consequences for the deaths.

The back-to-back scandals had rocked an insular, arcane world that had long viewed itself as either above the law or off its radar. Racing had for most of its existence in the United States been regulated, with varying degrees of rigor, at the state level—and in recent decades, most states had higher priorities for enforcement than a bunch of people who ran horses in circles. Meanwhile, as America's interest had dwindled in what was once among the most popular spectator sports in the country, national press coverage of racing had also grown increasingly spotty. The sport was a fiefdom unto itself, a cacophonous echo chamber of voices, often divided by class but united in the notion that it should be permitted to carry on as it had since the American breed registry was established in the late 1800s. The top strata of the sport had long been able to dodge questions about the ethics of its business model, cozily insulated as it was by money and prestige. (Some of the wealthiest people in the world—from George Soros to Mike Repole, the guy who created Vitaminwater—own racehorses.) At the lower levels, no one was paying attention anyway.

But the sport of kings was at last facing a uniquely American reckoning of conscience. Outside of the sport's closed-door, wood-paneled smoking rooms, beyond the graceful, tree-lined farms of the Kentucky bluegrass, average Americans with no exposure to horses or horse racing beyond the spectacle of the Kentucky Derby were asking: How is this allowed to continue?

"No other accepted sport exploits defenseless animals as gambling chips," wrote the *Washington Post* editorial board shortly after the 2020 indictments. "No other accepted sport tolerates the cruelties that routinely result in the injury and death of these magnificent animals. The rot in horse racing goes deep. It is a sport that has outlived its time."[5]

Baffert had always believed in fate. He and Medina Spirit had taken a bad step on racing's premier stage at exactly the wrong moment in history.

A decade before Medina Spirit was born, trainer Woodberry Payne had maybe two dozen young horses in his barn to be broken and shipped to trainers up and down the East Coast to begin their careers as racehorses. He also had a handful of older horses, layups that he would get fit for the track after a rest at the farm. When I was nineteen, he paid me fifteen dollars a head to exercise these horses at the little bullring training track in rural Virginia where his stable was based. Montpelier was the backwoods of a state whose racing industry was at the time dying a slow death. To me it was the pantheon, where men came every day to do immortal work. They came here to yoke their hands to nature's most intelligent, sensitive, and heartbreakingly noble creature, to use their bodies to speak to his, and, if they were skilled enough, brave enough, and wise enough, to bend him to their will. They came to ride Thoroughbred racehorses.

It was the most terrifying job I have ever done. Even today, I can feel the pulse of hard fear vibrating like a wire pulled too tight in my throat. The young horses didn't scare me—they were too young and too awkward to know yet how to really buck, how to drop a shoulder and squirt out from under you like ketchup from the glass bottle the second the knife releases the pressure. Besides, I knew how to ride a bucking horse. But the older horses scared me, the ones who wanted only to run faster and faster and faster, until the wind pulled the tears from your eyes and stopped the breath in your chest. Woodberry had a country boy named Jason riding for him at the time who used to say, every morning: "Welp, nobody's shooting at me!" Every morning, I felt like I was dodging bullets.

Woodberry did his best to teach me how to gallop a horse without getting run away with. It's not all about strength. It's about stillness and patience. At nineteen, I had neither of those qualities. He put me on a kindly bay horse named Mr. Hooker, a plain brown animal that at three years old had two years of training and experience on the babies in the barn. Every morning, Woodberry took the flat of my shin in his hand and lifted me like a bird into the tiny slip of leather that counts for a saddle in racing barns. I took the wide rubber reins in my hands and made a bridge against Mr. Hooker's neck, so that when he bowed his neck and made a perfect wheel of his body, he would pull against himself, not me. It is always January in my memory, sharp and bright and freezing cold.

Mr. Hooker—I called him Johnny Hooker—was kind. He would let me stand up in the irons and ease him into a gallop, gracious and gentlemanly. We would come around the first turn and into the backstretch as one, me perched lightly over his back, hovering with my hands fitted in the groove of his neck, my knuckles raw from the wiry hairs in his mane. (I had long since abandoned gloves after my fleece-lined leather work gloves slipped on the reins and I didn't have the sense to buy proper riding gloves.) When it was right, it was like carrying a hot stone in the center of your chest. But somewhere down the backside, my balance would tip in some imperceptible way. Johnny Hooker would start to lean against my hands. I tried a hundred things, over the months, to check him without stopping him—to keep him galloping steady panels. But always, Johnny Hooker got faster and faster. I would shift my butt back, my feet forward, set my hands against his neck. But it was no use. By the time we came around the far turn and into the stretch, my feet were on the dashboard and Johnny Hooker was screaming past Woodberry, who was standing on the rail, watching and shaking his head. It remains true to this day that I can't hold a horse for shit.

I eventually learned that there were jobs I could do in the racing business that didn't involve putting my life in the hands of fate six times a day and I wound up making a career on the supply side of the business, working for some of the big commercial breeding farms that create and sell the horses that eventually go on to run in races. But I never lost the sense of awe that I felt at nineteen for the Thoroughbred racehorse and the people who know how to speak to him. You will never convince me that the Thoroughbred horse doesn't love to run, that his soul doesn't thrill to it, and that when he is given a human partner who is sensitive, attentive, and—yes—affectionate, he does not grow more noble, more capacious, more giving of himself. I remember Mr. Hooker for his kindness, and I remember Mr. Hooker for the frank pleasure he took in running his heart out—"with no need / For voice or spurs or flailing whip / To guarantee he gets the trip."[6] I write these pages as a lover of horse racing; a lover of horse people in all their flaws, eccentricities, and outright weirdness; and, most importantly, as a lover of the horse.

I left the horse business when I was twenty-five. It was more than a decade later that racing came back into my life, this time in headlines from the *New York Times* and morning show interviews on my own network, CNN. They were covering a series of enormous scandals: the disqualification of a Kentucky Derby winner for a drug positive and the federal indictment of dozens of trainers and vets for doping their horses. The death of forty-two horses at Santa Anita, one of my favorite racetracks in the country. I found myself reflexively defending the sport I loved against the public perception that it was rife with doping—and that it was killing horses.

I knew racing had its problems. My own discomfort with some of the practices of the commercial sales side of the sport was one of the reasons I got out when I did. But I struggled with the image of the sport as depraved and evil. I needed to reconcile the horsemen* I knew with the horses I

---

* I use *horsemen* because the majority of public trainers in the United States are men. The leaderboards are dominated by male trainers. There are signs this may be changing—Jena Antonucci won the Grade I Belmont Stakes in 2023, making her the first woman to win one of the three races that constitute the Triple Crown—but it's indisputable that racing is a male-dominated industry. In addition, much of the language that the sport uses to describe different roles in the industry—like the plural *horsemen* to refer to trainers—defaults to the masculine even when referring to a female participant; throughout the book, I have chosen to use the language that the sport uses to speak about itself.

saw dying in headlines. I needed to understand what, exactly, was going wrong in racing.

Thoroughbred racehorses defy all attempts at categorization. They are certainly not pets—they are far too expensive and they have the potential to provide their owners with income. But they are not considered to be livestock either. Unlike cattle or pigs, they are treated as individuals by their handlers and owners rather than as an indistinguishable herd. And unlike cattle or pigs, they do not behave precisely as commodities: they have no intrinsic value in the marketplace. From a market perspective, they have more in common with fine art than they do with copper wiring or chickens. Their value, at least before they have raced, is almost entirely subjective: Is its pedigree in vogue? Does the animal appear physically to meet the criteria of a successful racehorse? What those criteria are, of course, is a matter of personal experience, opinion, and constant debate among equine professionals. Some preeminent buyers of successful racehorses, Baffert among them, are totally unable to articulate what it is, exactly, that they saw in a young racing prospect.

Neither can racehorses be termed pure athletes. That designation suggests a human agency that horses of any breed do not possess. Their fates as individuals are beggared to human whims. They are utterly at our mercy. And in any case, horses are stubbornly resistant to any effort to anthropomorphize them. Even the most beloved animal will disappoint its well-meaning owner by behaving, to the human eye, irrationally. They refuse to do what we expect or want them to do—like win a race—sometimes for no apparent reason. Generations of horsemen have spent decades of their lives trying, and often failing, to get inside the mind of a horse.

Horses remain, on some fundamental level, a mystery to us. The differences extend even to how we see the world: Horses are primarily monocular, meaning that the right eye doesn't see what the left eye sees. They see the world in panorama, unlike humans, whose eyes overlap to create a common picture and depth perception. Horses must raise and lower their heads to gauge distance and depth. The better horsemen learn to meet the horse on his own footing, to understand, through careful observation and study, what he sees and what he needs—and what it might take to bend him to our wishes. But the best of them will tell you that the process of learning is never done. They are a foreign species to us.

Still, they are a species that has captivated us and drawn our reverence and fascination long past the point of their utility in our society. There are no horse-drawn carriages or plow yokes any longer. We have an emotional connection to the horse, but what practical purpose does the horse serve now?

It has no purpose except for our entertainment, and therein lies the great paradox of the Thoroughbred racehorse. They have no value absent their ability to divert and amuse us—or, in the case of the truly horse-sick, to provide us some sense of physical purpose in a chaotic world that is migrating increasingly into the intangible metaverse. To some they are a calling: *for love of the horse.* To others they are a symbol of old-money wealth already possessed, or simply desired: Willy Wonka's golden ticket to a better life for the nouveaux riches. A pathway to *belonging.* For still others they are a simple job to prop up the irrelevant interests of a distant upper class. A way to send money back to family in another country. But it is their basic status as a plaything that makes the racehorse unique in the realm of animal-human interactions. The horse is beloved—but he is also a financial asset. In a market-driven economy, such a plaything must earn its keep.

For Thoroughbreds bred expressly for the purpose of racing, this means they must race—and win—to pay for the prodigious cost of their upkeep and give their owners, trainers, and other connections even a ghost's prayer of making any money on them. There are different levels of racing, meaning that horses that don't make it in the big leagues can drop down in "class" and compete in less competitive races at less competitive tracks for less competitive earnings, but the fundamental proposition remains the same. At the elite levels, the astronomical price of these horses means that even the highest-rolling owner expects *some* return on their investment to make the outlay worthwhile. At the workingman's track—the poorer facilities with cheaper racing that make up most of the tracks across the country—it's quite literally a question of livelihood.

The incentives to cheat, of course, are clear.

Like any elite athlete, the Thoroughbred is treated by a sports doctor who may prescribe therapeutic medication. Racing downplays this class of drug as the equivalent of giving aspirin to the horse after a hard day at the gym, but the reality is much more complicated. Horses receive everything from sedatives to joint injections to a deeply controversial drug designed to prevent spontaneous hemorrhaging of the lungs during intense exercise, sometimes in untested combinations with unknown outcomes.

These medications are governed by a constantly evolving set of rules about what is and isn't allowed in a horse's system on race day and at what threshold. In a perfect world, they are part of the humane management of an equine athlete. But some trainers and vets lean more heavily on so-called therapeutics than others, using them in place of rest or more time-consuming training techniques. They use them to help horses that shouldn't be running continue to run. They use them because they are willing to try anything that might help the horse win. They make little compromises to what's best for the animal, rationalized away in service of the business of the sport.

Then there are the truly banned substances: blood-doping drugs, literal snake venom, new so-called designer drugs made to be invisible on drug testing by tweaking a single molecule. It was this kind of drug that the FBI sought to crack down on in 2020.

These two very different practices are often incorrectly conflated in the public eye—and sometimes within the racing industry itself, where rumor and innuendo are so powerful that they can calcify into "common knowledge." But therapeutics and "dope" do share one important attribute: they are both given with the incentive of winning races. And it is racing's tolerance of drugs, legal and illegal, that has become the focal point of the debate over whether the sport has outlived its time.

These days, I have the luxury of not getting on horses that frighten me. What scares me now is not being run away with, but that there will be no more running horses left because racing has failed to heal itself. If Thoroughbred horse racing disappears, so does the Thoroughbred horse. There will be no more Secretariats to break the bonds of nature by running a mile and a half in 2:24. We petty mortals have ridden the horse into war and into strange, uncharted country. We have stood at the shoulder of giants and watched, suspended in time, as man and beast have, together, achieved purity of form. I may no longer want to ride racehorses, except in my dreams. But I want my son, if he wants, to have the opportunity to fold his knees to his chin, stretch flat across the neck of a galloping horse, and reach for something untouchable.

When I set out to write this book, I thought I would use what I knew about reporting and what I knew about racing to learn what was broken in the sport and speak frankly about it in ways that might offer a constructive path forward. I wanted to speak for the horse, this mute witness who is so often treated as little more than a symbol, used for maximum rhetorical effect by supporters and opponents of the sport alike.

But as I reimmersed myself in a world I hadn't visited for the better part of a decade, I remembered that it wasn't just the horse I loved about racing—and it wasn't just the horse who deserved a voice. Maybe because it revolves around a living animal, there's a realness to the racetrack that feels uncorrupted by social media and the flat homogenization of culture. There are no Starbucks at the racetrack: It's like Joseph Mitchell's New York, bursting with characters who feel too bizarre, too full of hope and striving, to be real. But they are. And if their little slice of America disappears, it will feel to me, at least, as if the world has lost a little of its color. I don't want to lose racehorses—and I don't want to lose racetrackers. Their fates are intertwined.

This is my love song to horse racing.

As Medina Spirit's dying body asteroided into the dirt, catapulting Ochoa over his head, Baffert sprinted down the steps of the grandstand toward the racetrack. Out of instinct, he called his wife, Jill, as he ran. She began to cry as he told her what had happened. *Medina has gone down.*

The scene had already played out by the time Baffert got to the track. The horse was dead. The palm trees shivered overhead. In the grandstand behind, the white railings and empty rows of Mediterranean green folding seats, relics of a grander era, looked on silently. Like everyone else by then, Baffert understood that the horse had succumbed to a cardiac attack. Ochoa was shaken but unhurt—a small miracle for a rider who had just been unexpectedly ejected from an animal hurtling along a metal railing at forty miles per hour. Baffert knelt over the horse, stunned. He removed Medina Spirit's bridle and stood up. He held it, uselessly.

Baffert would continue to fight the charges that he had inappropriately medicated Medina Spirit to win the Derby for more than two years after the horse died. He would lose, over and over again, both in regulatory battles and in the courtroom. Baffert's quest to claw back the victory in the Derby, and his own reputation, would nearly end his career. His was the sole face most Americans outside of horse racing recognized. Outside of the sport, and occasionally within it, he was made into the symbol for all its sins. But the true story of Bob Baffert—a tumultuous and controversial career that began long before Medina Spirit—was not a simple story about a singular sinner. It was a powerful illumination of how the sport had done business for decades. Baffert's story is the story of Thoroughbred horse racing.

Later, in his inarticulate way, Baffert would try to explain the shock and grief of the moment Medina Spirit died. "People don't understand what these horses mean to us—" he said, breaking off. The horse had been so gallant, his end so unfair, so tragic.

But it was a moment that, for Baffert, was all tied up in everything that had come before. The stinging betrayal he felt that the key masters of Thoroughbred racing hadn't given him the benefit of the doubt. The years of crushing, unrelenting media criticism, not only from the uninitiated outside his industry but from within it. The ignominious loss of his Derby win with a $1,000 horse, which he would later say had done more to satisfy him that he had really *done something* than any of the other wins with million-dollar colts. It was impossible to separate the loss of "that little horse," as Baffert called him, from the urgent and painful frustration he felt that people were still asking the question: Did Bob Baffert cheat?

PART I

CALL TO POST

◆

You could be walking around lucky, and not even know it.

—*Let It Ride* (Paramount Pictures, 1989)

CHAPTER 1

THE BEST AT WHAT YOU DO

B ob Baffert was born in 1953 in Nogales, Arizona, a dirt-scratch town
within spitting distance of the Mexican border. It was high desert country, four thousand feet above sea level.[1] The family's adobe house sat like a
belly button in the middle of acres of cattle fields. There were no neighbors
for miles around.

Boyhood in an Arizona border town sixty years ago had the sepia-toned
feel of a world already disappearing by the time Baffert was born into it.
But in the 1950s and '60s, it was all he and his six brothers and sisters knew.
They had no television because the cattle kept knocking over the antenna
in the field, and eventually the Bafferts said the hell with it. The only real
entertainment in town was a drive-in movie theater next to a swamp. Baffert's
mother would slather them all with oil to keep the mosquitos away while
they watched, then roll her grease-smeared children, already asleep, into
bed without baths.

Bill Baffert, Bob's father, was known by everyone who mattered as "the
Chief." He had retired from the army and wanted to live on a ranch, because
he loved horses and needed somewhere to keep them. When he first took
his wife to see the house, it was locked and she had to peer in through the
windows. Ellie Baffert, a schoolteacher born and raised in Nogales, saw
what she thought were gorgeous hardwood floors, but which turned out
to be linoleum that had rotted through and had to be ripped up. There was
no electricity and for a while, the house was lit only by gas lanterns. The
children—Bill Jr. and Bob, Penny and Nori, P.A. and DeeDee and, finally,
the surprise, Gamble—shared rooms even as the Bafferts progressively, and
one has to think with a certain sense of desperation, added new rooms to
the house. It was a close-knit family.

Baffert was a fastidious child, even by his own admission, a hangover from a stretch of time spent with a doting aunt who would wash his hands, dress him in a bow tie, and button his shirt to the top. He would come home from time spent with Aunt Ludie and correct his siblings' grammar and table manners over supper, until the Chief finally snapped at his wife: "What's the matter with your sister? She's going to make a sissy out of the kid."

That small addiction to neatness would prove problematic for a boy growing up in a ranching town. There were always animals around, mostly livestock that made up some of the family income. Baffert's father eventually ran cattle, but started out with a chicken business that topped out at about five thousand chickens in individual cages.[2] Chickens are, by anyone's measure, disgusting. There were 4-H lambs as well, which Baffert hated because they, like the chickens, stank. Occasionally the local ranch hands whom the Bafferts hired to collect and crate the eggs wouldn't show up Sunday morning, the sweeter libations of a night out in Nogales having proved too tempting, and the Baffert children had to collect the eggs. Baffert and his siblings walked the stinking, dusty rows of the henhouses, with the chickens raising unholy hell overhead, flapping their wings and stirring up the dust and chicken shit. They would come out of the chicken houses covered in a fine grain of filth. Baffert didn't care for that part of owning chickens, but he proved adept at the business side of the venture, selling and delivering eggs for his father in high school. He was a natural-born salesman, making his own deals and adjusting prices to move aging stock over his father's head—experience he would later credit with training him for a lifetime of making good business deals.

When he was about ten, Baffert was invited by a friend whose family owned a large ranch in Mexico to fly down on a private plane and spend three days on horseback pushing three thousand head of cattle on a hundred-mile drive across the border. It was a boy's dream, in an era when John Wayne was king: They slept on the ground under the stars and lived on canned tuna and tortillas. Baffert rode point—the lead position at the front of the herd—and learned horsemanship from the Mexican cowboys. They were excellent, and taught Baffert how to go after cattle, how to really *ride*.

But there was a problem. Baffert did not want to perform one of humankind's most important and private functions in the middle of the wilderness: he did not want to poop. In desperation, he asked the Mexican cowboys what they used to wipe. The cowboys soberly informed him that they used rocks. Ten-year-old Baffert, a forlorn Little Lord Fauntleroy left with no other options, held it in for three days.

◆

Nogales was about as far from the center of the horse universe as it was possible to get in those days. In Kentucky and New York, the 1960s and '70s were a halcyon age in Thoroughbred racing, an era of giants of the turf still remembered today. The year Baffert was eleven, one of the most important Thoroughbreds in the history of the breed won the Kentucky Derby— although no one knew it at the time. A small and fiery-tempered colt with a powerful engine, Northern Dancer had been underestimated from the start because of his size. He was foaled late in the season for a Thoroughbred and consequently stood a mere 14 hands as a yearling, when his owners held an annual auction to sell their stock. Horses are traditionally measured in "hands," or the breadth of a human hand, with a "hand" standardized to four inches in the modern era. Anything less than 14 and a half hands, measured from the shoulder, is considered a pony. Tiny little Northern Dancer failed to meet even the low reserve of $25,000 and, unwanted, remained to race for his breeders. In a sign of how little they thought of his long-term value, his trainer initially wanted to geld (castrate) the horse.

But the scrappy bay colt quickly showed himself. He blew away the field by eight lengths in his debut, then went on to trounce the best two-year-olds in Canada, often while carrying ten pounds more weight than his lesser rivals.[3] His first jockey, Ron Turcotte—who would later pilot Secretariat— had to be taken off the horse because Northern Dancer routinely ran away with him during races. "God knows how good he really was," Turcotte would later say, "for he was never a completely sound horse most of the time I rode him, and I still could not slow him down."[4] He won the Kentucky Derby in a blazing two minutes flat, a track record that stood for almost ten years until it was broken by Secretariat himself. As a breeding stallion, Northern Dancer proved even more undeniable: decades later, he is the dominant sire in the Thoroughbred breed. In the 1980s, his offspring routinely sold for more than $1 million at auction.[5] A privately negotiated breeding to the horse in the final years of his life—with no guarantee of a live foal—cost $1 million.[6] His sons and daughters appear wheeled out in the pedigrees of thousands of racehorses in America and Europe today.*

* In 2019, roughly half of the new stallions entering the market in central Kentucky were descended from Northern Dancer. https://www.bloodhorse.com/horse-racing/articles/231145/new-sires-of -2019-northern-dancer-fires-back.

The 1960s and '70s were a time of historic farms, owned by old East Coast money, farms steeped in gentility that bred regal, long-legged Thoroughbreds whose value was steadily increasing as the boom years of the 1980s ticked closer. Families like the Vanderbilts and their friends the Phippses bred blooded horses—Thoroughbreds—for the sport of it. The Thoroughbred was noble, refined, a work of art, his classic beauty immortalized in London's National Gallery in the form of the temperamental and heroic Whistlejacket, towering life-sized in George Stubbs's iconic 1762 oil rendering. This was the sport of kings. It belonged to artists like Federico Tesio, an Italian breeder who wrote an influential book called *Breeding the Racehorse* in the 1950s, and the particular class of person who had the time and leisure to read Tesio.

In Nogales, the Chief had gotten his son Bobby hooked on a very different kind of horse. Ironically for a breed now associated so thoroughly with the American West, the quarter horse has its origins in the East Coast dating back to the colonial era. As early as 1611, settlers had begun crossing their English stock with a faster, squattier Chickasaw pony believed to be the descendants of Spanish barbs brought to Florida by early Spanish colonists. They would come to be known as the "Celebrated American Quarter Running Horse," so named for their brilliant speed over a quarter of a mile. Later, an infusion of mustang blood would solidify the American quarter horse as the horse of the West. They carried cowboys and settlers alike across the harsh and unforgiving plains, and in Texas became the mount of choice for cutting and driving cattle. Their sturdy build and muscular haunches gave them not only searing speed over short distances but also the ability to cut and wheel, to change direction on a dime in pursuit of the Texas longhorn—with power and stamina left over to race up and down Main Street for a jug of corn whiskey on the weekends. This was the horse on which the West—at least for white Americans—was won.[7]

The Chief acquired a couple of quarter horses to race when Baffert was about ten or eleven. Bob won a couple of races with Baffert's Heller, a horse possessed of a terrible beauty for an eleven-year-old boy. Baffert was in awe of the horse, but he was afraid of him and the horse knew it. Baffert's Heller was cinchy, meaning that he would buck and sometimes throw himself on the ground when the girth was tightened around his belly. The boy spent months riding home on the school bus contemplating how to master the animal. By the time he had figured out the horse's proclivities and come to ride him without fear, he was sunk. Baffert was horse crazy. He would groom and exercise his father's horses and tag along to the races. By the time he was fourteen, the Chief had cut a quarter-mile strip in one of their hayfields and begun training their small string himself. There was a creek there, and the ground was loamy and soft. Baffert would exercise the horses for his father, riding them back and forth up the short strip. They weren't very good horses, but it was a good education. When he was a freshman in high school, Baffert was riding in unsanctioned match races for $50 or $100 pots and dreaming of being a jockey. He bought a pair of bell-bottomed pants with his winnings.[8]

The horses were a hobby for the Chief. For Bob they became not only a passion but the vehicle for a magical connection with his father. Baffert worshipped his father. In later years he would become his simulacrum.[9] Bill Sr. was *fun*. He was the kind of father who taught his son how to toss empty beer cans out of the window of a moving car without attracting police attention ("Hold the can down and keep your arm to the side of the car when you release it").[10] He let the boy sit around and listen to the old-timers' horse stories, tales of races won and lost, wisdom passed down of homemade liniments and tinctures to rub a horse's sore and ailing legs.

Nobody had any real money in horses in those days. The purse money for the top races was good—better, in fact, than for the big Thoroughbred races—and Baffert came of age with some of the greats in quarter horse racing. But most trainers were running just a couple of cheap horses for cheap purses, hauling them from race to race in a two-horse stock trailer attached to a pickup truck. Even the sanctioned racetracks were dusty, run-down affairs, nothing like the generous, tree-lined Thoroughbred ovals of New York's Saratoga or Kentucky's Keeneland. The famous El Paso tack-maker Johnny Bean once laughed off a persistent rumor that the now-famous Thoroughbred trainer D. Wayne Lukas, then training quarter horses, had stiffed him with a $20,000 bill: "Oh, that's ridiculous. Nobody had $20,000 in those days."[11]

The bush circuit for quarter horse racing was even poorer. It was part family picnic, part county fair, part illegal gambling ring, and it could be a rough-and-ready world with few rules: During one match race when Baffert was a sophomore in high school, the other horse in the race bolted from under his jockey, careening out of control off the dirt strip and into the crowd, running between the cars parked along the perimeter. Baffert kept riding, hollering all the way because the crowd had abandoned their barbecues and poured out onto the makeshift track to mill around on the finish line. They parted for him as he came blasting across the line first—but the instant he stood up in the stirrups to celebrate, the leather strap holding the footrest snapped. Someone had cut it in half, but it hadn't broken during the race as it was meant to.

Sonofabitch, what the hell did I get myself into? Baffert thought.

It was hard to say he hadn't been warned: The Chief had put $200 on his son to win, only to be told by a friend that it was a bad bet. The other horse had been "set up for a big race." Whatever that meant exactly, the horse was supposed to win.

Baffert rode back into the middle of an argument. A man who stood out in his memory mainly for his size—and the fact that he had clearly laid a lot of money on Baffert's opponent—wanted to call the race a no-contest because his horse had bolted off the track. The evidence that there had been a fix in on the race was mounting. The argument escalated, and pretty soon the big guy was whaling hell on two smaller fellas.

Other men stepped in to break up the fight. One of the smaller men ran off—and returned with a rifle. He fired a shot into the air as he approached.

Baffert's uncle, who was with Bill and Bob, yelled: "Hit the ground!"

Pandemonium broke out. Everyone panicked, leaping into their cars and hauling ass to leave. Drivers wrenched the wheel to whip their cars around, grinding gears and stirring up dust so thick it was hard to see. Baffert looked over and saw one driver barreling down the track itself. He saw what was going to happen seconds before it did: "Dad, he's going to hit the starting gate!"

The car plowed dead into the immobile metal starting gate with a sickening crash. The driver, who hadn't been wearing a seat belt, was bloody and dazed.

It was the man with whom the Chief had bet the $200. Somehow he was roused and in a condition that the Chief could address the outstanding wager between them. The man, convinced he couldn't lose, didn't have the cash. So the Chief took instead a pocket knife and a hundred-year-old reata, the kind of long, braided rawhide rope favored by Mexican cowboys.

As Bob and his father finally drove away, the Chief had a single instruction: "Don't tell your mother."

Ellie Baffert was no fool. She believed race riding was too dangerous for Bobby, and for a long time, the Chief and Bob conspired to keep what he was doing from her. They had a deal: Bill Sr. wouldn't squeal that Bob was riding races, and Bob wouldn't tell on his father for his beer drinking.[12]

Few endeavors are more dangerous than race riding. Piloting a half-ton animal with a mind of its own and a highly sensitive flight instinct at speeds of near to forty miles per hour, with nothing but the tips of the toes and a whisper of ankle and hands on the reins for balance, is a physical feat the best parallel for which is likely free climbing. Often referred to as the best athletes pound for pound, jockeys suffer a shocking number of injuries from on-track crashes. A fund started only in 2006 to help care for permanently disabled jockeys now supports sixty former riders who have suffered paralysis, brain injuries, or both.[13] Accidents happen both in the blink of an eye and in newly inventive ways every day. It takes only a split second for horses in a race to "clip heels": a following horse's front hooves grab a lead horse's back hooves in a rippling disaster that is likely to snap both animals off their feet, catapulting their riders over their heads. Perhaps the most dangerous moment in any race is the time that the animals spend confined in the metal ribs of the starting gate. A panicked horse might rear and flip, his rider still perched on his back. Today an ambulance is required to shadow the horses and riders as they compete in races, driving around the track just behind the racing field.

The races Baffert was riding in were particularly dangerous. His earliest experiences race riding were *en faja*, a traditional Mexican style of match race in which the jockey is literally tied onto the horse bareback by a long strap that hooks over the rider's lap and under the animal's belly. A pair of golf balls in the front pockets of his pants kept the *faja* from slipping down.[14]

It was terrifying. If a horse flipped, there was no way for the rider to bail out. He would be crushed under the mass of a thousand-pound horse.

The last time Baffert rode that kind of race, his horse "bolted," in the parlance of the track—running blindly and uncontrollable by the rider—and dove straight for the barbed-wire rail.

Somewhere in the back of his mind he remembered the counterintuitive wisdom given to all trackwork riders. If they're bolting, give them their head: release your grip on the reins and stop trying to steer the animal. It's the racetracker equivalent of "Jesus, take the wheel." For some horses, giving up the fight will short-circuit their flight instinct. In the worst-case scenario, it will at least allow the horse to see where he's going, and maybe he won't run right through the rail.

Baffert threw the horse his head and closed his eyes.

The horse at the last moment saw the rail and ducked to the outside. Baffert stayed on and somehow managed to pull up the horse.

Baffert wasn't any fool either. "I'm never gonna ride with that thing on again," he told his father. After that, he would ride in a saddle.

But even a saddle offered few guarantees of safety. In one race in Yuma, Arizona, Baffert picked up a mount on a horse that turned out to be dead lame. Baffert rode the horse on the outside of the field for the entire race just in case the animal broke down, so he would not go sprawling in the middle of a pack of other horses running at top speed. On that same trip, the cinch of his saddle broke while he was exercising a filly for some friends. The saddle slipped and sent Baffert shooting off the horse like someone had opened the passenger-side door of a racecar going around a turn. He hit the ground with his elbow and jammed it into his kidney. He urinated blood that night. It wasn't until a week later, when his older brother, Bill, caught him still pissing red, that Baffert was sent to the medical center in Tucson. He spent five days in a hospital bed with a bruised kidney.

Baffert didn't even bother going to the hospital when he fell from a horse he was breezing and the animal stepped on his chest. The impact of the fall knocked the heels off his boots.[15] He couldn't breathe, and after about a week of that discomfort, he asked a vet he knew to x-ray him. "Oh, yeah," the vet said. "You've cracked your sternum."[16]

It wasn't just the horses that were dangerous. He rode at the kind of track where the other riders would steal twenty bucks out of your pocket while you were out riding a race. "They were just a degenerate bunch of jocks who couldn't make it anywhere else," Baffert said.

There were some vestiges of the fussy boy who had refused to wipe his backside with rocks. Baffert was allergic to alfalfa, an occasionally convenient excuse to get out of barn work (and later, so legend has it, the reason for the trademark blue sunglasses).[17] Because he was riding races in the afternoon, it sometimes worked out that Baffert loafed around the night before a race while Bill did the chores.[18] But race riding was a real horseman's education, the rare kind that gives a person an intimate facility with the horse's body and his mind.

Ellie eventually found out that her son was riding in races. A friend noticed Bob's name on the entries at the local track in Sonoita and called her to wish her son luck. Bob tried to stammer his way out of it, to no avail. Ellie burst into tears, calling her son and her husband both liars and sneaks and begging Bob not to ride. After he wound up in the hospital, she kept saying, over and over, "You don't know what you've put me through."

It was no use: Baffert was desperate to ride. With the danger of race riding also came the thrill. And by that point, Baffert was a fool for horses.

Baffert stepped out of the hot box at Tucson's Rillito Race Track. He had been sitting under the burning red bulbs trying to get down to the 122 pounds he needed to weigh to ride races. The hot box is a feature at racetracks to help the riders drop weight. The professional jocks would slather baby oil on themselves and let the sweat run off them, but Baffert didn't sweat much. When he stepped out from under the bare bulbs, he fainted.

College-aged at the time, Baffert was really too big to be a jockey. He had been a scrawny kid, which kept him just under 122 pounds for a while.[19] But as he started to fill out, the problem of keeping his weight down became more acute. Although he was too squeamish to turn to bulimia—common enough in racing that jocks' rooms often have a dedicated toilet for "flipping"—he effectively starved himself down to a twenty-seven-inch waistline by eating nothing but protein. He was skin and bones, which made him weak.[20] He also wasn't making any money. The math was grim for a race rider in Arizona even if you were winning races: the purses at Rillito topped out at about $600 for a given race. Only about half of that went to the winning horse, and the jockey's cut of that was just 10 percent—$30.[21] And Baffert wasn't winning many races.

Still, he stuck with it for as long as he could. He deferred starting college at the University of Arizona for a year, in part because he knew his days riding races were waning. In the early 1970s, the Chief dropped him off at Los Alamitos Race Course, in Southern California, to spend the summer living on a cot in the tack room and breaking horses for a trainer there. Before long he had blisters on his ass from getting on horses from six in the morning to three in the afternoon. The blisters were worth it to Baffert because the horses belonged to Dr. Ed Allred, one of the legendary owners in quarter horse racing who later bought Los Alamitos. Baffert got to ride a few horses in the afternoons, in actual races. But the competition at Los Alamitos was stiff, and he eventually returned to Rillito.

In the end, it wasn't Ellie who convinced Baffert to hang up his tack. It was one of the top quarter horse jockeys in the country, Bobby Adair. Known simply as "the Master," Adair was the sport's superstar. He had ridden some of quarter horse racing's most famous horses to victory and shattered records for race wins. He famously remarked that he "thought he could ride anything that had hair on it," and Baffert idolized him.[22]

Around the same time that Baffert passed out trying to cut weight, Adair was in town to ride a big race at Rillito. He asked Baffert if he was planning to return to Los Alamitos the next summer to ride.

"No," Baffert said, honestly. "I'm not good enough." The competition at Los Alamitos was too tough, the races full of better horses with more experienced jockeys competing for bigger purses than Rillito and the local county fair tracks like Sonoita where Baffert was riding.

Adair gave Baffert some advice that he would carry with him for the rest of his life: quit.

"If you don't think you can be the best at what you do, you need to quit," Adair said. "Because if not, you're gonna kill yourself." The Arizona fair circuit was too dangerous, full of rough riders and rough horses.

Driving home from Rillito that night, Baffert knew that Adair was right. He was a good horseman, but he wasn't a great race rider. He couldn't "switch sticks" while riding—transfer the whip from one hand to the other seamlessly. His friend John Bassett, a hard-partying quarter horse trainer Baffert had met in California, once told him, "You can't ride a hog in a phone booth."[23] Privately, Adair was thinking the same thing, although he wouldn't tell Baffert that until years later.[24]

Reeling after the incident outside of the hot box, Adair's words ringing in his ears, Baffert decided he had had enough. He gave his tack to another jockey.

It was an early call of the true competitor in Baffert—or perhaps just a demonstration of the kind of boyish sense of entitlement to greatness held by restless young men who have yet to discover their ambition: a bone-deep belief that a thing isn't worth the effort if you can't be the best at it. In any case, Baffert would come to believe in Adair's advice with an almost religious fervor. He would set himself deadlines based on it, shape career decisions around it, and, in later years, reflect on it as a credo that has set him apart.

The decision didn't look nearly that fateful in the moment. In the short term, it mostly allowed nineteen-year-old Baffert to order a hamburger with impunity for the first time in a few years. He went to college, joined a fraternity, and, even as he continued to take jobs here and there fooling with horses, told people that he didn't want anything to do with the racing business.

But Baffert was about to discover what he *was* the best at.

CHAPTER 2

GO WEST, YOUNG MAN

Los Alamitos was plagued by rain almost from the beginning. The track, situated about twenty-five miles south of Los Angeles, began as just the corner of a ranch that belonged to a struggling Kentucky native named Frank Vessels. Vessels came to California with nineteen dollars in his pocket in the 1920s and limped along for decades before finally making a fortune building specialized drilling platforms for the oil business. He had long dreamed of building a racetrack, and now he had the money. By 1951 he had talked the state regulatory board into approving an eleven-day race meet, with wagering, for quarter horses.[1]

It rained for ten out of the eleven days of the meet.[2] Vessels and his wife, along with their son Frank Jr. and his wife, spent the bulk of their flagship race meet trying to repair the damage caused by the near-constant rain.

But Vessels wasn't a man to be put off his dream. He spent $100,000 on improving the facility and went back to the California Horse Racing Board (CHRB). The board allowed him another sixteen days of races in 1952, and quarter horse racing at Los Alamitos was off and running.[3] A superstar racehorse in the mid-1950s named Go Man Go—a hard-bodied, ferociously competitive animal described by his trainer as "jes plain mean as a bear most of the time"[4]—drew big crowds and the interest of sportswriters.[5] By the early 1970s, Los Alamitos was the glittering big leagues in quarter horse racing. The grandstand was packed on nights and weekends. A nobody like Baffert struggled even to get tickets to attend the races.

Baffert, then twenty-four and on break from the University of Arizona during the summer of 1977, wasn't doing much at Los Al. After he had hung up his tack as a jockey, he tried his hand at training, running a handful of horses mostly belonging to a friend. His own horses were losing.

It was raining at Los Alamitos the day that another trainer offered him a drug that he promised would help his horse win.[6] Baffert didn't know the guy well. But he desperately wanted to win a race at Los Al before the meet ended and he would have to go back to Arizona.[7]

The horse in question was a "claimer," a cheap horse that runs in races where he can be bought for a set price before the starting gate opens. Win or lose, the horse goes home with whoever "claims" him, while the original owner keeps any purse money from the race. Baffert had claimed the animal for $2,000 and planned to run him back quickly in another race, a risky strategy that might allow a trainer to capitalize on a horse's fitness from a past race—or could leave him running a tired horse before it's had a chance to recover.

Baffert had good reason to think he wouldn't get caught on a drug test. Quarter horse racing had a reputation for an enthusiastic culture of doping, and still does today.[8] But money for testing was tight, meaning that regulators likely limited the horses they tested to mostly winners. Baffert wasn't winning races.

Baffert told me that he allowed the other trainer to give the horse something called apomorphine, a morphine derivative used in human beings to treat advanced Parkinson's disease and in small animals to induce vomiting. Horses react very differently to morphine than humans or small animals. In horses, morphine and its derivatives act as a powerful stimulant, historically making it a very tempting performance enhancer.

There's some evidence that apomorphine was in vogue at the time— available if you were interested—and that regulators were aware of it. In a 1979 paper, one of the sport's most prominent pharmacological experts, Dr. Thomas Tobin, administered doses of apomorphine to horses confined to stalls and found that even a tiny dose of apomorphine would cause "locomotor stimulation," spurring the animals to move about rapidly. For the horse, it was probably an extremely stressful experience. Tobin found that apomorphine made the horses "apprehensive and uncomfortable"; they paced the stall and lunged at the ceiling in every corner, "as though seeking to escape."[9]

But for all its appeal as a potential stimulant, apomorphine was also unreliable. "The response of any horse to apomorphine could never be predicted or reliably repeated," Tobin found. Some horses had a "peak response" at smaller doses of between 18 mg and 30 mg, while for others it would take more than twice that to elicit a noticeable reaction.

It's not clear how much of this Baffert knew. He would have certainly known that morphine acted as a stimulant in racehorses. "You heard things," he told me. But how savvy he was to either the risks or the opportunities at the time is debatable. "I was sort of naïve," he said. In a 1999 memoir, he wrote that he didn't really know what he was giving the horse at the time.*

In any case, it didn't help him. The horse ran second, he told me.[10]

But Baffert got unlucky, not just in losing. The horse was tested. Of course, he came up positive for morphine.[11]

Baffert was humiliated. "It was like my guts had fallen out," he recalled.[12] He wasn't even planning on making a career out of training horses—yet here he was, getting caught for drugging a cheap, losing horse? *Man, this is not me. Screw this—I'm gonna do something else.*[13] The whole sordid episode put the terrible taste of being exposed, embarrassed, and stupid in his mouth. He never wanted to go back to Los Alamitos. Years later he would call it "a bad choice."[14]

Worst of all, he would have to face his father with the news. The Chief was the listed owner of the horse. And because the meet was over, he was on his way to Los Alamitos with the horse trailer to pick up his son and bring him home to Arizona. Instead, they would have to drive that night first to Hollywood Park, on the other side of Los Angeles, to address the positive test with state regulators. The Chief reamed out his young, dumb son. Then he went silent.

"It was a long, quiet ride home. I'll never forget that," Baffert said.[15]

But once the lecture was out of the way, the Chief moved to protect his son. "All right," he said. "Let's deal with this."[16] Standing in front of the regulators that night, Baffert wrote in his memoir, "I do the usual deal: 'I don't know what happened.'"[17] (He told me that he didn't want to throw the other trainer under the bus.[18] The racetrack has a certain code of omertà when it comes to drugs, legal and illegal.)

Sour on racing, Baffert skipped his initial hearing in the matter. Months later, unable to leave the racetrack behind, he flew to Sacramento for a make-up hearing to try to keep his license. He had a layover in LA on the way from Tucson to Sacramento and he almost missed his connection

---

* Throughout these pages, when a trainer has directed the administration of a drug—legal or illegal—I have chosen to describe them as "giving" or "administering" that drug. However, particularly with legal medication, it's important for readers to understand that while it's the trainer who makes the decision that the horse should have a drug, with few exceptions, a licensed veterinarian physically administers it.

out of pure naïveté. Baffert had never been on a commercial plane before. Believing he had to claim his checked bag during his layover, he went down to baggage claim. He panicked when he couldn't find it and begged for help from an airline employee, who explained that his checked bag would be sent automatically to his final destination. Baffert, country as a hayseed, had no idea that was how it worked.

In the end, the hearing at the state capitol wasn't much. Regulators suspended Baffert for a year but made it retroactive. With a few months still left to go on the penalty, Baffert asked if he could attend the races as long as he stayed off the backstretch of the racetrack. They agreed.

Baffert didn't quite abide by those terms, though. He and the Chief still had a few horses in training at the ranch in Nogales, and whenever his father hauled a horse to run at Los Alamitos, Baffert would stow away in the trailer when they came to the entrance gate. He would get the horse ready, then stay hidden by hanging around the barn during the race. Afterward, he would cool out the horse, get back in the trailer, and he and the Chief would leave.[19]

It was the first positive drug test of Bob Baffert's career. He was still a long way from thinking of horse racing as a serious career prospect. But when he did eventually become a public trainer—a professional training for multiple different owners—he would remember the episode vividly. "I never wanted to put myself in that situation again," he said.[20]

Baffert continued to take odd jobs around horses, in between other gigs in his early twenties, including one job as a substitute teacher in Nogales that became full-time when the regular history teacher showed up at the school one day with a carload of rifles and a plan to start shooting.[21] He worked at a veterinary supply company in Tucson, played a lot of *Pac-Man*, and loitered around a restaurant that two of his siblings ran. He had become his father's son, always joking around.[22] He would do things like float Big Macs in the lobster tank or cut the rubber bands holding the claws so that he could laugh at the servers trying to fish them out without losing a finger.

Horses continued to have a pull on him. Occasionally he would train a few horses for the Chief. He came close to success with a horse named Pete Hoist, who would run blisteringly fast qualifying times in trial races but would find a way to lose in the finals. The horse almost ruined Baffert for good as a trainer. "I felt I couldn't win the big one, so I got the hell out."[23] Bobby Adair's advice was still ringing in his ears: *If you can't be the best, quit.*

Then, in 1981, fate came for him. He was working at a small breeding operation in Prescott, Arizona, but he was starting to get itchy locked away on the farm. It gnawed at him that he still hadn't won a big race. It felt like a void, a missing piece of his life. If he just went back to win that one big race, then he could quit and do something else with his life . . .

It was drugs that handed Baffert his first big break.

Two other trainers in Arizona had just had horses test positive for banned substances. One of them was Ray Yeigh, a friend of Baffert's. When Yeigh was suspended for his positive, Baffert took over Yeigh's stable. He borrowed $1,000 from his grandmother—and $600 from the cocktail waitress he would later marry—to get started. He hung out his shingle at Rillito Race Track with eight horses to begin with. He figured he could win the big one and then get out.

Rillito, then and now, was a blue-collar track. A chain-link fence surrounded the paddock, where horses were saddled before walking onto the hard dirt course to compete. It was quirky: the PA system played the famous "Colonel Bogey March" from *The Bridge on the River Kwai* at post time. The grandstand was a ramshackle plate-glass hangar with red metal siding that looked more like a run-down train station to nowhere than a racetrack.

But it had a certain romance to it too. The track sat in the shadow of the Catalina Mountains in Tucson, rough-hewn and browned in the background of every race. Spindly palm trees and lost-looking desert shrubs dotted the racecourse. Rillito had a storied history in quarter horse racing. In the 1940s, the original owners of the course built a straightaway, forty-five feet wide and three-eighths of a mile long, that became known as the "chute system." That layout became the foundation for how regulated quarter horse racing is run today—in a straight line.[24] The oval racecourse was added only later to allow for Thoroughbred racing. Rillito's original owners were also the first to develop the technical method still used today to determine the winner of an extremely close-run race, combining a high-speed clock with a movie camera at the finish line—a "photo finish."[25]

Baffert was successful there immediately. One of his horses, a filly that he had broken in for the breeding farm owner in Prescott, turned out to be a superstar. And Yeigh's horses could run too: he won three races, including a stakes race, on his first day out.[26] So-called stakes races are racing's upper level of competition, where higher-quality horses vie for bigger purses. Baffert had an epiphany: the reason he hadn't been able to win "the big one" was that he had only been training his dad's horses, and the Chief, as it turned out, didn't have very good stock. Once Baffert got his hands on some better horses, he was flying. By the end of his first season as a public trainer, he was the leading trainer at Rillito.

Baffert loved it. He was working as hard as he ever had in his life, but he was thriving on the competition and the thrill of winning. Plus, he was in love. He had moved in with Sherry Buffett, the waitress who had loaned him the $600 to get started. They had met while Baffert was working at the veterinary supply company and hanging around his siblings' restaurant, a joint called the Vineyard. She was the worst waitress Baffert had ever seen, but she knew how to give him a hard time. Baffert and his buddies would come to the Vineyard for free lunches and Sherry would come over while they were drinking and carrying on: "You guys don't want *another* drink, do you?" Later, she would remind Baffert: "Remember, buddy, I'm the one who lent you money to get started." They would get married in 1984, although not before Baffert had spent the money earmarked for her engagement ring on a horse.[27]

There still wasn't any money. A stakes race was worth at most $20,000, he recalled later,[28] and the regular races were still only worth that paltry $600. As his success snowballed and his stable ballooned to thirty horses, Baffert started to think of the unthinkable: going back to California. With a taste of success, he was ready for a bigger stage.

As Baffert began to win races at Rillito, he started to become aware that people were talking about him.[29]

Some of the gossip was de rigueur for any winning trainer. The backstretch of any racetrack has a lot in common with the small halls of the local high school: full of petty jealousies and unfounded rumor. Trainers have to explain to their owners—and themselves—why their horses are losing and someone else's are winning, and sometimes the easiest explanation is that the other guy is cheating. That was what people were saying about Bob Baffert: that he was "helping" his horses, as he had already done once before, with the apomorphine. What other explanation could there be for this kid from nowhere who had never been able to win more than a handful of races suddenly emerging as the leading trainer at Rillito? He must be giving them something.

In hindsight, Baffert blamed his own personality for the gossip. He behaved exactly like any other brash thirtysomething whose career is suddenly taking off—which is to say, he was obnoxious as hell. "I might have rubbed people the wrong way," he acknowledged.[30]

It's impossible now to know if there was any truth to the allegations. Baffert admits only to giving that one horse a performance enhancer, one time, the kind of stupid mistake that you make when you're painfully young and ambitious. But that murky suspicion would come to dog him for the rest of his career.

Baffert got off to a rough start in California. He brought ten of his best horses, and it still took him weeks to win his first race. He might have been top dog at Rillito, but California was much more competitive. With Bobby Adair's words nagging at him, he almost packed up and went home.

In Baffert's telling, he studied other trainers while learning to trust his own instincts, and it gradually paid off.[31] He caught his big break when a new owner sent him a flashy palomino named Gold Coast Express to train. The yellow horse was tough. He would come whipping out of the starting gate on the lead and turn one beaded eye to stare down his competitors in the stretch until they knuckled under. His other horses started winning too. By the time Baffert won quarter horse racing's premier year-end race with Gold Coast Express, he had cemented himself as one of the top trainers in the sport.

The horse's success came with a price. Every time the palomino won, Baffert recalled, his brand-new Ford Bronco would get keyed. The night he won the Champion of Champions at Los Alamitos in 1986, Baffert rolled out of the bar across the street from the track and headed for his car in the parking lot. *Am I drunk or does my car look like it's leaning off to one side?* he thought. Someone had slashed both tires on the right side of the vehicle.

Baffert was in his midthirties. His hair was turning white and he was beginning to settle into his adult form, a strange mix of personality traits that would later make him something of a Rorschach test when his history became a matter of public debate. There were two curious sides to Baffert: He had natural charisma, a buoyant and infectious confidence that everything was going to work out. He could be cocky.[32] He was quick to kid around. The only thing he really took seriously was winning races. But he had been almost shy as a boy, and as an adult, he sometimes came off as aloof. He wanted—maybe even needed—to be liked.[33] He seemed to view horses, these animals that he had grown up with and understood, as a place of belonging.

Horses, he said to me several times, are "therapy for me."

CHAPTER 3

THE COWBOY HAT

affert had never seen anything like the Las Vegas suite that his new client had booked on a whim. He and the client, Mike Pegram, had missed out on a few horses they both liked at a public auction and, sour, had driven to El Paso, Texas, to catch a flight back home to Los Angeles. When there were no flights, Pegram turned to Baffert: "I might end up in Dallas, or I might end up in Chicago. I might have to go the wrong way to get where I want to go, but I sure as hell ain't staying here."[1]

Baffert didn't have to be convinced. They wound up in Vegas, in a suite with a baby grand piano and a Jacuzzi—which Baffert was now sitting in with an aspiring rodeo queen, drinking Budweiser and wearing his cowboy hat.[2] It was fun to be with Pegram, who had made a lot of money on McDonald's franchises and liked a good party.[3] Baffert had already watched him blow five grand in his first five minutes shooting craps at the casino and, in the mysterious economy of Sin City, still walk away with a voucher for fifty grand. That was eye-popping money to Baffert, who lost twenty dollars and quit.[4]

He did at least have the good sense to call his wife and tell her where he was headed, categorizing the trip as business travel. *I'm with a new client and he's going to be really big*, he told her. Sherry didn't buy it. ("She never believed shit I told her anyway," Baffert said.)[5] But Baffert had a sense that Pegram was going to be the kind of owner who could change your career. He looked up from the Jacuzzi as Pegram came in from the other room where he had been doing some business on the phone, beer in hand.

"I think this is going to turn out to be a good relationship," Pegram said. "The two of us are going to go places together."

Pegram convinced Baffert to try his hand at training Thoroughbreds. By the mid-1980s, Baffert had won every major race there was to win with quarter horses. There was a ceiling to how much money you could make in the quarter horse business, and by this time, he and Sherry had four children and lived in a house by the beach.

"The quarter horse industry was very limited," said D. Wayne Lukas, who had by then made the jump to training Thoroughbreds. "There are just not that many tracks. The purse money, other than the big, big races, wasn't there on a daily basis; the Thoroughbreds at Santa Anita at that time had strong purses and the best horses."[6]

To run in the Kentucky Derby and the Breeders' Cup in the United States, or the Epsom Derby and Royal Ascot in England, or any of the other elite races from Asia to Australia, a horse must be a registered Thoroughbred. The breed is descended from three so-called foundation sires initially imported to England from the Middle East and Turkey in the 1600s and 1700s. A son of one of those three foundation sires was imported to Virginia in 1730, thus establishing the breed in the New World. Today the bloodlines of every Thoroughbred alive or dead are meticulously tracked by the breed registry, the omnipotent Jockey Club, which has its executive offices in Manhattan.

If the quarter horse is the cowboy's horse, the Thoroughbred belongs to the landed gentry. He is the gentleman's horse. The Vanderbilts and the Mellons bred Thoroughbreds. Physically, the two breeds are as different as marathon champion Eliud Kipchoge is from sprinter Usain Bolt. Quarter horses, which specialize in running shorter distances of no more than a half a mile, are built for short bursts of speed: they are short coupled with massive, muscle-bound hindquarters. The Thoroughbred, which typically runs races of anywhere from just over half a mile to a mile and a half, is bred for stamina. He is longer, leaner, more refined. There is a grace and elegance to the Thoroughbred that true snobs will say is denied his western cousin.

Another quirk of the Thoroughbred that differentiates it from the quarter horse: he must be conceived "live cover." In blunter terms: his parents have to do the deed. Thoroughbred breeders have long disavowed artificial insemination, in large part to keep the value of their stock elevated. Although prices in the breeding shed have waxed and waned over the years, for decades now the top stallions in the country have commanded hundreds of thousands of dollars per mating and are asked to breed more than two hundred mares a year in some instances.

The Thoroughbred and quarter horse worlds have little to no overlap. They have different racetracks, different players, different rules and races. It's a different society. All of this made training Thoroughbreds a foreign proposition for Baffert. He might have been a hot ticket in the quarter horse world, but when he started training a couple of Thoroughbreds for Pegram, he was a nobody—a rube in a cowboy hat. No one knew him. To top it off, the glossy, moneyed world of Thoroughbreds intimidated the hell out of him.[7]

He was so green that he once asked one of the country's top jockeys, Gary Stevens, how he should train his horse. His first faux pas was that he asked Stevens to gallop the horse: give it a slower, routine workout as opposed to a fast, sharp one, known as a "breeze" or a "work." Jockeys will breeze a horse for a trainer in the morning but typically do not stoop to gallop them—that is labor for an exercise rider. But Stevens, amiable, agreed. He asked Baffert what he'd like him to do with the horse. How far should he go?[8]

"I don't know," Baffert confessed. "What do they usually do here?"

If Stevens was nonplussed, he was gracious enough not to show it. "Usually, they back them up to the half and then they'll gallop around one," he explained.

"All right, do that," Baffert told the leading rider.

Even once he learned the basic rules, most of the time Baffert couldn't even get a rider to breeze his horses. One morning in the late 1980s, he took a horse he had claimed for Pegram up to the racetrack to breeze. He saw Alex Solis, another of the top jocks, loitering around what's known as the "gap," the entrance to the racetrack where horses come on and off. Much like other elite athletes, jockeys have agents to help them hustle the best mounts in different races. Most jockeys aren't associated with a particular stable and instead earn their living on a 10 percent commission of the winning cut of the purse. Baffert, spying Solis's agent, asked him if the jock would work his horse a half mile. If he liked the horse, a cheap animal named Hidden Royalty, he could have the mount in his next race. The agent agreed to ask Solis.

Baffert stood there holding the horse while the agent ambled over to his rider. Hidden Royalty was disintegrating, spinning around Baffert in circles. Baffert could see them all looking over at him in his cowboy hat and laughing. *I probably look like some dumb shit to them.*[9]

The agent came back to Baffert.

"Alex said he's too busy right now, and he doesn't want to ride him back anyway," he said.

Of course, the rider wasn't busy. He was just there drinking his coffee, leaving Baffert standing like a jerk on the end of the shank. Hidden Royalty whirled around him like a moon knocked off its axis. Baffert never forgot the moment. "That shit stays in my head," he said. He went back to the barn and found an exercise rider to breeze the horse. When he eventually ran Hidden Royalty in a race, he lost.

The basic business model of the Thoroughbred industry is this: Public trainers, like Bob Baffert, prepare horses on behalf of clients—almost universally referred to as "owners"—to run in races for a percentage of purse money won. In the small industry of training racehorses, owners can be fickle, moving their horses from trainer to trainer. When a trainer is young, he needs owners to take a chance on him. He is dependent on them. Larger, successful trainers exert a power of their own. There is a famous racetrack adage: "Owners are like mushrooms: Best kept in the dark and under a lot of shit." The owners have the money, but the trainer has the expertise. There's a strange power dynamic at the top levels of the sport, one where the client is often deeply deferential to the man he's paying to perform a service for him. Some trainers develop an almost mystical reputation for their work, so that it's the billionaire owner whose image is aggrandized by his association with the trainer, not the other way around.

But getting there is tough. The economics of the business are brutal to smaller trainers. Trainers charge a "day rate" of somewhere between $75 and $150, but that only just covers the expenses of caring for the horse. An owner might expect to spend $50,000 a year to train and maintain a racehorse, but none of that is profit to either the owner or the trainer, both of whom only make money when the horse wins races. For most owners, this is discretionary income. (Another old joke in the horse business has it that if you want to make a million dollars, start with two.) But this is a job for horse trainers, who are essentially small business owners. Caring for horses is labor-intensive, requiring salaried grooms, exercise riders, even hot-walkers whose sole responsibility is to walk the horse until he is cool after exercise to free up the grooms for other work. Then there are the hours trainers spend developing a training program, managing injuries, and poring over the "condition book"—the list of upcoming races—to find appropriate spots for their horses to run. (Another old saying: "Never let your owner get a hold of the condition book." They might start getting ideas about what races a horse should be entered in, and those ideas might include running a nag that can't run its way out of a wet paper bag in a stakes race that it has no business even contemplating. Owners have been known to become possessed of delusions of grandeur.)

For all of this, trainers typically receive a 10 percent cut of the winning purse. Whether that amounts to a living depends on the size of the purses. Ron Faucheux was the leading trainer for the third year running at the Fair Grounds Race Course in New Orleans in 2023, but he decided to quit training and become a jock's agent instead. "I was just breaking even doing what I was doing," Faucheux said. "I love training horses, but I wasn't getting the kind of day rate trainers in places like New York and Kentucky get and our expenses are pretty comparable to theirs. This was a lot of work and, in all honesty, over the last several years, I wasn't making any money doing it."[10]

The racetrack, meanwhile, makes its money by withholding a certain percentage ("the takeout") of all dollars wagered that day ("the handle"). The state also takes a cut of the takeout. In parimutuel wagering on racing, gamblers are betting against one another, not the house. The more people gamble—the greater the handle—the more money the track makes, no matter who wins or loses. New York tracks, for example, keep about 6 to 8 percent of all dollars wagered for its own operations.[11] From the racetrack's perspective, the most important thing is that it can offer full, competitive fields, which are the most attractive gambling product. Takeout money goes in part to funding purse money.* Racetracks are in the gambling business, not the horse business.

There is one more part of the Thoroughbred industry: the bloodstock business. Horses that perform well in top races—stakes races—are bought and sold as breeding prospects. Their untried offspring are bought and sold as racing prospects, and the cycle continues. An entire industry exists to facilitate the breeding and trading of racehorses. There are bloodstock agents who identify racing and breeding prospects for clients and then

---

* Some racetracks are also able to supplement purse money with revenue from casino operations in the state. Racing used to be among the only legal forms of sports wagering in the United States. That has gradually changed in recent years, and racing has not only lost its monopoly but lost popularity against football and other sports. Purses suffered as a result. At the same time, an uncomfortable marriage between casinos and racetracks has arisen. To get around the concerns of "sin industry" critics who opposed the legalization of casino operations, some state legislators have yoked them to existing laws permitting gambling on horse racing and mandated that part of casino revenue be earmarked for racing purses. This has given a huge boost to purses in some states, but it's a tenuous arrangement. The casinos are often far more profitable than the racetracks and are, effectively, propping up a dying product. There is no inherent business connection between them, and how long state legislators will keep this arrangement in place remains to be seen.

purchase them on commission (and sometimes with a little kickback from the seller).[12] Some bloodstock agents study pedigrees and plan matings for wealthy owners. Some prepare untried yearlings and sell them as part of a consignment at public auction. Others buy yearlings and then resell them as two-year-olds. The most impressive money is made by horse traders who select a young colt at an early age that performs well enough to be sold as a breeding stallion, usually under a "syndicate" agreement made up of forty or more individually sold shares. Trainers who are able to help their owners play *that* game successfully aren't trying to scrape by on their day rate.

Around the time Baffert began running a few Thoroughbreds for Mike Pegram, the top trainer in the country who was also an old quarter horse trainer. D. Wayne Lukas was a former high school basketball coach from Wisconsin who now flew around the country in a private jet, wearing $3,000 bespoke suits and a Stetson. Lukas had done more to change the business of training Thoroughbred racehorses than any other horseman before him, pioneering a business model that became known as the "super trainer." Instead of training a string of horses based at a single racetrack or in a single region, Lukas kept satellite stables run by assistant trainers at racetracks around the country, a model he frequently compared to a McDonald's franchise. He shipped horses from barn to barn, seeking out the most favorable race conditions for each individual horse to run under. In its heyday in the 1980s, D. Wayne Lukas Racing Stables boasted close to two hundred horses in training across the country.[13] Before Lukas came around, even the top trainers might have just thirty horses in training at a single racetrack.[14] This new business model made Lukas fabulously wealthy: In addition to the private jet, he also shared a helicopter with one of his top clients and kept a fleet of cars emblazoned with the stable logo. One entire room of his large and immaculately landscaped home in Arcadia was devoted to his flashy and expensive wardrobe, which at the time included more than two hundred sport coats.[15]

Lukas had stepped into the Thoroughbred game at a moment of profound transition in the sport in the 1970s. Racing had long been dominated by old families with old money, who campaigned Thoroughbreds mainly for the sport of it. Horses offered at public auction—like Northern Dancer—were the rejects. Between 1930 and 1970, Fasig-Tipton, one of the leading auction houses, sold only four Kentucky Derby winners.[16] But by the 1970s, some of those old dynasties had begun to die off, making room for younger sportsmen—and opening access at auction to some of the brilliant pedigrees long hoarded by the old families. Buying and selling racehorses became an increasingly commercial business, and in the 1970s, Fasig-Tipton sold four Derby winners in a single decade. (Keeneland, the other major auction house, sold two others.)[17] As a speculative fever took hold, the price of bloodstock began to skyrocket. New money entered the sport, in particular a conglomerate of buyers, led by a British bookmaker, an Irish stallion manager, and an Irish trainer, a group that would eventually become known as "the Irish mafia."[18]

Robert Sangster, the bookmaker, recognized that the price of bloodstock was rising. He recognized also that the real money was to be made in syndicating stallions. Leaning on the brilliant eye of John Magnier, the stallion manager, and Vincent O'Brien, a horse trainer of legendary talents, Sangster amassed huge sums of money to sweep the Thoroughbred sales in Kentucky for well-bred, well-made colts. He called it buying "baby stallions."[19] Those that raced well would be syndicated for millions. It had never been done before, at least not at the scale that Sangster did it. He almost single-handedly pioneered a business model that upended the purpose of buying a racehorse. No longer was the point to *buy a racehorse*. The point was to make millions investing in a stallion prospect.

In the 1980s, a group of Arab royals also began shopping in earnest at the same horse sales. By the middle of the decade, head-to-head bidding wars between Arab and Irish buyers would drive yearling prices into the tens of millions. One of those yearlings, a $10.2 million colt named Snaafi Dancer, never raced and turned out to be infertile—but it hardly slowed down the frenzy. Suddenly, there was *real* money in racing.*

It was a prime time for an upstart quarter horse trainer to break into the hidebound world of Thoroughbreds.

Lukas professionalized the world of racehorse training. His immaculately landscaped barns—bright peacocks among the sea of modest jerry-rigged affairs scattered across the backstretch—bespoke of a slick operation catering to the rich. He made racing attractive to high-dollar businesspeople who wanted to treat it like an investment rather than a sport. The pure simplicity of racing, the unspoken gentleman's bet that *I can breed a faster horse than you*, was an archaic holdover in the shamelessly acquisitive decade of the

---

* This inflated market would eventually crash, losing over 30 percent of its value by 1992. But prices for well-bred yearlings and stallion prospects would never go back to what they were before, and the larger commercial industry built around producing sales horses remained—albeit with tighter margins. https://www.thoroughbreddailynews.com/pdf/oped/oped120921.pdf.

1980s. The days when racing was a sign of class and generational wealth, not profit, were gone. Lukas and Sangster helped usher out an old way at the racetrack, and fashion a new way of thinking about the horse.

Unlike the old guard of owners, Lukas's top client, Gene Klein, a long-time owner of the San Diego Chargers, had no interest in breeding horses. Klein shocked the racing world in 1987 when he offered to sell his champion racing mare, Lady's Secret, for $5.7 million. (He didn't get his price, but she eventually sold two years later for $3.8 million.)[20] The idea of selling a mare rather than breeding her struck many horsemen at the time as not only bad business, but disloyal to the animal.

"When a horse has been that good to you, you don't peddle her like some piece of meat," Eddie Gregson, a California trainer, told turf writer William Nack at the time.[21] "Everybody was shocked when he sold Lady's Secret. You can't sell a horse like that. It destroys your karma."

Horses had never been pets. But neither had they been seen as strict commodities, to be traded on the virtue of their market value alone. The selling of Lady's Secret was "revolutionary," Gregson said. "It's a new notion of attacking the game. There is no loyalty to any of your retired champions. Let them go; let someone else breed them. This approach is so different."

As Thoroughbred racing was changing, its traditionalists looked askance at this brash cowboy from the quarter horse world who wasn't just buying and selling in new and shocking ways—he was also whupping everyone's ass in California. Lukas didn't exactly help himself: he made a number of public statements questioning the horsemanship of established trainers and he steadfastly refused to blend in, sporting his Stetson and western chaps while riding his stable "pony" to the track to watch his horses train. ("Ponies" at the racetrack aren't actually ponies, but rather horses of a variety of breeds with quiet dispositions used to accompany high-strung Thoroughbreds to the track.) Lukas was a natural-born showman, a carnival barker in a world that valued quieter, more exclusionary demonstrations of wealth.

"People didn't like Wayne when he first changed over," his assistant trainer at the time said. "He made some statements about trainers that get stuck in ruts and the world passes 'em by."[22]

Thoroughbred racing had always had an upstairs and a downstairs. But as in any society, the floors can become jumbled during times of great economic upheaval. The old families in Kentucky and New York who had been the center of gravity for racing and breeding for the better part of a hundred years had connections to an old-world understanding of "society" and how it should be organized. When Queen Elizabeth II, an avid breeder of racehorses, visited central Kentucky, she stayed at the private home of the owner of Lane's End Farm. Lukas—and in Europe, Robert Sangster—upended the domination of racing by aristocrats.

This world in flux is what Baffert had stepped into, backed by a free-wheeling McDonald's franchiser.

At an annual two-week-long auction for yearlings in Kentucky, the top prospects are sold during the first week. The second week, so the old saw goes, is when the cowboy hats come to town to kick the tires on less expensive horses. "When the cowboy hats come in, you're not going to be getting a lot of money for your horse," Baffert said.[23]

Baffert was a cowboy hat.

Baffert was standing outside the bidding ring at Keeneland, in Lexington, Kentucky, in the fall of 1988. It was the third day of the two-week September yearling sale, and so far Baffert was agog at the money being spent. He still only had one Thoroughbred in his stable—Hidden Royalty—and the idea of paying hundreds of thousands of dollars for a one-year-old horse that had never seen the racetrack seemed absurd to him. He was looking for a horse for a client at around fifteen or twenty grand.

The horse racing calendar is punctuated with different sales throughout the year, for every kind of horse: breeding stock sales for mares and wean-lings, two-year-old sales, yearling sales, sales for older horses in training. But Keeneland September is the grandest of all of these, in the cradle of the sport's breeding industry. Its auctioneers and executives all don a "Keene-land green" blazer, as does the man whose job it is to hold each yearling while it stands on a raised dais to be auctioned off, his arm outstretched as rigidly as a lawn jockey to show the horse.* Until very recently, Keeneland was the exclusive purview of men; the men who held the horses in the ring

---

* Ringmen are among the most skilled horsemen at any sale, capable of taking the shank of any one of hundreds of strange horses under profound stress, leading them into a tiny ring amid the hubbub of a crowd, the shouts of the bid spotters, and the rapid-fire patter of the auctioneer. They not only keep the horses safe but "show" them to prospective buyers. Cordell Anderson and Ron Hill, whose work I have admired since I was nineteen years old, are artists. They "vanish next to the horse," another fan of their horsemanship said to me recently, and that is the correct way to put it. https://paulickreport.com/news/bloodstock/its-a-gift-the-calming -influence-of-cordell-anderson.

were Black. (Lawn jockeys—or hitching posts—were historically racist caricatures of Black horsemen,[24] that, even as the statues came to have white faces and were embraced by the racing community as a way for owners to celebrate their racing silks, served as a subtle signifier of class, evocative of antebellum racial and social hierarchy; in particular, the period of time in which jockeys were enslaved people riding on behalf of their enslavers—and sometimes, riding their way out of slavery. Now lawn jockeys are increasingly understood as a racist symbol of an old power structure—not, of course, that they are seen that way within horse racing.[25]) For years, European horsemen would also quietly whisper that the bathroom attendants whom Keeneland hired to hand you a hand towel after you had washed your hands were always Black too. It was never discussed openly. But there was no mistaking the "Keeneland green" and the country club air it represented. This was the power center of Kentucky and, in some ways, of the entire industry. Central Kentucky had the stallions. It had the yearlings that would become stallions. It had the mares that would be bred to the stallions to make more yearlings, and, one hoped, more stallions. Central Kentucky was where the *money* was.

There is an order to the apparent chaos at Keeneland September. Yearlings are led up and down the granite dust yards between the barns in endless parades for prospective buyers, always turned to the right at the walk and observed standing from the left, with the feet positioned just so. Assistants for each buyer run ahead to the next consignment to mark down which horses their boss wants to see. Buyers will have spent days sorting through a "catalog" of the horses on offer, studying their pedigrees and the race records of their parents and siblings and then, finally, studying the horses themselves for clues about how well they might perform on the racetrack. Are their limbs "correct"—straight, without fault? Do they walk well, with the strong but easy gait of a natural athlete? (Fillies who possess the trifecta—who have, to borrow another racing bon mot that would never survive contact with the outside world, the "face of a lady, hips like a washer woman, and a walk like a hooker"—are prized as potential broodmares. Colts are the most valuable because they are stallion prospects, capable of breeding hundreds of mares annually, in some cases for hundreds of thousands of dollars apiece.) Finally, do X-rays of their limbs show any barely perceptible defect that might become a soundness problem down the road? Does a camera threaded down their throat show a paralyzed larynx, a naturally occurring defect that could limit a horse's performance on the racetrack?* Every buyer will have different opinions about which flaws are acceptable and which are not.

There's a certain insanity to the whole enterprise. Not only must a horseman be able to peer into the future of a living animal to judge the shape that this immature and unformed creature will take at a specific point, but he or she also has to keep it alive. Another famous racetrack adage is that Thoroughbreds—flight animals—are born trying to kill themselves, so infinite is their capacity to do things like get spooked by a pleasant spring breeze rustling the leaves near their paddock, panic-gallop and acquire a small cut from a fallen branch, then develop a subsequent life-threatening bacterial infection that makes the whole leg blow up like an elephant. For this reason, it is perhaps not a surprise that most horsemen are affected with the sort of punchy sense of humor that comes with living so close to catastrophe. One must be possessed of a certain fatalistic bent to make it in the horse business, where an investment of $100,000 or $300,000 or $1 million may suddenly run itself through a board fence or begin to exhibit latent neurological symptoms that will render it practically worthless overnight. Horsemen of all stripes—the old "hardboots," or native Kentuckians, the cowboy hats, the come-here Irishmen, the skilled Black grooms from Virginia who are vanishingly rare but still around—have adapted to this constant threat of disaster by developing a pathological attention to detail and a bottomless appreciation for gallows humor. The particular breed of Thoroughbred horsemen found at sales tends to be, as a type, incredibly uptight and extremely funny.

Baffert always liked to get a feel for something before he jumped in, to make a proper study of it. Otherwise, how could you become the best? He had thrown himself into learning about Thoroughbreds, picking the brains of the old masters at Santa Anita, trainers like Laz Barrera and Charlie Whittingham. He visited the historic Claiborne Farm to study the physical conformation of their stallions, which included Secretariat. He moved only reluctantly to spend his clients' money, aware of all he didn't know.

Finally, after days of looking at horses he couldn't afford or didn't like, he saw a gray colt that he absolutely loved. Best of all, the horse was a ridgling—a colt with a testicle that hasn't descended. Because undescended

---

* This kind of presale diagnostic work is far more prevalent today than it was in 1988 and, some sellers say, detrimental. Buyers turn down horses based on minor imperfections on an X-ray or a scope that may never result in a clinical presentation. https://paulickreport.com/news/back-80s -era-easy-selling.

testicles can sometimes cause an animal discomfort and require surgery—and because at one time, people believed that it could impact a colt's fertility down the line[26]—the horse would likely be cheaper because of it. He spoke to Bill Mitchell, another client, and said, "Bill, I just saw this beautiful gray sonofagun. You need to buy this horse."

Bill Mitchell was in at $20,000. But the bidding on the gray colt quickly jumped to $22,000, then $25,000. Baffert urged Mitchell to stay in, but it was too rich for Mitchell's taste. "You got other clients," he told Baffert. "If you like him that much, buy him for them." Baffert raised a hand for the colt at $30,000. The bid spotter's voice rang out in a shout indicating to the auctioneer that he had a bid: *Heey-up!*

Baffert immediately regretted it. "Man, I hope someone ups the bid, so I can get out of this deal," he thought.[27]

From the podium, the auctioneer banged the gavel. "Sold, $30,000."

Someone from the auction house came over with the ticket for a shell-shocked Baffert to sign. He was "shaking like a leaf."[28] How the hell was he going to get out of this one? Here he was, holding the ticket for a ridgling by a sire he had never even heard of, a young stallion off to a slow start named Slewpy. Until he got the horse sold, he, Bob Baffert, was on the hook for $30,000, money he could hardly afford. He and Sherry were trying to buy a house back in California.[29] When he cut the check to Keeneland—he didn't have an established credit line, like most buyers—there was barely enough money in the account for it to clear.[30]

R. D. Hubbard, the head of Hollywood Park, offered Baffert a ride home from the sale on his private jet, and Baffert tried to sell the colt to him on the way back to LA. Hubbard was a self-made millionaire to whom "winning is everything,"[31] and he had money to spend. He took one look at the pedigree and told Baffert he was on his own.[32] By the time Baffert got the horse to California, the situation had not improved.

"What's the matter with his head?" his assistant, Laura Pinelli, asked him when the horse arrived. "He's got some big indentation." Baffert hadn't even noticed. His immediate fear was that the horse had a fractured skull that he had somehow neglected to see. In the end, Baffert recalled, it was only a natural and harmless depression that young horses get from lying down on their side in their stall.

Pinelli asked Baffert what he had paid for the horse.

"Thirty freakin' slews," Baffert said, and the horse was christened: Thirty Slews.

Baffert at last found some old quarter horse clients to buy the horse, who continued to underwhelm. Thirty Slews took a long time to come to hand. He was big and what horsemen call "backward," or physically immature. Two years later, when the horse turned three, he still hadn't seen the races yet. He was also slow. The undescended testicle was bothering him, so Baffert had him cut. Finally, exasperated and needing the stall space for other, more promising horses, Baffert sent Thirty Slews to a trainer in Tijuana, Mexico, named Pepe Magana, who would get the horse in shape for the rock-bottom price of twenty dollars a day.

One day, Baffert got a phone call from Magana.

"Hey, Bob," he said. "This big gray horse is a runnin' sonofabitch. He's way too much horse for down here. You got to get him out of here."[33]

Baffert brought the horse back to California and stabled him at Del Mar, the palatial resort racing oval built by Bing Crosby in 1937 in San Diego. Baffert, a nobody, was stabled in the worst barn on the premises, a hodgepodge of portable stalls known as the chicken barn, because it was used for poultry during the county fair. Big old Thirty Slews could barely turn around in the tiny stalls and one day, he rubbed against the siding and the entire construction collapsed.

But the horse was ready to run. His first time out, he won by daylight, running easy.

People took notice. R. D. Hubbard came down to the winner's circle. "This isn't that same sonofabitch you bought at that sale, is it?"[34]

The second time Baffert ran the horse, in an allowance race, Thirty Slews won again. It was the first time the man who would become the undisputed Kentucky Derby king experienced a particular, tingling excitement known only to a select few every year in horse racing: Derby fever. He might have a horse for the big show.

The sensation didn't last long. Baffert, coming from the quarter horses, made his first big mistake with a Thoroughbred. He sent Thirty Slews to Kentucky for the Grade II Lexington Stakes at Keeneland, a prep race for horses pointed at the Derby, and before the race, Baffert told his exercise rider to work the horse five-eighths of a mile. The horse wound up working the distance in a blistering 57 and 4/5 seconds. He came off the track "coughing and gagging."[35] The rest of the week, the horse was quiet and listless. "I cooked him right then, and he never got back on his toes," Baffert said.[36] Horses, just like a human runner training for a race, can overdo it during training and have no reserves left for the main event. Thirty Slews went to the lead in the Lexington, but by the time the field turned for home, he had run out of gas. The horse put in a gallant effort to finish third, but Baffert's Derby dreams were done.

Baffert had set himself a huge task in shifting from quarter horses to Thoroughbreds. Not only was the human environment in racing challenging, but training a Thoroughbred compared to training a quarter horse was as different as training a human to run a marathon rather than a 100-meter dash. "I think it's much more difficult to train a Thoroughbred," Lukas has said. "You can take good care of a quarter horse, get the right bloodlines, good conformation, give him the ultimate in care, and he probably will run four hundred yards effectively. . . . But you take a good conformation Thoroughbred with bloodlines, and if you don't have him dead fit he's not going to run a mile and quarter."[37]

Baffert had to learn not to lean on his Thoroughbreds as hard as he could lean on his quarter horses to get them fit. Trying to strike that balance—to get the horse fitter than its competitors without burning it out or injuring it—was like standing on a knife's edge. He learned quickly with Thirty Slews that you can't make up for a too-fast work. You can always make up for a too-slow work by upping the training intensity for the rest of the week.

In retrospect, Baffert realized he hurt a lot of horses in the early days. They would get a little shin problem and Baffert would try to train through it as he would have with one of his sturdier quarter horses. The Thoroughbreds would crack under the strain, and Baffert would have to put surgical screws in the shin.

"It took me a few years, but I finally realized that if these horses were going to last, I had to get rid of that Quarter Horse mentality," he said later. "When you turn them out and bring them back, the money is still going to be there."[38]

Baffert had made some mistakes. He might not fit in with the sockless-loafer-and-Barbour-jacket crowd in Lexington. But the Kentucky boys would take anybody's money, if they wanted to spend it on a horse—and Baffert was about to start spending some money on horses.

CHAPTER 4

DERBY FEVER

In the paddock before the Kentucky Derby, surrounded by a jumbled mosaic of bright, elaborate hats, Baffert gave the jockey his final instructions: "Go out there and make me famous."

Baffert wasn't actually expecting to win. It was 1996, and he had been training Thoroughbreds full-time for less than five years. His horse, Cavonnier, was California-bred—most of the horses that run in the Derby are bred at the blue-chip farms in Kentucky—and won his first race at a fair track, not one of the big racetracks. Cavonnier was the kind of horse known around the sales as a "plain brown wrapper": an uninterrupted brown with very little white on him, just a single star pinned to his forehead, nothing flashy to look at. But he had an expressive eye that made him appear almost earnest when he pinned his ears and ran. The horse was training well, and he went off as the second betting choice behind the slate-gray phenom Unbridled's Song. Baffert told jockey Chris McCarron to give the horse a big ride at the three-eighths pole (three-eighths of a mile before the finish) and see if he could get lucky when the cavalry came running at the end. It's an almost superstitious ritual among horsemen with a runner in the Kentucky Derby: you can only claim to be "happy to be there." Anything more, and you'll jinx it. The Derby belongs to fate.

The Derby is an indisputable dash for commercial value. A colt that beats the nineteen other best colts in the country over the so-called classic distance of a mile and a quarter is a colt that is worth money as a stallion. Few other races offer the same opportunity for instant appreciation. It's also the oldest continuously run sporting event in the United States, with a rich and romantic history, and so for a muddled combination of reasons— some pure, some less pure—the Derby is racing's most treasured prize. It has an almost religious standing among horsemen. It's not uncommon to see one tear up when the band plays "My Old Kentucky Home" over the loudspeakers before the big race. (The song is actually tremendously sad, written from the perspective of an enslaved person sold south. The original 1853 lyrics included the line "the darkies are gay"; the Kentucky legislature officially changed the words to "the people are gay" in 1986.)[1]

The field size is huge and the race, especially the start, can be a free-for-all as twenty young horses bump and jostle each other in a frantic scramble for position. Because the field is so large, a horse's post position, determined by the luck of the draw, can have a dramatic impact on the outcome of the race. And because only three-year-old horses can run in the Derby, meaning that a given horse can only run in the race once in its life, the pressure of having a horse enter the starting gate is enormous.

The Derby is a race where anything can happen. The odds-on favorite, bred from the right bloodlines by the right connections and trained by the top trainer, can prevail. Or the race might be won by a horse like Rich Strike, who in 2022 won the Derby for his obscure connections at 80-1—the second-longest shot in history. In 2009, Mine That Bird captured the race at 50-1 for another trainer in a cowboy hat, Chip Woolley. Woolley drove the horse to the race himself from New Mexico, hauling him behind his Ford pickup truck rather than using one of the sleek commercial shipping companies favored by larger trainers.[2] That the Derby can be anyone's dream to come true is something of an article of faith in racing.

The noise at the start of the Derby is overwhelming, an inchoate roar from a drunken crowd that drowns out every other sound except the low, inexorable rumble from somewhere deep in the earth of horses running. The sensory overload of the day narrows down to a single frame.

Cavonnier broke cleanly and cruised midpack during the early stages of the race. Pressed by Unbridled's Song, a horse named Honour and Glory established a quick early pace—22.34 seconds for the opening quarter and 46.09 for the half—setting up the race for closers to conserve their energy and then charge home fresh. Baffert, in the stands, was elated. Cavonnier got around the first bend in the oval in a perfect position and then settled down the backstretch six or seven lengths off the pacesetters. The mysterious biomechanics of the year's most unpredictable horse race were setting up exactly in his favor.

The field reached the final turn. At the three-eighths pole, Cavonnier was moving easily and Baffert had begun to think he would hit the board in his first try at the Derby. To "hit the board" refers to the top four finishers in a race, which are generally posted on the giant tote board in the infield that tells bettors the finishers, odds, and other information about a race. It meant that Baffert would pick up a bigger check: the purse money in 1996 did not all go to the top finisher but rather paid out in graduated portions through fourth position. (In 2005 the payout was extended to the fifth position.) To hit the board in a race then worth $1 million, that would be something for the quarter horse guy just starting out in Thoroughbreds. It would show folks what he could do.

By the quarter pole, the marker measuring a quarter mile from the finish, the metallic gray Unbridled's Song had taken the lead. Honour and Glory had collapsed into fifth position, unable to sustain his blistering speed for longer than a mile. Cavonnier had moved smoothly into third position, just two and a half lengths in Unbridled's Song's wake. Then, the unthinkable happened: Unbridled's Song began to drift out into the middle of the track, a signal he was giving way. Cavonnier began to close the gap between them. It was as if Unbridled's Song were standing still on a treadmill. With an eighth of a mile to go, Cavonnier seized the lead in the Kentucky Derby.

Baffert was not prepared. It was a dizzying, disorienting moment. He found himself praying: *I'll start going to church every day.*[3]

Horse races are measured in furlongs. One furlong is an eighth of a mile, a distance that the quickest Thoroughbreds can cover in ten seconds—or even a tick less, if they are only running a single furlong. Inside of a race, twelve-second panels are what separates the pretenders from the ones that can really run. The final two furlongs of the 1996 Kentucky Derby was run in 25.9 seconds. But as a lived experience, the final furlong of a race is elastic. Time can balloon out painfully as you pray for your horse to hang on or catch up. *Come on, get there already*, Baffert prayed. Somewhere in that endless moment, he looked back at the rest of the field. He could see one other horse that was charging for the finish line, not staggering home weary-legged and fading. He didn't know who it was, but the jockey was wearing the white and green silks that belonged to Overbrook Farm, one of the best farms in Kentucky, so Baffert knew it was a good horse. It was Grindstone, a rich bay animal, powerfully built with a powerful closing kick, and now eating up ground in massive strides. He was reaching forward with his muscled forelegs, grabbing the track and pulling it beneath him, driving his body up to Cavonnier's hip, then to his shoulder. McCarron didn't look back and he never stopped riding Cavonnier, scrubbing at his neck and urging him forward toward the wire. The two horses hit the line together, Cavonnier on the inside and Grindstone hung way out in the middle of the racetrack.

It was too close to call.

Baffert thought Cavonnier might have hung on. But Sherry, somehow, knew better.

"I think we ran second," she told her husband, who wanted to shake her. *What the hell do you know? You don't even go to the races!*[4]

There was an interminable delay as the racing judges deliberated over the finish, the red letters reading PHOTO frozen on the tote board.

It was the closest finish in the Derby since 1959, just a sliver of open air separating the flared nostrils of the two horses on the stretched, black-and-white image that the judges were studying. But it was unmistakable: Grindstone, the Overbrook horse in the white and green silks, trained by Wayne Lukas, had won. Cavonnier had lost.

As it turned out, it wasn't enough for Baffert to run in the money in the Kentucky Derby. The narrow loss devastated him. To have come so close, only to get nipped at the wire, broke his heart. He was convinced he would never have another horse that would bring him to Churchill Downs on the first Saturday in May.

"I had never seen Bobby so disheartened," his friend Brad McKinzie said. "Cavonnier's loss haunted him for a year. . . . That thing ate at him and ate at him. To get that close and get beat a nose . . . He never got it out of his system. In his mind, he was never going to get back there again."[5]

Horsemen call it having "the big horse"—the one that changes everything.

Baffert had bought a dark gray two-year-old colt at an auction in central Florida the same year he lost the Derby with Cavonnier. The colt's pedigree was a little weak and he was a little toed-out, a mild conformational flaw in which a horse's front feet appear duck-footed—but one that most horse buyers will accept, especially when a horse does like this one did and worked a quarter mile in 21 and 4/5 seconds. Baffert paid $85,000 for him and sold him to Bob and Beverly Lewis, major Thoroughbred owners at the time known for spending money and frequently shifting trainers. The Lewises had most of their expensive horses with Lukas, and Baffert was on his last chance with them. Bob Lewis had warned him a year earlier: Baffert was winning races for other people but not for him. That's the kind of death knell that no trainer wants to hear from an owner like Bob Lewis, who, as the magnate behind the second-largest beer distributor in California,[6] you did not want to lose.

The horse came with a name: Silver Charm. Baffert briefly tried to convince Lewis to change the name to "Poker for a Buck," a raunchy nod to his sire, Silver Buck, and his damsire, Poker. Lewis, while amused, demurred.[7] Baffert brought the horse back to California and started training him. He was lazy in the mornings, big and slow, and he could look stiff in the back galloping.[8] But at Del Mar that summer, the horse worked six furlongs out of the gate in 1:10 and 3/5 seconds.[9] The middling-bred gray horse was flying. By the fall, Baffert was already thinking about the Kentucky Derby again.

Silver Charm officially turned three on January 1, 1997. He kept beating another, more expensive two-year-old of the Lewises' named Gold Tribute, an impeccably bred bay colt who was in training with Wayne Lukas. Lukas and Baffert weren't exactly friends. They had a stiff rivalry on the track and Baffert, with his big mouth, had made a few remarks to the press that had rubbed Lukas the wrong way. After Silver Charm beat Gold Tribute in the Grade II Del Mar Futurity, Lukas told Baffert sourly: "Do you realize what you did? You just cost Bob Lewis about two or three million dollars."[10]

His point was that Gold Tribute, as a son of perhaps the most dominant stallion of his generation, Mr. Prospector, with a physical conformation that had commanded $725,000 as a yearling, would have been worth several million dollars as a stallion prospect had he won a prestigious graded race. Silver Charm, with that same Grade II to his name, likely couldn't command that kind of money.

Baffert was unmoved, perhaps because for him, the point of the game wasn't the money. Not exactly, anyway. The loss of the purse in the Kentucky Derby, or the possibility of a rich stallion deal, wasn't what had eaten at his most private, tender ambitions for months. (Cavonnier, as a gelding, could never have become a stallion anyway.) What Baffert wanted was to *win*. He wanted to be the best there was—just like Bobby Adair had said—and to be accepted as the best there was. He shot back at Lukas: "Well, if you want to make your horse worth two or three million dollars, you better get him the hell out of California."[11]

Silver Charm didn't have Gold Tribute's pedigree, but he had drawn enough attention on the merits of his racing ability alone to attract some money. Not long after his victory in the Del Mar Futurity, Bob Lewis received a $1.7 million offer from Michael Tabor, a wildly wealthy British bookmaker who had joined the same commercial racing and breeding partnership started by Robert Sangster. At first Baffert told Lewis that he should accept the offer. But by the time Tabor's representative, David Lambert, arrived to watch the horse gallop, Baffert had changed his mind. He could feel it: Silver Charm was his chance to get back to the Kentucky Derby. Lewis didn't commit one way or the other and so Lambert came to the barn, not knowing that Baffert had privately decided he wanted the horse to stay with him.

Baffert got to the barn ahead of time. He was armed with one crucial piece of information that Lambert didn't know: the horse was lazy in the mornings. Baffert pulled his exercise rider aside, telling him, "Larry, I want you to make him look real shitty today. Don't even carry your stick. I don't want to sell this horse, but I want them to be the ones to back out.

"When he comes back, I'm going to ask you how he went, and I want you to say he felt okay, but not like he did at Del Mar. Maybe it's the track here. Say it usually takes him about a mile to warm out of it."

But don't go overboard, Baffert warned. "I don't want it to sound too obvious that we're trying to talk them out of it."

The horse did exactly as expected: he galloped like shit. Lambert turned a gimlet eye on the horse and said skeptically to Baffert that the horse looked a little stiff.

"I think it's the track here, David," Baffert said coyly. "It always takes him a while to warm out of it. You should have seen him at Del Mar. But he's okay. He's sound."

The exercise rider came back. "So Larry, he went good?" Baffert asked.

"Yeah, like usual," Larry said, innocently. "It took him about a mile to warm up. He wasn't like he was at Del Mar. Maybe it's the track."[12]

Lambert passed on the horse. It was the kind of light chicanery that horse traders delight in. Even at the top levels of the sport, with millions at stake—maybe especially there—a little roguishness isn't just expected, it's seen as part of the charm. Perhaps it's the ghost of Damon Runyon, that iconic chronicler of gamblers, hustlers, and gangsters, hanging over racing. Or perhaps it's simply that to gamble millions on four matchstick legs and a flight instinct, you have to be imbued with a certain twisted sense of humor.

Still, it was a risky move on Baffert's part. In his enthusiasm to get back to the Derby, he had potentially risked what, for Lewis, might have been the better financial deal. Lambert later told Baffert that it was Silver Charm's pedigree that had spooked them off the deal, not Baffert's sales job. Thoroughbreds' pedigrees are printed, in sales catalogs and elsewhere, with the best accomplishments of the progeny on the mother's side listed back through several generations. (It is assumed that the stallion's progeny and accomplishments are known.) Names of horses that have won stakes races are printed in blocked, bolded letters, so-called black type. There might only be room for two or three generations on a single page in a good pedigree, the black type thick as a dense ground cover. Silver Charm's page was "all white." It made him a potentially perishable investment: because of his unimpressive pedigree, Silver Charm's only path to value was on the racetrack. His Grade II win wasn't enough to make him a stallion, yet, so if something happened to him, Lewis would be kicking himself for passing up $1.7 million when he had the chance. Baffert had even said as much to Lambert: "He can really run, but I just hope that goddamn pedigree doesn't show up. I even told Bob Lewis, one bad step and this sonofabitch is worth twenty-five hundred bucks."[13]

But Baffert had always been an incurable optimist, even when it meant he couldn't see the future clearly or glided over all the ways that his own actions might come back to haunt him.[14] He always thought everything was going to turn out okay.[15] The risk was worth it. He wanted to win the Kentucky Derby. That, not $1.7 million, was the game.

Baffert really screwed up the Grade I Santa Anita Derby—one of the major prep races for the Kentucky Derby—but in the end, it didn't matter. He had never been so thrilled to lose a race.

Wayne Lukas was running a filly that he had done a good job of convincing the world was Derby material. Sharp Cat was a daughter of the legendary stallion Storm Cat, and she already had four Grade I wins to her name. She was expected to get loose on the lead in the Santa Anita Derby and, the idea was, no one would be able to catch her. Baffert had other ideas. He told jockey Gary Stevens—the same rider he had once asked to gallop his horse—to take Silver Charm to the front early and battle Sharp Cat for the lead. He wanted to get a hard race into Silver Charm to get him fit for the Derby. Plus, he figured the gray horse could grind down the filly through sheer cussedness.

"I want you to go toe-to-toe with her and run her into the ground," he told Stevens in the paddock before the race.[16]

Silver Charm hooked on to the filly out of the gate and the two burned down the backstretch like the rail was catching fire behind them. The elbows of their two riders moved lightly but as if locked together, contracting and relaxing in sync as Silver Charm and Sharp Cat went stride for stride. They sizzled out fractions of :22 and change, :45 and change, and then, impossibly, 1:09 and change for the opening three-quarters of a mile. *Oh my God, what did I do?* Baffert thought.[17]

Coming out of the final turn, Sharp Cat had no more left to give. Her jockey urged her to hang on, but she was done. Only then did Baffert see the threat. Another gray horse, almost white, was driving for the lead from the middle of the pack. Free House linked up shoulder for shoulder with a tired Silver Charm, then muscled a head in front. In a desperate move, Stevens switched his stick to his left hand. Silver Charm had just run viciously fast early fractions and put away a tough rival; there was no way he would be able to hold off another challenger who had merely drafted behind his fast pace.

Then, something miraculous happened: Silver Charm came back at Free House. In a supreme display of will, he dragged himself level with the other horse. It wouldn't be enough to win—Free House would best Silver Charm by a head—but that didn't matter. One more jump and he would have had Free House too, Baffert thought. The way he had dug in to take on a fresh rival was something to behold.

"We may have lost the battle, but we're gonna win the war," he told Stevens after the race. "I've never had a horse who came back like that."[18]

Baffert had gotten attached to the horse. All horses have their own personalities and private worlds, but just like people, some of them stand out more than others. Silver Charm was a character. He was a sensible horse, settled in his own skin, rarely ruffled by the constant hustle and bustle of the racetrack. He was a cool customer around the barn. But on the racetrack, he was a tenacious competitor. There was something achingly noble about Silver Charm. Later in his career, in a race long after the Derby, Baffert failed to get the horse fit enough for the distance. Gary Stevens, his regular rider, knew coming down the backside that he had "no horse" under him. But "because the horse is so gutsy, Gary knew he'd keep on trying to hook those horses even though he was tired," Baffert recalled.[19] The rider had to "wrap up" on the horse—use the reins to discourage the horse from running on. That was who Silver Charm was.

Of course, he would also give you a heart attack. Perhaps because he rarely got excited, Silver Charm would rouse himself to provide only the exact amount of effort required to win and no more. He had to have someone to beat. *If you couldn't be the best,* he seemed to say, *what was the point in putting in all that effort?*

As they always do, the band played "My Old Kentucky Home," and twenty three-year-olds entered the starting stalls of the 1997 Kentucky Derby, each freighted with the dreams and ambitions of their human connections. Free House, a white blur out of the gate, seized the lead early. Silver Charm, darker than his old rival, settled fourth on the outside of the pack. The favorite, Captain Bodgit, was somewhere behind him. As the field came around the final turn, Stevens made his move on Silver Charm, asking him to run down the lead horses. At the same time, Captain Bodgit was accelerating out of the middle of the pack. Silver Charm flew past a tired Free House and seized the lead as Captain Bodgit charged him from behind in the final jumps of the race. He had his head at Stevens's knee, both riders in a desperate drive. But the favorite was no match for the $85,000 horse with grit to spare. Silver Charm refused to yield, crossing the finish line a head in front of Captain Bodgit.

Bob Baffert had won racing's most sought-after prize.

The next morning, Baffert was at Churchill buying Derby '97 T-shirts at half price when he got a phone call from Mike Pegram, who was in jail. Incredulous, Baffert asked him what the hell had happened.

"Ah, that damn goofy broad," Pegram said.[20]

Pegram and Baffert's exploits hadn't cooled in the years since their spontaneous Vegas trip. They were winning big races and flying high. After Thirty Slews won the Breeders' Cup Sprint, Pegram got caught by track security fooling around with a woman on the track at Gulfstream Park, in South Florida. He had lifted her up against the rail by the eighth pole when the security guard started flashing his lights on them. Pegram, with a wink, infamously named a horse Loveontherail after the incident.[21]

Pegram had remained Baffert's most steadfast and loyal owner, and his greatest cheerleader when Silver Charm won the Derby. Even though he didn't own the horse, they cried on the track together after the race. Baffert had dedicated the win to Pegram, thanking him on national television for getting him into Thoroughbreds in the first place. It had been a perfect weekend. Now Pegram was supposed to be on his way to Turf Paradise in Phoenix to watch one of his horses run. He hadn't gotten further than the airport.

"Remember I told you she gave me a gift?" Pegram said of the woman. "Well, I never opened it and it turned out to be a goddamn gun, so they locked me up."[22]

Pegram, incidentally, had also won a significant sum betting on Silver Charm, paid out by the racetrack in cash. Security had caught the man red-handed with a wad of cash and a gun on his way out of the state. Baffert was his one call.

"Did it have any bullets in it?" the trainer asked, stunned.

Baffert could think of only one person to call who might be able to help. Conveniently, one of the top owners and breeders in the state of Kentucky was its former governor, Brereton Jones. He owned Airdrie Stud, 2,500 acres of rolling bluegrass just outside Lexington. Baffert caught him just as he was fixing to leave for church and the governor promised to make some calls.

In the way that racing has of making its most inconvenient problems disappear—not always through money but sometimes through the who-do-you-know that powers small, insular communities—Pegram's salvation was engineered not by the governor but through yet another stroke of good luck. As soon as Baffert got off the phone with Jones, he ran into the director of horsemen's relations at Churchill Downs, Buck Wheat. He told him the story.

"Don't worry, I'll take care of it," he told Baffert. "I got a buddy down there."[23]

Wheat, as it turned out, knew the chief of police for the city of Lexington, a Captain Steve Thompson. Within thirty minutes, Pegram was out of the clink.[24]

Baffert still had to convince Pegram to break up with the woman, who Pegram was convinced was responsible for a recent string of successes on the racetrack. "We're on a roll because we're on a roll," Baffert told him. "If you think it's because of some girl, you're crazy."[25] Superstition is a powerful force at the racetrack.

Racing at all levels is an addicting life. A day at any racetrack in America offers an opportunity for redemption every half hour, when the next group of horses enters the starting gate. At the top level of the sport, its sheer decadence is part of the seduction. The Taittinger champagne is flowing. Trainers and owners travel on private jets. There are sports and music stars at the big parties. Suddenly Baffert was running in a crowd that rubbed elbows with celebrities—and, even more alluringly, the kind of millionaire and billionaire whose name stayed *out* of the nightly news.

He still kept company with his old friends, people who made him laugh, like Pegram, and John Bassett, the friend who once told him he was a terrible jockey. (One time, at a dinner party with Reba McEntire, Baffert asked Bassett if she had a big hit. "Yeah, Reba's got a monster," Bassett said. He told Baffert, who listened to rock and roll, the name of the song. Baffert, at the end of the dinner, congratulated a startled McEntire on her success with a tune called "Big Ball's in Cowtown," an existent tune but not, it appears, one McEntire has ever recorded.)[26] He exasperated the old-school trainers by showing up at the track at eight or nine o'clock—heresy for a horse trainer, who the old rules dictated should be in the barn by 6 a.m.[27] He had an irreverent sense of humor: whenever he bought a horse at sale without a particular buyer in mind, he would sign the ticket "Morning Wood Stables."[28] A gifted storyteller, he also was a spot-on mimic of some of racing's bigger personalities. "I haven't really changed," he said.[29]

Silver Charm almost took Baffert all the way on his first try. He won the second leg of the Triple Crown, the Preakness, by a head, running down his rival Free House in the stretch, and he came up short by just three-quarters of a length in the Belmont, the third and final race in the series. Baffert didn't blame the horse. He blamed Free House, who was between Silver Charm and the winner, Touch Gold. Had the Charm been able to see Touch Gold flying up his tail, Baffert believed, he would have dug down and found what it took to beat him. The horse was that noble.

But the loss didn't sting like Cavonnier's defeat in the Derby the year before. Even that pain had been wiped away by the Charm. For the rest of his career, Silver Charm would be special to Baffert. It wasn't just that he had won him the Kentucky Derby for the first time. It was something in the horse's character that moved Baffert. When Silver Charm retired from stud duty to a farm in Lexington, Baffert would drive the hour down Interstate 64 from Louisville every year to visit the old horse when he came to Kentucky for the Derby. He missed seeing the horse's alert eye and broad, intelligent forehead hanging over the stall webbing every morning. Seeing the horse again always choked him up.

"He was like my fifth child," Baffert said. "I wanted that Kentucky Derby win so badly, and he gave it to me."[30]

The next year, Baffert did it again, with another horse of equally obscure origin. He almost didn't get up to look at the colt that would take him back to the winner's circle of the Kentucky Derby. He was sitting on a wall at Keeneland and sent an associate, J. B. McKathan, over to examine him.

McKathan came back and reported that the colt looked okay, but that he had crooked front legs. He was also extremely narrow through the chest, nothing like the strapping powerhouses that were leading the sale. Baffert eased off the wall anyway to check out the horse himself. He decided he would bid up to $50,000 or $60,000 for him.

Real Quiet didn't bring nearly that much. Baffert signed the ticket under Pegram's name for $17,000. When the three men met for dinner at an upscale steakhouse in Lexington later that night and Baffert told him what he'd paid for the colt, Pegram asked, "What does he have, cancer?"

"No, he's kind of aerodynamic," Baffert said. "He looks good from the side, but there isn't a lot to him from the front."

"I'll tell you what he looks like," McKathan said. "You know when you look in a fish tank and you see a fish that's so beautiful from the side? Then, he turns and swims toward you and there's nothing there?" He held up a menu and turned it edgeways toward Pegram. "That's what this colt is like."[31]

Real Quiet, ever after, would become known in the barn as "The Fish." He would go on to win the 1998 Derby and the Preakness.

If Silver Charm was cheap, Real Quiet was a giveaway. The Fish cemented a reputation that the Charm had begun: Baffert was now known for his uncanny ability to find diamonds in the rough. The cowboy hat had now two years in a row bought an underrated, imperfect horse for a song and won racing's most prestigious prize. It would make him famous among horsemen. In this Baffert was, and is, indisputably the real deal.

Buying cheap horses was an intentional strategy. Baffert and Pegram would usually spend half a million dollars at a sale, but they wouldn't pay more than $100,000 for a single horse. "We'd go for numbers and try to pick up little freaks," Baffert said. "That's where we had most of our success."

As a strategy, it sounds easier than it is. Very few horsemen have Baffert's natural eye for talent, especially when that talent is buried in a weedy, immature frame with crooked knees. Baffert could somehow see through the obvious imperfections and find the athlete underneath. He could never articulate what it was that he liked about a horse; it was all gut feel. While some trainers and bloodstock agents have a grading system that they use to rate horses, Baffert would simply wait to be impressed. He particularly liked to watch a horse right before it went through the auction ring, when it was surrounded by a crowd. If they became so nervous that they "washed out"— sweated profusely—or did something foolish like rear or flip over, Baffert would know that they couldn't handle the stress of race-day crowds. Pass.

His ability to see what others couldn't had vaulted Bob Baffert, a farm boy from nowhereville Arizona, into the stratosphere. Pegram, somewhere along the way, told him he had to lose the hat. But it was a strange juxtaposition, this glamorous high life in what was effectively a livestock industry. Baffert is never more confident than when he is talking about the routine care and management of animals. He learned how to judge conformation, he told me, by looking at cattle when he was a boy in 4-H. But even now, he name-drops the rich and successful in a way that betrays a sense of wonderment that he has found himself in this world.

As Baffert rose, Cavonnier faded into obscurity. After his near-miss in the Derby, Baffert ran the horse in the Preakness and the Belmont in 1996. Cavonnier broke well in the Belmont and, coming out of the final turn, started to make a bid for the lead. But something happened in the stretch. Chris McCarron pulled the horse up, stopping him on the track and jumping off him before the finish line. The horse ambulance carried him to the backside. McCarron, returning on foot with his saddle in his arms, told Baffert the injury was bad.

Baffert prayed all the way back to the barn that the injury was in the soft tissues and delicate sinews of the animal's legs, not the bones. Specifically, he prayed the horse hadn't shattered his sesamoids, the equivalent of the human ankle. Shattered sesamoids are a death sentence for a racehorse.

At the barn, the vet was already examining the horse's right foreleg below the knee. "It's a high bow," the vet said. Baffert was flooded with relief. A bowed tendon—so named because the damaged tendon curves outward like a bow—might end the horse's career, but it wouldn't end his life. Cavonnier stood calmly and patiently as they packed ice on his injured leg. Baffert stayed for a long time petting him. The horse had been tired after the Derby. Baffert had wanted to skip the Preakness. But the horse's owner wanted to run in all three races, and he paid the bills.

"Buddy, I'm sorry I put you through all this," Baffert told Cavonnier as he patted him.[32]

He blamed the track at Belmont. A loose, deep track can cause the kind of tendon injury Cavonnier had suffered in the same way running on a sandy beach might cause a human being to strain a tendon. Belmont is notoriously deep, known as "Big Sandy." On top of that, Baffert believed that the way the track maintenance team had managed the track going into the race had exacerbated the issue.[33] But a tired horse will also bow a tendon, even in good conditions.

Cavonnier would eventually return to the races more than two years later. By then, Baffert had had a falling out with the owners, who sent the horse to another trainer. Cavonnier won a lower-level stakes race in his first race back, in December 1998. But that was the last stakes race he won. His new trainer continued to try him in stakes races, but Cavonnier couldn't quite find his way to the winner's circle. By 2000 he was dropped down to the allowance level, where he won. He was eventually retired and lived out his days as somewhat of a local hero on a ranch near where he was born.[34]

This is the lot of most racehorses. The year Cavonnier ran in the Derby, there were 32,000 Thoroughbred foals born in the United States. Only a very small fraction of those horses would win races of high enough caliber to justify a breeding career. The rest must earn their living on the racetrack, for as long as they remain sound and competitive. Cavonnier was unusual. He ran in the biggest races in the country as a gelding, something you don't often see. It meant that his owners could never cash in on his unlikely success on the Triple Crown trail by retiring him as a stallion. Like the tens of thousands of other horses running each year, his only value was as a racehorse.

This isn't an inherently cruel fate. Many of these mid- and lower-level horses wind up in happy second "careers" as trail horses, fox hunters, and show jumpers when they are no longer able to earn money as racehorses. Some wind up as beloved backyard companions or doted-upon pensioners like Cavonnier. But some, of course, also wind up in kill pens, bound for Mexico or Canada, where slaughter is legal. An ancillary economy has sprung up "based around selling horses online at escalated prices under the threat that if the kill pen operator doesn't get his demanded price, he'll ship the horse across the border," the *Paulick Report* has reported.[35] There is a patchwork of nonprofits dedicated to Thoroughbred aftercare, but these organizations are often strained and at capacity.

And so it's worth keeping those numbers in mind. The top stallion prospects, the kinds of horses identified by Robert Sangster and raced by Wayne Lukas and their competitors, have an enormous impact on the market gross in Thoroughbred racing, and its image as the playground of the superrich. But in raw numbers, those horses represent only a small percentage of the racing population. Those horses have more in common with a high-dollar art investment—a risky commodity—than they do with a backyard pet. The rest, at least so long as they are running, are more akin to livestock. But nearly all horses running in America share one important attribute: they represent a way of making money for the people involved in their day-to-day care. They are understood within the sport—even if it is occasionally squeamish about saying so—as an economic asset.

Dr. Robert Hunt, one of the most widely respected veterinarians in central Kentucky, gave an interview with one of the major racing papers in 2023. He said that his interest in farm practice arose because it was "the one thing I can do that's going to help a guy put bread on his table."[36] Hunt described emergency interventions during foaling, when a mare or a foal's life is on the line, as an opportunity to ensure that the animal lives "and stay[s] in production." His language is the language of the dairy farmer or the cattleman raising beef. He talked about the decision to euthanize primarily in the context of financial, rather than emotional, loss.

"If everything works out, you may have a million-dollar commodity at the end," Hunt said. "But we also need to recognize early, hard as it is, if this is not going to be a viable individual and you need to cut your losses now."

It's a staunchly practical way of thinking of the animal. The standard of welfare that it implies is similar to that applied to other animals that are used for the benefit of humans: dairy cattle, chickens, and other livestock. Over the years, Americans have become more cognizant of industrial farming practices and the potential harm it does to individual animals in the name of cheaper chicken in the grocery store, sparking occasional welfare-driven reform and some small consumer-driven market shifts—as well as a related debate over how best to support the farmers and other agricultural workers who depend on a functioning market for chicken. But the basic argument about the ethics of the practice of raising food animals has remained static: we will accept the broad use of cattle, chickens, and pigs in this way to feed ourselves at a price we consider affordable. As a result, the standard of care that farms must meet still allows for a herd-based approach to animal husbandry, rather than one that emphasizes the quality of life of individual animals. The fate of a single chicken is rarely discussed, even if the welfare of "chickens" is.

Of course, Americans don't eat horses. And no one steer is making a cattleman a millionaire.

It invites an obvious ethical question: Should the standard of care that this foundationally agricultural industry is held to for the individual animals that it uses be higher than the standard that the food industry must meet for its own?

During the course of Baffert's career, that unanswered question would come to imperil the sport of racing. But in the cheery hedonism of the 1990s, Cavonnier—whose fate Baffert ultimately had no say over anyway—had simply done his trainer a good turn. Just getting the horse to the Derby, where he had run such a gutsy race, "doubled" Baffert's business, he said.[37]

CHAPTER 5

FREE FROM EVERY MORTAL SIN — INCLUDING BUTAZOLIDIN

In the days leading up to the 1997 Kentucky Derby, a rumor circulated on the backstretch of Churchill Downs that the Baffert horse, Silver Charm, was a bad bleeder. It's a common affliction in Thoroughbreds. Intense exercise can cause the small blood vessels in a horse's lungs to bleed, sometimes enough for blood to trickle out of the nostril. In less severe cases, blood pools in the horse's windpipe. Veterinarians can snake a scope down the horse's nose to assess whether he has bled during exercise. So-called exercise-induced pulmonary hemorrhage (EIPH) isn't life-threatening, but it can hinder a horse's performance, so the rumor was of great interest to everyone trying to predict the outcome of the Derby.

The talk was true: Silver Charm was a terrible bleeder. Baffert was constantly having to manage the horse to prevent it. He never bled out of the nostrils—it was never that bad—but when he bled, he would run a temperature. Baffert would give him antibiotics to try to prevent that, a common practice.

On the Tuesday before the big race, Baffert planned to give the horse an easy five-eighths work. He called his vet to the barn to scope the horse afterward to see if he had bled. But he also wanted to quiet down the gossip that was circulating at the racetrack.[1]

"Doc, I want you to scope him, but when you take it out, I want you to say, 'It looks good,'" Baffert said. "I'll talk to you later about it, and you can tell me what you saw."[2]

The vet did as instructed. He pulled the long, black snake of the scope out of Silver Charm's nostril and said, "Looks good." Baffert walked him to his car and the vet, who had never treated Silver Charm before, told him the truth: "It looked terrible. He bled, he's got mucus, I mean it looked horrible."[3]

Baffert reassured him. "Relax, will you," he said. "He always bleeds. Don't worry, I've been through this before. He'll run big."[4] He put the horse on some antibiotics for a day to prevent him from getting sick, obsessively took his temperature for the next four days, and then sent the horse to the post to win the Kentucky Derby. He bled during the race.

Four hours before post time, Baffert also gave Silver Charm a medication to help with the bleeding. It was a legal medication, permitted on race day at every major racetrack across the country. All of this was very routine. The drug had been around for decades and virtually every horse in America ran on it. It was noted in the public program purchased by bettors.

But its use was also arguably the single most controversial issue in the racing business, because the drug straddled the line between a safe and effective therapeutic treatment for a medical condition and a performance enhancer. This one medication has been the subject of multiple congressional hearings across decades, countless research papers, and passionate columns by turf writers in major publications like the *Washington Post* and *Sports Illustrated*. When it became legal, beginning in the 1970s, it quite literally changed how horsemen thought about medication and how the sport regulated it.

The drug was called Lasix.

The first known instance of a veterinarian treating a racehorse with Lasix was in the 1964 Kentucky Derby. Dr. Alexander Harthill knew track security was watching him. He was planning on administering a new drug known as furosemide—trade name Lasix—to Northern Dancer, the fiery little colt from Canada that would go on to win the race later that day and become the breed's most important modern stallion. At the time, it was against the rules to administer Lasix on race day. Harthill had a solution to that inconvenient problem.

"I got a vet I knew from out of town to come along with me," Harthill told the *Daily Racing Form* in 2002, three years before he died.[5] "I told him I was going to turn to the right, and would he go that way and take this little syringe down to barn 24, stall 23, and give this to that horse. There would be a guy there called Will. He'd be waiting.

"So he did it, while the gendarmes followed me."

Harthill was already a legend by the time he treated Northern Dancer. A charismatic man with a "twinkle in his eye,"[6] he was one of the most skilled veterinarians to ever ply his trade at the racetrack—a skill that included the aggressive and novel use of drugs. Harthill didn't hide how he practiced: by helping horses run faster through the latest, cutting-edge medication that he had gotten his hands on. He traveled widely, often overseas, to procure the hot new thing.

Drug-related scandals dogged Harthill's career almost from the moment he began practicing in 1948 and continued throughout his life.[7] In 1955, he was arrested for bribery in New Orleans related to an alleged racetrack doping plot.[8] There are several versions of an infamous incident that took place in 1980—all unproven, of course. In one version, thieves stole Harthill's Cadillac. An anonymous caller later claimed to the sheriff that a satchel was found in a parking lot containing Harthill's racing license and vials of an anti-inflammatory drug recently found in post-race drug tests. The drug, Voltaren, which is now available over the counter for arthritis, wasn't legal at the time in the United States. In another version of the story, the police were simply tipped off that Harthill had illegal drugs in his car. Harthill claimed the car had been stolen and that he had never seen the drugs in question.[9] In 1995, the Drug Enforcement Administration found sleeping pills, narcotic painkillers, and amphetamines in his office in Louisville—all drugs not used in horses and none of which Harthill had maintained the proper documentation to have and dispense. A civil suit appears to have been settled out of court.[10]

Harthill isn't remembered as nefarious so much as taking a mischievous pleasure in outwitting the other guy, "the other guy" usually being hapless regulators and his competition on the racetrack. Harthill appeared to delight in the practice.

"Alex was a real Damon Runyon character," according to the late Hall of Fame trainer John Veitch. "He was a brilliant vet. But he'd rather make a dollar on the sly than a hundred bucks on the level."[11]

Harthill was deeply secretive about his sources, Veitch said.

"He loved the edge," the trainer went on. "I don't care where the medication was made, whether it was in Europe or Canada or Mexico, Alex was right on it—and often before it was legal to be used in the United States. Day or night, if you called Alex, and if he liked you, he was there for you."

At the time Harthill gave it to Northern Dancer, Lasix had only recently been synthesized in a lab in Germany and had not yet been approved for use in humans. The first trials appear to have been for patients with heart conditions.[12] It's not clear how Harthill obtained the drug or what gave him the idea to use it on a racehorse.

He didn't appear to administer the drug to prevent bleeding in the lungs, for which the drug is prescribed today. Northern Dancer had several documented problems going into the Kentucky Derby, but bleeding doesn't seem to have been among them. He suffered from a quarter crack, a painful split in the hoof wall between the toe and the heel that can be incredibly difficult to resolve. He was also notoriously hot, shedding energy like a downed power wire and burning needless calories just before a race. Veitch said the vet told him years later that he thought Lasix would help settle the horse by lowering his blood pressure.

But Harthill's treatment would gradually become mainstream for bleeders in the United States. It was effective. Unlike in other countries, where racing is run seasonally, there is live Thoroughbred racing run year-round in the United States, with different tracks running overlapping "meets" made up of a set number of contiguous racing days. As the length of race meets grew, it put pressure on racetracks to fill races—their betting product—year-round.[13] That, in turn, put pressure on horsemen to run horses that might in the past have been given a rest or a different career. Unlike many of their European counterparts, American horses are often housed in stables in the middle of cities, where air quality is poorer. They run on a dirt surface, rather than grass, which is kicked up during races and can be inhaled. All are thought to be aggravating factors for bleeders. Trainers wanted access to a drug that many saw as an effective way to overcome these environmental challenges and keep a horse on the racetrack.

Another popular medication that most states allowed for training but was not permitted for use on race day was phenylbutazone, known by its trade name, Butazolidin, and referred to universally by trainers and veterinarians as "bute." It was one of the first nonsteroidal anti-inflammatories developed, similar to aspirin, but more powerful. In 1968, a horse named Dancer's Image tested positive for bute after winning the Kentucky Derby. He too had been treated by Harthill, who said he had given the horse bute six days before the race—long enough, theoretically, for the drug to clear his system. The horse was disqualified, and the positive became the subject of years of litigation.

Let's get this out of the way right now: Drug use at the racetrack is not a new phenomenon. The sport of horse racing has never been "clean." In fact, it's far from clear that drug use, both legal and illegal, is higher now than it was in earlier decades. It may even be lower.

People have been giving drugs to racehorses to make them run faster at least since the 1890s and the invention of the hypodermic needle. Purses were small and the main motivation for doping horses was to cash in on a bet. Horses were sometimes doped to ensure a loss. Some trainers would run a horse "cold" so that his odds would be longer in his next start, then give him a hop and make a huge wager. Cocaine, morphine, and heroin were all available and, it appears, routinely administered to horses. (Morphine was so commonplace inside and outside the horse business that it was found in a patent medication known as Mrs. Winslow's Soothing Syrup, marketed as a cure for teething pain and fussy children. The morphine content was so high that the drug came to be known as the "baby killer.") Horses sometimes died: In 1903, a horse called Dr. Riddle was out of control in the paddock before the second race at a track in the Bronx. "The man in charge of him had a hard time of it trying to hold him," one report read. "At times as he walked around the paddock with his eyeballs distended and the perspiration running off him, he would rear, carrying the man off his feet and swinging him around as if he had no more strength than a child."[14] The horse was somehow negotiated to run in the race, which he lost. When he returned to the barn, he went into convulsions and dropped dead. Newspaper articles pinned the horse's death on an overdose of "dope."

The main objection to the practice was that it corrupted the gambling product, and in 1897 the Jockey Club stepped into this Wild West frontier and instituted the country's first rule prohibiting doping. That, of course, stopped no one. The Jockey Club, a private organization made up of the era's most august men of the turf, had little means by which to uncover dopers. Inconsistent performance—a horse that ran well in one race and poorly in another—was seen as evidence of doping. In the 1930s, the Federal Bureau of Narcotics (the Drug Enforcement Administration's predecessor) seeded undercover agents into at least fifteen racetracks, an investigation that spanned eight states and claimed to find over three hundred cases of alleged doping.[15] But it wasn't until 1934 that a saliva test capable of detecting a few prohibited drugs was introduced at Hialeah Park in Florida. Trainers were so opposed to what became known as the "spit box" that they nearly boycotted.[16]

In 1951, a New York court transferred the authority to write and enforce the rules of racing from the Jockey Club to a state racing commission, making the regulation of racing an official government function. The number of drugs that state commissions tested for gradually increased over the years. But the basic structure of regulating drugs in racing remained in place. There was, effectively, a zero-tolerance standard for drugs of any kind in a horse's system on race day—if you got caught. There has never been a time when Thoroughbreds raced on just hay, oats, and water.

But then, as now, it was incredibly difficult to judge exactly how widespread "doping" was. A successful doping scheme is necessarily secret. It must evade the scrutiny of regulators and, most importantly, bookmakers. The cocktail of drugs is a secret. The administration is a secret. The use of medication at the racetrack, both legal and illegal, is and has always been talked about obliquely, or not at all. This fundamental uncertainty about the scope of the problem remains one of the sport's greatest challenges. The endless recriminations, wild accusations, and convoluted and ineffective regulatory schemes that have sprung up in the face of that uncertainty today threaten to tear the sport apart from the inside, a peril just as profound as waning public support.

Ten years after Harthill administered Lasix to Northern Dancer, Maryland would become the first state to allow Lasix to be given on race day to prevent horses from bleeding.[17] Kentucky, Florida, Pennsylvania, and several other racing jurisdictions quickly followed suit. Eventually only New York remained a holdout; it did not legalize Lasix on race day until 1995.[18] By the time Silver Charm hit the racetrack, more than 95 percent of all starters in the United States were running on Lasix.[19] At the same time, many racing commissions also dropped the old zero-tolerance standard for other drugs in favor of testing for allowable thresholds of different commonly used medications.

Two things had happened to lead to this general relaxation of the drug rules in Thoroughbred racing.

The first was that labs had started making more effective medications. For years, the traditional plant-based narcotics and stimulants—cocaine, ephedrine, heroin, morphine—had been the drugs of choice at the racetrack. But by the time Maryland and other states moved to legalize Lasix, those drugs had been replaced by potent and effective synthetic drugs developed in laboratories. Amphetamine, for example, was one of the first drugs to be synthesized in a laboratory, in the late nineteenth century, and it was used by US troops during World War II to combat fatigue. It, along with anabolic steroids and testosterone, had already been used in horse racing for decades by the 1960s. Labs had also started synthesizing different categories of drugs—drugs like Lasix and bute, which had obvious applications for a performance athlete, but less obvious applications as a performance *enhancer*. It was still against the rules to have any of those drugs in a horse's system during a race—racing commissions had begun testing for bute in the 1950s, for example—but it was legal to train on them.

The second thing that happened, beginning in the 1960s, was that drug testing became increasingly sophisticated.[20] Suddenly, post-race testing could pick up minute traces of drugs in a horse's system long after the medication had ceased to have any impact on the horse. Trainers began to agitate that the old zero-tolerance standard was now a trap. They were being penalized for the lingering presence of drugs given outside of the context of racing and, many would later claim, entirely for the benefit of the animal.[21] (To this day, trainers who receive a positive test often complain that they have been the victims of too-sensitive testing—something that is likely a convenient excuse in some instances and the God's honest truth in others. Telling which is which is the great challenge.)

When racing regulators began to allow the use of certain medications on race day, and regulate allowable thresholds for others, they were making an argument that there are two fundamentally different kinds of drugs: those designed to enhance a horse's performance beyond its natural ability and those designed to humanely enable a horse to perform at its natural best. The former class was "doping"; the latter, "therapeutics." The differentiation works better in theory than in practice.

When Dancer's Image tested positive for bute in the Kentucky Derby, racing scribes of the era moved to defend against the prevailing public opinion that bute was "dope," in the same way an amphetamine or morphine, which acts as a stimulant in horses, was dope. Dope, these writers argued, either stopped a horse or made him run faster than he was otherwise capable of doing. Bute did neither.

"Phenylbutazone is not a stimulant and not a narcotic," David Condron, a writer for the *Chicago Tribune*, asserted. Thomas Rivera wrote that equating bute to dope was "one of racing's greatest public misconceptions."[22]

Regulators eventually came up with a class system to rank "controlled therapeutic substances."[23] In Class 1 were drugs that had "the highest potential to affect performance and that have no generally accepted medical use in a racing horse"; Class 5 drugs were "therapeutic medications that have very localized actions only, such as anti-ulcer drugs." The era of technocratic regulation of Thoroughbred racing had arrived.

The problem, as regulators have discovered in the intervening decades, is that no bright line separates performance enhancers and therapeutics. Is a mild sedative, given to keep a horse calm and allow him to train effectively, good management—or a "performance enhancer," at best replacing more time-consuming and expensive training tactics, at worst, enabling an animal to perform that could not have otherwise? Lasix has lived between those two worlds since Alex Harthill first gave it to Northern Dancer. The debate over which category it most appropriately belongs to has raged unabated for the past sixty years.

Lasix is extremely effective at preventing exercise-induced pulmonary hemorrhage in racehorses.[24] But whether it has an additional, performance-enhancing impact on a horse is murkier. Academic studies into the performance-enhancing capabilities of Lasix have reached contradictory conclusions.[25] Anecdotally, it certainly appears to. Bettors at the racetrack have long observed that horses get a hop the first time they are administered the drug on race day. It seems to give them a little one-time added oomph. There is also long-standing suspicion that Lasix can mask the presence of other drugs in routine testing, although lab experts say that's unlikely.[26]

The Jockey Club in 1988 commissioned a study on its performance-enhancing efficacy that found horses running a mile on Lasix ran an average of 0.48 seconds faster than those not on the drug, regardless of whether they were bleeders. Later studies would contradict that finding.[27] Some other studies have suggested that the drug's impact on performance has more to do with the fact that Lasix is a diuretic and thus causes dehydration and weight loss in horses.[28] A horse might drop as much as thirty-two pounds when given the medication.[29] A 1996 study, meanwhile, found that it takes longer for horses to reach fatigue while running on Lasix by reducing the oxygen deficit during exertion.[30]

That element to how Lasix impacts the horse's body raised the possibility that not all of the 95 percent of runners on Lasix were strictly on it to prevent pulmonary hemorrhage. There is, horsemen almost universally acknowledge, an incentive to put every horse in the barn on whatever you can that might help maximize their performance.

"We know it exists," Dr. Dionne Benson, the chief veterinary officer for the company that owns Santa Anita, told an industry reporter in 2020.[31] "I'm not sure how you draw the line for those that need it for EIPH and those that are using it to keep up with the other horses."

Even setting aside whether Lasix is a performance enhancer, there is the question of whether horses that bleed should be "enabled" to run at all. Animal welfare activists argue that to push a horse to run in the first place is inhumane, much less an animal whose lungs may bleed under the pressure of maximum effort. Certain breeders in Kentucky argue that Lasix has weakened the breed by allowing horses that can't run without it to remain in the gene pool.

Some trainers, on the other hand, believe that doing away with the drug will have the practical impact of putting smaller trainers out of business. The larger trainers with top-shelf stock—trainers like Baffert—are so in demand by wealthy clients that if a horse is a bleeder, they can sell the animal or send the horse to the farm for extended rest, and another will quickly fill the empty stall. But smaller trainers with fewer horses owned by clients who do not have a bottomless bank account don't have that luxury. Their livelihood depends on getting the horses they have to the track.

"I can deal with [running without Lasix], but I'm afraid I'm not gonna have anybody to run against, because it's gonna affect field size," Baffert told me. "If I have [a bleeder], I can turn it out, forget about it, and bring another one in. But the little guy . . ."[32]

The United States became the only country in the world to allow Lasix to be administered on race day, although other countries allowed it to be used for training, which trainers routinely do. Those in favor of banning Lasix on race day often point to Europe's and Australia's rules as evidence that the drug is not, in fact, indispensable; those opposed point out that it makes little sense to allow the drug for training but withhold the drug on the day when a horse is likely to need it most. (The increased stress and maximum effort of a race can contribute to bleeding.) Besides, training on Lasix still allows bleeders to remain in the gene pool and, because bleeding is iterative—preventing the horse from bleeding during training may help the horse avoid bleeding on race day—the rule still acknowledges the need for the medication.

In 2020, under increasing public scrutiny of the use of medication, the racing industry in the United States began to phase out the use of Lasix on race day. But Alex Harthill had already opened the proverbial barn door. By the 1990s, many veterinarians were now acting—perfectly legally—not only to cure ailments but to maximize performance through constantly evolving chemical means.

Trainers had always reached for whatever the latest medical advancement was to try to manage, or promote, their horses.* But now there was an explicit

---

* Tom Smith, the trainer of Seabiscuit, used the bronchodilator ephedrine on some of his horses in the mid-1940s to help them breathe better; the Jockey Club subsequently suspended his trainer's license for a year. Milton C. Toby, *Unnatural Ability: The History of Performance-Enhancing Drugs in Thoroughbred Racing* (Lexington: University Press of Kentucky, 2023), 42.

legal framework that condoned the use of medication. By the 1990s—and perhaps long before—the prevalent attitude on the backstretch was that as long as a drug wasn't explicitly disallowed in regulations, and as long as a horse didn't test positive, it was legal. The use of anabolic steroids, for example, was widely permitted for training until 2008. Rick Dutrow, who trained Kentucky Derby winner Big Brown, acknowledged publicly that he gave all his horses a shot of the anabolic steroid Winstrol on the fifteenth of every month.[33] California didn't explicitly ban the use of the blood-doping agent erythropoietin, or EPO, for training until 2002.[34] In 1999, the trainer Bobby Frankel was rumored to have given a high-profile filly a "milkshake"—a high dose of baking soda intended to increase endurance—before a race in Kentucky.[35] (Racetrack gossip also had it that Frankel used EPO, which he denied in an interview shortly before it was banned in California.)

"Keeper Hill . . . wasn't there some story about her getting a milkshake before the Spinster?" turf writer Ray Paulick asked Frankel in the same 2001 interview. That "might not have gone over very well with [owner] Alice Chandler, who had been leading the fight to tighten Kentucky's then-lax medication rules," Paulick noted.

Frankel "didn't say yes or no, but his answer told me all I needed to know," Paulick wrote. "'It wasn't illegal,' [Frankel] said, stretching that last word out in a way that only a native New Yorker could."

Frankel was right. Milkshaking wasn't declared against the rules in Kentucky until 2001.

Frankel summed up the attitude toward medication, talking to Paulick about a different race: "'If I lost by that much,' he said, holding his thumb and index finger an inch apart, 'and didn't take advantage of whatever was legal, I wouldn't be able to sleep.'"

After the Preakness, Baffert stopped scoping Silver Charm altogether. Bleeding didn't seem to bother him enough to stop him from winning races. And, Baffert said, "it was driving me crazy."[36]

Silver Charm also performed at the top of his game without Lasix. In 1998, Baffert took the horse to the United Arab Emirates to run in the $4 million Dubai World Cup. The UAE did not allow race-day medication, and Silver Charm ran without Lasix. Silver Charm put in a gutsy performance to hold off Swain and win by a nose. But in 1999, when he returned to run in the same race again, he bled and finished sixth.[37]

Baffert had gotten in trouble in 1991 for another therapy sometimes used to prevent bleeding. He had given one of his horses Robinul, which relaxes the smooth muscles of the airway, to clear up some mucus in his bronchial passages. The horse was a $32,000 claimer that had never won a race, hardly one of his better prospects. "A lot of guys were using it, so we didn't think it would be a problem," Baffert recalled. But it was: Baffert received a two-week suspension from state regulators when a routine drug test revealed the medication in the horse's system. Baffert took Sherry to Hawaii for a vacation.

There is a less generous interpretation of this story. Some racetrack insiders have long alleged that sharp veterinarians—vets like Alex Harthill—have been able to "teach the trainers how to cheat," by learning what state labs were testing for and medicating with whatever *wasn't* on the list. Or by "figur[ing] out that if they cut the Robinul dose and gave it [intravenously] instead of [intramuscularly] it wouldn't test and they'd beat the lab," one racing scribe wrote in 2017.[38]

Once again, Baffert became aware that there were rumors about him circulating on the backstretch.

"I vowed right then and there, I would never help one of these horses out like that again. It always seems to happen with the cheap ones. I told the investigators after it was over, 'Boys, that's the last shot you'll ever get at me,'" he said. "After that Robinul incident, it seemed as if every time I started winning races, people thought I had to be using something."[39]

Bob Baffert was king in the late 1990s. He had won the Kentucky Derby two years in a row. He had won the Eclipse Award for Outstanding Trainer, racing's top annual award, in 1997, 1998, and 1999. In 2002 he won the Derby again with a horse named War Emblem, owned by a son of Ahmed bin Salman bin Abdulaziz, who would later become king of Saudi Arabia. (He reigns still; Mohammed bin Salman is his son.) But Baffert felt acutely that the old-school power brokers of East Coast racing did not care for him. He was brash, a showman, a huge personality—and he came east for the big races and ate their lunch. They denied it, but it surely grated on these bastions of the turf.

Baffert came to understand that they believed he was cheating. Not with Lasix, or bute, or any of the other legal therapeutics that virtually every trainer in America now used. The suspicion that he was using something else, some illegal secret sauce, trailed Baffert whenever he shipped horses East. In 1999, when he ran a hard-knocking older horse named

River Keen in a pair of prestigious Grade I stakes races at Belmont Park in New York, he said the horse was tailed by security the entire time he was there. Later, he said, a senior track investigator told him that the New York Racing Association and the Jockey Club—two of the most powerful institutions in racing—had warned him: "You gotta watch that guy. He's doing something."*[40]

---

* A source close to the Jockey Club denies that it gave any such instruction. The New York Racing Association did not respond to a request for comment on this allegation.

CHAPTER 6

IT WAS THE POPPIES!

Baffert's cell phone jingled. It was the day before the 2000 Preakness and he was in Baltimore with a Pegram horse called Captain Steve, so named in honor of the police captain who had gotten Pegram out of jail in 1997.[1] Tim Yakteen, Baffert's assistant at Hollywood Park, was calling with news of another kind of police story: investigators with the California Horse Racing Board were searching the barn.

"We had a positive," Yakteen said grimly.

Baffert was flummoxed. "For *what*?" he asked. His first guess was bute.

"It's for morphine," Yakteen said.

"Morphine?"

The horse in question was a filly named Nautical Look, who, unusually for Baffert, was running on the grass. Most of the horses in Baffert's barn were dirt specialists. In the United States, dirt racing is where the money is. The Kentucky Derby, the Breeders' Cup Classic, and most other stallion-making races are run on dirt. Baffert, who by the year 2000 was in the business of winning stallion-making races, did not generally attract or take on very many turf runners. He once joked to Yakteen that he had experience training grass horses because one time he had a horse dump its rider, jump the inside rail, and run loose around the turf course.[2] That the positive test should arise from a grass filly—and one who had only just won her first race—was exasperating.

"Of all things, it was a turf horse! *A turf horse!*" he would recall, years later.[3]

Baffert's life was in a bit of turmoil at the time. His marriage to Sherry was ending. Baffert was constantly on the road with horses and Sherry preferred to stay at home with their four children. They "drifted apart,"

Baffert said, adding that "there was no way to drift back."[4] In the meantime, he had also gotten involved with Jill Moss, an ambitious local TV news anchor in Louisville, sometime after they met in 1998. He had a "star quality" that drew her in, she said, and they began a very public on-again, off-again affair that lasted for years. They broke up eighteen times during that time period, she recalled later.

"I could always tell when he was getting ready to do it," she told Bill Nack in 2003. "The guilt would overwhelm him. He'd go home, break up with me, and two days later he was back: 'I'm so sorry. I can't live without you.'

"I would send him off. I told him, 'Leave me alone until you get your life straightened out. Make an honest woman out of me.' In his heart he wanted to do what he thought was right for the kids.

"My mom said, 'What are you thinking? This man is forty-six years old, and he has four kids? He's in a midlife crisis.' I took a lot of heat at work. There was a time when they were threatening to take me off the air."[5]

Baffert would eventually divorce in the fall of 2001 and propose to Jill later that year, but at the moment Tim Yakteen called him about Nautical Look, the situation was still a mess.

According to Baffert, the positive was mystifying. The use of morphine as a performance enhancer has a long history at the racetrack but was not seen much by the year 2000, because authorities were routinely testing for it. It had also gradually faded from use as a performance enhancer as laboratories began synthesizing more effective drugs—including morphine mimetics that were invisible to testing.[6] By 2000, the use of traditional morphine at the racetrack was practically unheard-of. It was simply too easy to get caught.

Morphine positives still occurred, however. They were largely viewed both in the United States and Europe as cases of accidental ingestion or feed contamination, likely arising from grain grown or processed alongside poppy plants. Some people also claimed that positives could originate from baked goods kept around the barn—for example, if poppy-seed bagels were brought to the barn and a groom shared a muffin with a beloved horse. Some racetrack vets are less likely to credit that explanation than others, but it's possible. Queen Elizabeth II's stakes-winning filly Estimate tested positive for morphine in 2014, amid a spate of positives in the barns of multiple trainers that year.[7] Trainer Bobby Frankel had gotten a morphine positive in California in 1996. The CHRB still disqualified the horse in that race,[8] but Frankel was able to successfully argue that the test result could have come from the ingestion of poppy seeds.

In the past, it had been difficult for labs to differentiate between morphine and pharmacologically similar but distinct morphine derivatives. These drugs were like cousins of morphine and, like morphine, could act as a stimulant in a horse. In the old days, track regulators had to rely on rumor and word-of-mouth investigation to try to pin down exactly which derivative trainers were using on their horses in order to know what to look for on a drug test. One of these mimic drugs was a dangerous synthetic opiate called etorphine, more commonly known as "elephant juice" because its legitimate use is as a tranquilizer for elephants and other large exotic animals. But like other morphine derivatives, it can act as a powerful stimulant when given in tiny, tiny doses to racehorses. The 1980s saw a handful of documented etorphine positives in the Midwest that led to widespread suspicions that the drug was in use at tracks across the country, spreading like an insidious flame from barn to barn as greedy trainers sought an edge and their desperate competition tried to keep up.[9] The suspension that a twenty-four-year-old Bob Baffert had earned for administering apomorphine to his quarter horse was for morphine.[10]

As lab testing has become more sophisticated, labs can now differentiate between morphine derivatives fairly easily. The big question is whether the morphine a horse has in its system is naturally occurring, suggesting it came from a poppy seed or contaminated feed, or is made in a lab, suggesting a performance enhancer has been given. According to Rick Sams, a former director of the lab used by the Kentucky Horse Racing Commission, it's technically possible, but incredibly difficult, for labs to distinguish "morphine from a poppy plant and morphine from an injectable preparation that is used in human medicine."

The CHRB's search of his Hollywood and Santa Anita barns struck Baffert and his team as unusually aggressive. Dr. William Bell, the CHRB veterinarian, arrived at Yakteen's barn during morning training hours with a team of investigators who interviewed every employee and searched not only the barns but the dormitory-style rooms of Baffert's grooms who lived on the backstretch. Baffert alleged that they broke locks to enter the grooms' living quarters. "They raided [both barns] like they were looking for El Chapo," Baffert said.[11]

"They were looking for something," confirmed a source with firsthand knowledge of the search.

◆

Baffert chose to exercise his right to have what is known as the "split sample" tested to confirm the positive result for Nautical Look. When regulators obtain urine or blood samples from a horse, they reserve part of the sample to be tested by the laboratory of the trainer's choice. Baffert sent the vial of urine to the Texas Veterinary Medical Diagnostic Laboratory at Texas A&M University, where analysts confirmed a morphine concentration of 73 nanograms per milliliter in Nautical Look's sample, a low but easily detectable amount. (A nanogram is one-billionth of a gram.) A month later, three more horses tested positive for morphine in separate races: two trained by Frankel and one trained by another trainer, Jesus Mendoza.

"Obviously, it's a contamination thing," Frankel said at the time.[12] "One horse had 19 nanograms and the other 95. . . . I was told that when an airline pilot flies a plane, up to 350 nanograms is considered legal. I just don't understand what the hell is going on. If I'm giving something like morphine to these horses, then I'm either a real moron or I need to be committed."[13]

Baffert would ultimately spend years fighting the charge. He testified at the time that he believed the positive had come from baked goods in the barn. According to Baffert, Yakteen had told him that he had brought bagels to the barn. Poppy seed, Yakteen told him, was his favorite. It was the sort of convenient, if plausible, explanation that made Baffert's critics roll their eyes. But other trainers in Southern California rallied around him, arguing that the suggestion that Baffert had given morphine to Nautical Look to gain a competitive edge made no sense. For one thing, it was a grass filly running in an allowance race. Why on earth would Baffert risk his reputation over such a relatively low-level horse?

"Why would Baffert choose that horse in that race?" Ron Ellis, another trainer, said at the time. "If you're going to use [morphine], you're not going to use it in an allowance race with one horse."[14]

In a hearing on the matter before the Santa Anita stewards,* a veterinary chemist testified on Baffert's behalf that such a tiny concentration of morphine was unlikely to be the result of intentional doping because it would not impact a horse's performance, an assessment that other lab

---

* "The stewards" are the top regulatory officials at any racetrack. They act as referees during races, enforce track rules, and on a day-to-day basis, are the most direct point of contact that horsemen have with the regulation of the sport. The structure varies from state to state, with some stewards appointed by the state and some appointed by the track itself; in New York, the Jockey Club also has an appointed steward.

directors familiar with the case echoed to me separately. Although Baffert maintained that Tim Yakteen's bagels were to blame, his bedding and feed provider also testified at the hearing that the majority of grains and feed provided to Santa Anita came from the Antelope Valley, where some alfalfa fields were adjacent to poppy fields. Harvested feed, Citrus Feed owner Larry Bell said, is never 100 percent pure. This was the explanation largely accepted in Europe when the queen received her positive for morphine.

According to Baffert, the CHRB's own vet had even reassured him at the time of the raid that the positive was almost certainly the result of accidental contamination. *It's just like Frankel*, he said Dr. Bell told him on the phone. *It's environmental.* And the trainer called Baffert himself, he recalled. The whole thing was bullshit, Frankel said, and he'd be happy to testify on Baffert's behalf if it would be helpful.[15]

Yet the people who mattered—the California Horse Racing Board— didn't seem to believe that this was all a random and insignificant piece of bad luck, at worst an innocent mistake by barn staff for which Baffert himself bore no responsibility. Baffert felt distinctly targeted, a feeling that he would return to time and again as the years passed and he received more positive test results. He felt he knew who was coming after him: Roy C. Wood, the executive director of the board, and Ingrid Fermin, then a steward. He struggled to understand why, beyond a vague sense that he simply wasn't seen in the same league as the legendary horsemen of the backstretch— specifically Frankel and Charlie Whittingham, another older trainer known as the "Bald Eagle." Both were thought of as maestros of their craft, imbued with a kind of magical sixth sense about horses.

The word *horseman* carries a special significance when applied to some men.* True horsemanship is part art, part science, and part decades of experience. It is accrued by men who have put their hands on thousands of different horses across the span of their lives and whom the animal has allowed to learn its secrets. Some of those best remembered for having the touch have leaned into the more mystical performance of the job, aging into gruff, terse personalities and communicating almost exclusively in aphorisms that are more like a game of Mad Libs than actual guidelines for training a Thoroughbred racehorse. ("Horses are like strawberries, they can

---

* Women, for whatever reason, never quite seem to gain this storied reputation, although there are signs this is changing. There are a few extremely good horsewomen who are breaking barriers in the sport.

go bad overnight," is one turn of phrase widely attributed to Whittingham.) Occasionally, some hot new outfit claiming to have used biomechanical measurements or electric sensors or some other newfangled technology to standardize the production of a more perfect racehorse will splash into the industry, backed by a few big-money clients with the same hubris. Horses, as they always do, will eventually make fools out of the technocrats with their glossy brochures and calipers. In racing, it is always the old oracles, the sages of the turf, to whom the real respect is given. Their authority is unexplained and thus unimpeachable.

There was nothing mystical about Bob Baffert, but he was a good horseman, and the thought that he was underestimated for that ability galled him. He was being penalized, he thought, for being *too* successful. If you were more successful than the old masters, you must be doing something shady. Someone as wide-open, as talkative and impolitic, as Bob Baffert could not soar higher than the Bald Eagle.

"I think if you win at a certain [rate]—not too much—then you're going to be considered . . . 'a great horseman' and all that," Baffert complained to me. "I've never gotten that. These guys will say [of other trainers], 'Well, oh, he's such a great horseman.' I never get that. [I get:] 'Oh, he does well because he gets all the best horses.'"

Baffert believed with an almost talismanic faith in old-fashioned horsemanship, so not to be considered a great horseman touched a sore spot in his pride. He had grown up listening to aging quarter horse guys talk about mixing their own liniments to patiently work into a sore tendon. He had tried to adopt some of this horsemanship of the plains. "I could have a little ankle with a little wind puff and I could rub it until it was gone," he said, referring to swelling that is usually benign but should be managed to prevent injury. "You could rub and rub, and now we just slap mud [commercial clay poultice] on there. I still believe in icing." The ancient tools of horsemanship held a seductive power for Baffert.[16]

Racing is a small world. Few sports are more viciously—and more personally—competitive. On the backside, where the racing gods bestow their favor and then take it away with caprice, envy is a natural human by-product of success. Baffert chalked up the miasma of mistrust hovering over him to jealousy. As a man of pride—a man who needed to be liked, needed to be the best at what he did—it was perhaps the only way he could stand the charges.

"Jealousy on the backside is at an all-time high and it's the fault of the trainers who aren't doing well. When someone is doing well, they start rumors that somebody ain't that good—they got to be doing something wrong," he told the *New York Times* at the time.[17] "What I want to know is how old you have to be before you're considered a good, solid horse trainer?"

For the regulators in question, this was all a lot of bullshit. Ingrid Fermin knew that Baffert believed she was out to get him—because he told her so—but she had to roll her eyes at it. "I said, 'Come on, Bob, you're not the only fish in the pond,'" she recalled.[18] "Certainly, the focus was not on Bob Baffert." The investigation was legitimate, she said, because routine testing had showed a positive result for a forbidden drug. It was as simple as that.

Even as states were testing for more drugs than ever, there were indications that trainers across the country were still experimenting to try to gain an edge. A few suspected practices qualified as barbaric. In 2007, Kentucky trainer Patrick Biancone was suspended for a year after cobra venom, given to deaden pain, was discovered in his barn.[19] A lab in Colorado conducted multiple rounds of research in the 2010s to identify and develop a test for dermorphin, an opioid that occurs naturally on the backs of some South American frogs and is colloquially known as "frog juice." It acts as a stimulant in racehorses.[20] In 2012, post-race testing found dermorphin in samples from more than thirty horses in Louisiana, New Mexico, and Oklahoma.[21] The possibility that a horse trainer, even one as high-profile as Bob Baffert, might try to use illegal substances to win races wasn't something regulators were going to dismiss.

How to handle positives that result from accidental ingestion or exposure has long presented a tricky balancing act for regulators. In a world where it's simultaneously true that some trainers do use illegal drugs *and* that it is impossible to prove how a particular drug entered a horse's system, it is hard for investigators to prove conclusively that a given positive has come from doping or an unavoidable accident. The stubborn reality is that horses are barn animals operating in an impossible-to-sterilize environment. They are exposed to contaminants constantly. Before a race, many horses are shipped in and out of a "receiving barn" that has been temporarily inhabited by countless prior horses, horses that likely rubbed sweat and saliva against the walls and defecated. Horses have been known to nibble on their own manure. It's plausible that a trainer could be charged with a positive in one horse arising from a substance given by a different trainer to a completely different horse that had merely occupied the same stall. A horse could also plausibly pop a positive for a substance ingested by a human being who only handled the animal in the final moments before it raced—one of the crew that loads horses into the starting gate before each race, or a staff member working for the racetrack in the receiving barn, for example. One 2017 study conducted by researchers at the University of Kentucky found twenty-eight substances—including cocaine and the diabetes drug metformin—in a review of twenty-one stalls at Charles Town in West Virginia.[22] Horsemen tend to call these positives "environmental contamination," although some lab experts feel this is an inaccurate term of art because most drug positives *do* have a specific point of origin, even if it's not known.[23]

In part to get around the tricky question of intent, racing has relied on a nearly ironclad principle known as the absolute insurer rule. The rule, which has its origins in the early days of modern doping enforcement in the 1930s, stipulates that the trainer bears unequivocal responsibility for the animals in his care. In other words, if a horse is found to be running on a prohibited substance, it doesn't matter how the substance got into the horse's system: the trainer is liable. The rule has been the subject of litigation for decades over the "constitutionality of the rule's most basic and controversial concept: trainers are guilty until proved innocent of doping, sometimes without any meaningful opportunity to defend themselves," writes racing historian Milt Toby in a history of drug regulation in racing.[24] But the principal tenet has survived basically untouched since its inception at Hialeah Park almost one hundred years ago.

At the time of Baffert's positive, some other states had so-called thresholds for morphine to allow for accidental exposure—concentrations under which a finding of morphine in a sample would not be recorded as a positive. In 2000, the cutoff was 75 nanograms per milliliter in Louisiana and 50 nanograms per milliliter in Ohio,[25] meaning that Baffert would have received a positive in Ohio, but not in Louisiana. This approach has done little to settle the debate over how to adjudicate accidental positives. In the court of public opinion, guilt or innocence still hinges on whether you think the trainer in question can be trusted.

This wouldn't be the last time Baffert would claim that a positive had arisen from "environmental contamination." In later years, he would accrue other positive test results that he also pinned on forces outside his control. He claimed, variously, that a positive test for dextromethorphan was the result of a groom who had taken cough syrup urinating in a stall; that a lidocaine positive came from a back patch worn by his assistant trainer. None of his explanations were novel. Horses periodically test positive for meth, caffeine, and cocaine, all potential performance-enhancing substances that are also used by human beings—including, potentially, the grooms who handle these horses on a day-to-day basis. In a world where the testing had evolved to be carried out at the picogram level (one-trillionth of a gram), these explanations had gained some legitimate credibility.

Where Baffert lost credibility, according to some racetrack vets and lab experts, was in the torrent of dubious explanations. The poppy-seed excuse was reliant on far too many one-in-a-million factors. Not only would the horse have to have ingested the poppy seeds, but those seeds would also have to have been consumed proximate enough to the time of testing to be detectable. And how much morphine might be in a given poppy seed is impossible to know. It depends on how long the seed was stored and whether it was exposed to light, moisture, or other conditions that might degrade it, among other factors.

Still, it was possible: Sams, the Kentucky lab director, was part of research that arose out of Nautical Look's positive. Researchers purchased the kind of bulk poppy seeds available to American bakeries, fed them to horses, and tested the results. They found that "commercially available poppy seeds contain substantial amounts of morphine, and that when administered to horses, they can produce concentrations in the urine that are higher than what was observed in the Baffert horse," he said.[26]

But that bought Baffert little credibility inside racing for an explanation that was a perfect echo of a *Seinfeld* episode in which Elaine tests positive at work for opioids after eating a poppy-seed bagel.[27] To his critics, it reeked of the desperate excuses of a child who has gotten caught in a lie. Baffert could make all the grand proclamations he wanted about the basics of horsemanship, they believed; there was no way he had gotten where he was on nothing more than homemade liniment and a bucket of ice.

After the hearing, the CHRB moved to suspend Baffert for sixty days for the positive, on the grounds that the absolute insurer rule made all this quibbling about whether the positive test was the result of accidental contamination irrelevant. Baffert wasn't planning on ceding the point. He was granted a stay on the suspension pending appeal and sued in federal court, arguing that he stood to lose millions of dollars in purse money. Challenging a state administrative action in federal court was an unusual move, and what followed was years of winding proceedings as the case bounced back and forth between federal and state courts. Baffert and his legal team were stubborn in the pursuit of what Baffert felt in his bones was justice due him.

The federal case largely turned on the fact that the CHRB had destroyed blood samples drawn from Nautical Look the day of the race that Baffert felt certain could have exonerated him. Urine samples show that a substance has been metabolized and excreted; blood samples show what is circulating in a horse's system in real time. If a substance isn't present in the blood, said Sams, it can't have an effect on the horse. Often when there's a low concentration of morphine in the urine sample, Sams said, "little or none of it is actually present in the blood."[28] That's what Baffert was hoping for.

Truesdail Laboratories, the CHRB lab, had tested the horse's original urine sample, and Texas A&M had tested the split urine sample. Both vials of blood, one held by Truesdail and one held in a CHRB evidence locker in Sacramento, were destroyed after Truesdail had notified the board of the positive result—but before administrative proceedings had been launched against Baffert.[29] Baffert learned that the samples had been destroyed during his initial hearing before the board. Dr. Steven Barker, chief chemist of the Louisiana State Racing Commission, testified in federal court that if the blood samples had been tested for morphine and the result was negative or showed extremely low levels, then this might have "presented conclusive proof that there could not have been an intentional administration of morphine to the horse prior to the race."[30]

The federal judge agreed, writing that the CHRB had "secretly discarded and destroyed the official and split blood samples, thereby depriving [Baffert] of his right to defend himself in the disciplinary hearings with scientific exculpatory evidence."[31]

For Baffert, even years later, the destruction of the samples was a clear sign that the board was out to get him. The board maintained that it was an unfortunate coincidence that the samples were discarded, part of a cost-cutting measure by the CHRB, which in 1999 had directed Truesdail to randomly discard some of the daily blood samples from each track to save on storage costs. It was just bad luck that Nautical Look's had been among those that were thrown away that day. The CHRB in its initial decision to suspend Baffert called it "perceptually unfortunate that a portion of the blood was discarded."[32]

While the federal court decided the case in Baffert's favor, an appeals court overturned the decision on the grounds that the case should have been handled in state court. The case would eventually be heard by an administrative law judge charged with providing a recommended course of action to the CHRB. By now, it was January 2005, almost five full years since Nautical Look's race. This time, Baffert's attorney was able to present testimony by the CHRB veterinarian, William Bell, that the amount of morphine found in Nautical Look's sample was "pharmacologically insignificant and most likely due to environmental contamination." Baffert's barn, Bell said, was the "most secure" he had ever seen.[33]

More to the point, Baffert's lawyer said, was the fact that between May and June of 2000, 13 out of 95 samples drawn from the barns of multiple trainers were found to be "suspect" for opiates. Barker testified that such a rash of apparent positives was unusual and suggested environmental contamination.[34]

In the end, Baffert was victorious. The administrative law judge recommended that the CHRB drop the whole thing, finding that "these facts and [Baffert's] success as a trainer support the conclusion he had nothing to gain and a great deal to lose by the use of a banned substance on this horse." The CHRB in spring of 2005 accepted the recommendation and dismissed the case.[35]

The five-year ordeal was an object lesson in how positive tests were adjudicated on the racetrack. For decades, the well-worn pattern used by trainers and the small cottage industry of lawyers hired to defend them has been to challenge the ruling and delay adjudication. In 2022, the New York Gaming Commission attempted to disqualify a horse named Forte and suspend his megastar trainer, Todd Pletcher, after the horse tested positive in a Grade I for a small amount of meloxicam, a nonsteroidal anti-inflammatory used to treat arthritis in people. The positive test was kept private by the gaming commission for more than nine months—it was eventually revealed only by the *New York Times*[36]—and two years later, it was being fought in state Supreme Court.*

Trainers may have legitimate reasons for challenging a positive test. The ultimate-insurer rule does defy the basic precept of the US justice system that you are innocent until proven guilty. But the practical impact of this tactic is twofold: The bad press associated with a positive test fades into the

---

* Pletcher and one of Forte's owners, Mike Repole, argue that the horse was not intentionally administered meloxicam and that the drug got into the horse's system through "environmental contamination."

background as a parade of other positive tests from other trainers become public. And as the penalty is delayed, it means the trainer can keep entering horses in races and earning purse money and stallion-making Grade I wins. A horse might, theoretically, pop a positive test in a Grade I, be permitted to run in additional stakes races, win, and be syndicated as a stallion—all while the challenge of the original positive test remains mired in adjudication. A trainer can then take his seven-day or his fourteen-day suspension at his leisure after the moneymaking is done.

Of course, that wasn't an issue with Nautical Look, a turf filly whose value in the breeding shed was limited compared to the dirt colts in Baffert's barn.

The case was also a lesson in the limitations of drug testing, one that challenges the perception that testing is the ultimate judge in a case of potential doping. In fact, testing can do as much to cloud the issue as it can to illuminate the truth. Modern testing can reveal information that would have seemed extraordinary to the scientists who invented the saliva tests first used at Hialeah. But it still offers few, if any, direct answers about the intent of the people who have the responsibility to care for horses. That remains the purview of those flawed arbiters of human nature: the courts, public opinion, and occasionally journalism. Only the horses know the whole truth, and they keep their own counsel.

The lesson that Baffert took away from the experience was that if you wanted to clear your name, you had to get litigious. You had to get your case heard before a "real" judge, he said. The commissions that governed racing—which were state government bodies—had too much discretion. And, in Baffert's mind, they weren't fair to him. That, above all, was what he learned from the episode.

It left a sour taste in Baffert's mouth. He felt vindicated—but abandoned by a sport to which he felt he had given a great deal. It wasn't just that he was successful. Baffert took seriously his role as an ambassador for the sport, a showman. In his telling, he is constantly acquiescing to requests from Churchill Downs and other racetracks to parade his horses and himself to fans, for the good of the sport. Yet the sport, he felt, had kicked him to the curb in his time of need.

"I do all this stuff trying to promote our sport and I get all this cross-examination," Baffert told the *New York Times'* Joe Drape in 2001. "I'm not going to become a turtle [and] go in a shell. I'm not going to get sour. I have thought to myself—'Where did everybody go?'"[37]

What he gave less thought to, years later, was the origin of the positive itself. Generally, he still claimed that Tim Yakteen's poppy-seed bagels were to blame. But he left open the possibility that morphine got into Nautical Look's body in some other way. "We'll never know where it came from," he said to me.[38] The hard facts of the case seemed no longer important, diluted by memory. What mattered was that Bob Baffert was an innocent victim of the whims of regulators.

It marked Baffert's first high-profile run-in with state regulators, but it wouldn't be his last. Within a decade, Baffert would find himself the single focus of a special-ordered investigation. Horses were dying at an alarming rate in his barn. And no one, including Baffert, could explain why.

CHAPTER 7

SUDDEN DEATH

Irrefutable, a five-year-old son of Unbridled's Song, trotted briskly back to his groom after finishing second in a Grade III stakes race in November 2011. A striking dappled gray with black hair gathered on his knees and hocks like a heat map, Irrefutable had never been a top-flight stakes horse, but he was stolid and dependable at his level. Earlier that month, Baffert had given him a shot in the Grade I Breeders' Cup Dirt Mile, only to watch the horse finish dead last in racing's year-end championships. Now he had wheeled him back to lower-level company and Irrefutable had redeemed himself, passing a rival in the stretch and closing well to finish in the money. It was an ordinary Saturday at Hollywood Park, the kind of workaday card that makes up most days of Thoroughbred racing in the United States. The Vernon O. Underwood Stakes was worth only $100,000 all up.

Irrefutable's groom took hold of the horse's bridle as his jockey, Mike Smith, slid off, undid the girth, and slipped the racing saddle off his back. The groom sloshed water over Irrefutable's head to allow it to run down his neck and over the jugular vein to cool him. It was a pleasant afternoon without a breeze to stir the air and everything seemed fine.

The groom turned to lead Irrefutable to the barn, where he would be given a proper bath and walked until he was cool. The gray horse took five or ten steps under the bright California sun and then collapsed in a heap of black and gray on the racetrack.[1] He was dead.

So-called sudden deaths like this one happen to Thoroughbred racehorses from time to time and aren't, in and of themselves, suspicious. Like the high school track star who suddenly drops dead of a heart arrythmia on the field, this kind of death was maddeningly mysterious. It was awful, but it happened—and vets couldn't explain why. But Irrefutable's death was unusual. He was the second horse from Baffert's barn that had suddenly dropped dead in less than a month. The other horse, a two-year-old colt that had collapsed while galloping in the morning, had belonged to the same owner, Kaleem Shah. It was strange enough that the California Horse Racing Board's on-track veterinarian called Dr. Rick Arthur, the equine medical director, to flag the death for him.

That phone call would mark the beginning of the crucible. By the time it was all over in 2013, seven horses would be dead. And Arthur would spend the next two years investigating, looking for something, anything that could explain why.

Rick Arthur had been around horse racing for more than three decades by the time he gave up private practice to become the CHRB equine medical director in 2006. Direct, intimidatingly no-nonsense, with a soft, square face and inscrutable eyes that seemed perpetually narrowed, Arthur had become one of racing's foremost experts on the tangled issues of racing injuries, medication, and drug testing. Over the course of his fifteen years as equine medical director, he would become among the regulators most intimately acquainted with Bob Baffert's operation. Even today, Baffert sees him as a menace.[2] (Arthur, like other CHRB regulators whom Baffert has accused of targeting him, appears wryly amused by the allegation.)

Within a few hours of Irrefutable's death, Arthur had contacted the leadership of the CHRB to notify them of the two deaths. The two-year-old that had died three weeks previous had been handled routinely: a necropsy had been performed, and it was found that there had likely been a failure of the cardiac conduction system—a misfire of the electrical signals that direct different parts of the heart to relax and contract. Officially, however, the death was considered unexplained by the pathologists at the California Animal Health and Food Safety Laboratory at the University of California, Davis—a fairly routine finding given the mysterious nature of sudden death. It was the last Baffert sudden death that would be treated in a routine manner.

The necropsy for Irrefutable showed mild inflammation in his heart and signs of chronic bleeding in his lungs. He was diagnosed with likely "heart failure and/or exercise-induced pulmonary hemorrhage"[3]—something that fit his veterinary record. Irrefutable had been a bleeder who was routinely treated with Lasix during both his workouts and his races, although that didn't necessarily cause his death.

The two horses had little in common to suggest why they might both have died in such a short period of time. They were different ages, under completely different training regimens. The two-year-old had just returned to training after a rest period to allow a tendon injury to heal. Irrefutable was an older horse in the midst of an active campaign. And their necropsies showed two vastly different pathologies.

Then, on January 6, a four-year-old named Uncle Sam collapsed halfway through a five-furlong workout at Hollywood Park. Mike Marlow, Baffert's assistant trainer who ran his Hollywood Park string at the time, thought the horse had been a little "weak behind" and Baffert's vet had treated both his back and his hocks. The necropsy suggested that the horse had been misdiagnosed: it showed that he had a neurological disease known as equine protozoal myeloencephalitis, or EPM. EPM, which is caused by a parasite originating in opossums, inflames the horse's central nervous system and in its later stages causes a horse to stagger drunkenly behind. In its early stages, it can present like general hind-end weakness that can be confused with musculoskeletal lameness. Neither of Baffert's vets thought that Uncle Sam had shown any signs of a neurological condition. They had treated the horse as if he were simply lame.

But in any case, EPM was not recognized as a cause of sudden death in racehorses. Uncle Sam's death was puzzling—and once again, seemed to bear little resemblance to those of the other two horses except that he too was owned by Kaleem Shah and trained by Bob Baffert.[4]

Because all three horses belonged to a single owner, investigators were almost certainly considering the possibility that the horses had been killed for insurance money. It wasn't unheard-of: In 1991, the FBI arrested a contract horse killer named Tommy Burns, who for decades had murdered show horses for 10 percent of the insurance payout. Known as "the Sandman"— because when he entered a stall, the horse "went to sleep"—Burns helped sometimes already-wealthy owners defraud insurance companies by electro-cuting horses that were more valuable dead than alive. In an interview with *Sports Illustrated*'s Bill Nack, he described slicing an extension cord down the middle into two strands of wire, attaching a pair of alligator clips to the bare end of each, and attaching the clips to the horse—"one to its ear, the other to its rectum."[5] Then he would step back. It would appear as if the horse had died of colic, a common intestinal disorder that can be fatal in horses.

The specter of insurance fraud also hung over perhaps the most famous mystery in the history of modern horse racing. In 1990, one of the most valuable stallions in the country, a horse named Alydar, snapped his right hind leg in the stall in the middle of the night. Alydar was insured for more than $32 million, a function of the fact that he stood for $250,000 a pop and covered ninety-seven mares in his last season at stud. Unbeknownst to the racing world at the time, the farm that owned him was also drowning in debt. Calumet Farm, with its white board fences and iconic red-trimmed stables, had been one of the giants of the turf but under the management of a ne'er-do-well son-in-law would be forced to file for bankruptcy the following year. One of the premier veterinary surgeons in the country, Dr. Larry Bramlage, operated on Alydar in an effort to save his life, but the injury was catastrophic and Alydar could not cope with the recovery. When he tried to stand on the casted leg, he staggered, fell back on his haunches, and snapped his femur, the main weight-bearing bone connecting his hock to the hip. He was euthanized immediately. Many in Lexington, Kentucky, to this day believe that J. T. Lundy, the son-in-law responsible for the storied farm's financial demise, broke the horse's leg in the dead of the night to collect on the insurance money. Lundy eventually served four years in prison on charges that he defrauded the First City National Bank of Houston of $65 million in loans to Calumet, but despite the FBI's best efforts, he was never tied to the death of Alydar, and his role—if any—in the horse's death remains disputed.[6]

But that pat answer could not explain the three Shah-Baffert horses that had died in the space of two months. Investigators quickly established that none of the three were insured.

By the time Uncle Sam had dropped, Baffert was aware that the CHRB was watching him closely. Arthur had been in and out of his barn to ask questions, gather records, and try to get to the bottom of what had now become a swirling mystery in California racing. There are no real secrets on the backstretch, and by this point, Hollywood Park and Santa Anita were abuzz with the deaths.[7] The rumor mill was working overtime—and few of the rumors were friendly to Baffert. Eventually, the prevailing theory that developed was that Baffert had been administering rat poison, an anticoagulant, to his horses to counterbalance the thickening effects of blood doping. Erythropoietin is believed to cause heart attacks by packing a horse's blood with so many red blood cells that it becomes sludgy. Even today, more than ten years later, people cited this theory to me as if it were a fact.

The suspicion that had always hovered over Baffert had now roosted permanently in the eaves of his barn. And his brash, big-mouthed personality had left him with few friends to defend him against those smug and self-assured chatterers who haunt the gap at every racetrack, coffee steaming in their hands as they trade back-fence hearsay with the confidence of prosecutors. Baffert suffered a heart attack in 2012 that softened him some, and Arthur would later say teasingly, "If he would have had a heart attack ten years before, he probably wouldn't have so many enemies."

"Bob was pretty obnoxious," Arthur said. "Lorded it over his colleagues. Didn't have many friends except Tim Yakteen and . . . a few guys that worked under him."[8]

Arthur was stumped. After Uncle Sam died, he performed out-of-competition testing on many horses in Baffert's stables at both Hollywood and Santa Anita, even though all three of the horses that had died had been stabled in a single barn at Hollywood Park. The testing—including blood tests specifically looking for EPO[9]—found no evidence of any illegal drugs. There went one backstretch theory.

"I think trying to balance polycythemia, caused by EPO administration, with rat poison is stupid," Arthur told me, referring to a condition where the blood is packed with too many red blood cells. "It would be impossible to try to balance those two and I don't know how you'd do it."

For a while, the crisis seemed to be over. Months passed, and training and racing continued as usual in the Baffert barn. Mike Marlow, in charge of the Hollywood Park barn where all three horses had lived, allowed himself to breathe a cautious sigh of relief. A true cowboy in shit-kickers and a ten-gallon hat, narrow-framed and known for delivering his blunt opinions even to the boss, Marlow had hardly relished having to pick the phone up to tell his boss that another horse had died. Hollywood Park was where most of Baffert's horses were stabled, around 60 percent, but it was the second string. Layups, two-year-olds not yet ready for the big leagues, and older, blue-collar types. This was supposed to be the drama-free string. As spring crept into summer, things seemed to have returned to normal.

Then, in June, Mike Pegram's homebred four-year-old colt CJ Russell collapsed and died shortly after finishing sixth in an allowance race at Hollywood Park. He did not even make it back to be unsaddled and had to be vanned off the racetrack. The necropsy listed his cause of death as apparent heart failure. Two months later, another two-year-old colt was coming back from a routine morning gallop, wobbled, staggered, and tipped over.[10]

That necropsy also showed a little bit of inflammation in some parts of the heart, but nothing severe. The horse had been diagnosed with a systolic heart murmur shortly before his death, but according to his veterinary records he had not been showing any signs of exercise intolerance or cardiac insufficiency—and in fact, he had comfortably breezed up to a half-mile at that point in his training.

These five horses had just one thing in common: all were stabled in the same barn at Hollywood Park.

The deaths clobbered Marlow. There seemed to be no warning, no way to predict when death would return.

"They got fed the same as all the other horses, they got treated all the same, there was really no clue," Marlow recalled. "In the morning, I go through all the horses. They ate up that night, they looked healthy. That wouldn't even have crossed your mind, something's gonna happen to him today. It was just crazy."

The Baffert operation was drawn as tight as a wire. Marlow felt certain that Baffert had to be wondering what in the hell he, Marlow, was doing to the horses in his barn.[11] And other trainers were starting to confront Marlow about it directly. Peter Miller, a relatively modest California trainer who is seen as something of an antagonist in the Baffert barn, rode up next to Marlow one day on the pony and started talking shit. *I know you have to do what Bob tells you*, he told Marlow.[12]

"I said, 'You know what you need to do is get away from me, right now,'" Marlow said. "'You just need to get away from me.'"

The sixth death didn't come until December 21, when a three-year-old gelding galloping in the morning collapsed. He had died of internal hemorrhaging in his abdomen, but, strangely, there were no major burst vessels. Liver sampling during the necropsy found a trace of diphacinone, an anticoagulant rodenticide, but the amount was so low that the toxicologist wasn't sure whether it could have contributed to the mysterious hemorrhaging.

Still, it was a clue. Rat poison had not been part of the standard toxicology screen prior to this sixth case. Equine internal medicine specialists at UC Davis thought that the finding was significant enough that they moved to test the liver samples of the first two Baffert sudden deaths, which were still available in UC Davis stores. It was another dead end: rodenticide wasn't found in either sample.

The final death came in March 2013, a five-year-old mare named Miner's Daughter who also died during training hours. She too was screened for rodenticide, but none was found. Later that year, rat poison would be found in two other sudden deaths caused by internal hemorrhage—one racehorse at Santa Anita and a lead pony in the postparade at Los Alamitos—but neither was connected to Baffert. And crucially, none of the other Baffert cases outside of that one horse had hemorrhaged.

Arthur had been conducting a rolling medical review of the deaths since Irrefutable's death. Now, after the seventh death—with no way of knowing if it would be the last—Arthur recommended that the CHRB conduct an official investigation. He emphasized to the board that his investigation had suggested no hint of improper activity in the Baffert barn. But something had gone deeply wrong at Hollywood Park.

In 1983, Baffert had trained a dogged old gelding named Wheelin Ernie for a small syndicate of first-time owners. Wheelin Ernie was a tough old bird that Baffert had claimed for $2,500, the kind of gutsy campaigner that you had to like even though he would never be a big stakes horse. Still, the owner wanted to run the horse in a small stake on the undercard of a big day, and Baffert reluctantly agreed. He knew the old boy would have to run hard in a race like that. Ernie "ran his guts out and finished third," Baffert said, but dropped dead when he got back to the barn.

When Baffert returned to the grandstand, he still had two other horses to saddle in the big race that night. And the various partners who had a piece of the horse were there with their families, including a passel of little kids who wanted to go back to the barn and see Ernie. Baffert tried to put them off, not wanting to break the news to these kids that Ernie was dead. The kids started yelling, "We want to see Ernie! We want to see Ernie!" The owner who ran the syndicate was getting impatient and insisted that they be taken to see the horse. Baffert, harried because he had to go saddle his two horses in the Futurity, couldn't "take it any longer," as he recalled in his memoir, "so I just snap back at the guy, 'Hey, buddy, Ernie's dead, okay?' All the kids started crying and I felt terrible."[13]

Most Thoroughbred trainers globally have some experience with sudden death, defined as the acute collapse and death of an otherwise apparently healthy racehorse. Sudden death is often referred to as a heart attack on the racetrack, but as the rash of Baffert deaths illustrates, necropsies show a variety of different pathologies. Those that are suspected to be cardiac are not, in fact, a "heart attack" caused by a blocked artery. Instead, sudden death is often attributed to a cardiac arrhythmia, a misfire of the electrical signals that keep the heart pumping in rhythm. It is precisely because arrhythmias are electrical that it is almost impossible to pinpoint their cause after the fact. They are a silent assassin that leaves no evidence of the crime behind.

In 2013, when Arthur completed his final report, sudden death was reported to account for somewhere between 3.5 and 19 percent of all fatalities, depending on the country in question. In the preceding six years in California, sudden deaths accounted for an average of about 7 percent of all fatalities[14]—meaning that it's common enough that trainers don't necessarily question them.

"We probably have one or two a year—and I could not tell you why it's happened," one large US-based trainer said. "There's no rhyme or reason. I had a two-year-old pull up from a gallop in the spring. It had been here for a month or two, it pulled up from a gallop and had a heart attack.

"I always wonder if I'd missed something with a horse. But you know, normally with those cases, it's pretty random," this trainer said. "I've never tied it to anything."

But the number of deaths Baffert had racked up in a four-month period was extraordinary. Arthur's final report looked at sudden death over a six-year period beginning in summer of 2007. There were twenty trainers stabled at the facility during that time who had a horse die during racing. Three of them, including Baffert, had two die during racing, while the other seventeen trainers had only one each.

But the number of deaths that happened during training hours was truly stark. Forty-three trainers had a horse die this way in the morning between 2007 and 2013. Six of the horses—including the five that died at Hollywood Park, plus another that died during training at Santa Anita in July 2010—were in training with Bob Baffert. By comparison, during the same period, only one other trainer came close: Steve Sherman had three. Three other trainers lost two horses. The rest lost only one.

Using the number of racing starts as the denominator—the common metric by which racing judges most of its statistics—in the state of California, Baffert-trained horses had a nine times greater incidence of sudden death during racing or training than horses not trained by Baffert.[15] It was staggering.

Somehow, word about the rash of fatalities hadn't appeared in the press. Sometime shortly after the final death, Arthur got a phone call from Joe Drape, the racing reporter for the *New York Times* and bête noir of the racing industry.

"'I hear Bob has lost a lot of horses there,'" Arthur recalled Drape saying. "I said, 'What did Peter Miller say?'"

Arthur looked carefully at the medications that the seven dead horses had received, as well as what was found in their systems at the time of their death. Because California requires that medications given to racehorses be recorded with the CHRB in near-real time, there was a detailed official history for each of the horses that had died. Each showed the administration of a host of common therapeutic medications, all unremarkable on the backstretch. Almost all of Baffert's horses received the anti-inflammatory phenylbutazone—bute. His staff gave it orally the morning before a race. They were given GastroGard, the horse equivalent of Prilosec, to treat ulcers. Irrefutable had received bleeder medications and a common antiarthritic. Uncle Sam had received Robaxin, a muscle relaxant that could be legally administered forty-eight hours before a race, and Banamine, another commonly used anti-inflammatory. Several of the horses had received Lasix. About a quarter had received clenbuterol, a bronchodilator.

It was a long list. Yet none of these medications were unusual, much less illegal. Clenbuterol has some steroid-like effects and had long been speculated to be a potential cause of sudden death. But while it had been associated with changes in equine cardiac muscle, there was no scientific proof linking it to heart arrhythmias. And in any case, it was in such common use across the backstretch that, alone, it didn't explain why Baffert's barn had seen so many deaths. You couldn't race on clenbuterol, but in California until 2012, there was an allowable threshold level that could be found in a horse's post-race sample that made it an enormously popular training tool.

The toxicology reports were similarly unsatisfying. Four out of the seven found no foreign substances in the dead horses whatsoever. The rest found only traces of the legal therapeutic medications that the vet record showed the horse had received.

"Bob Baffert's use of medication and veterinary services, at least in the 7 horses examined, can best be described as moderate and, with the exception [of] prescription medications and supplements dispensed somewhat routinely by his veterinarians, his medication and veterinary services were not out of the ordinary," Arthur wrote in his final report.[16]

One thing stood out to Arthur as potentially significant: all of Baffert's horses were receiving a prescription medication, called Thyro-L, that was supposed to treat hypothyroidism. In practice the drug speeds up a horse's metabolism and it was commonly prescribed to help animals coming in fat from the farm lose weight. But Baffert was giving it more like a supplement than a medication. None of the horses were tested to see if they had hypothyroidism. It was given so routinely that Baffert's vet prescribed the drug for Uncle Sam a week after he died. Baffert told Arthur in an interview that he was giving the drug because he thought it helped "build up" his horses—a comment Arthur found "surprising since the drug is most commonly used to assist weight loss."[17] Baffert told me in 2023 that he failed to finish his thought in that interview and that he had intended to say that he believed the drug "built up the thyroid"—a plausible explanation since Baffert is almost congenitally incapable of completing a sentence.[18]

Most importantly, there was some reason to believe that Thyro-L could cause cardiac alterations, although there was limited scientific literature on the subject. Baffert was allowing grooms to administer Thyro-L in the feed, raising the possibility that dosing recommendations weren't strictly followed. "When the barn personnel are administering the same material to dozens of horses at feed time, I question whether they level off every teaspoon, but I don't know that wasn't the case," Arthur said.[19]

Yet again, Arthur ran into a dead end. Like clenbuterol, Thyro-L was used by other trainers at the time. Baffert was hardly the only one giving it to his horses. After talking to other racetrack vets, Arthur found that "prescribing thyroxine without evaluating thyroid levels is consistent with the standard of care for prescribing and dispensing thyroxine at the Thoroughbred race tracks in southern California."[20]

Plus, Baffert had kept all of his horses on Thyro-L—not just those at Hollywood Park—for at least five years, he said. The deaths had only occurred at Hollywood Park beginning in 2011. If the drug were to blame for the rash of deaths, horses across his operation at Santa Anita and Del Mar should have begun dropping dead five years earlier.

When it came to drugs, in other words, it appeared that Baffert was running a garden-variety racing barn. It could read as an exoneration of his approach to medication or a searing indictment of the norm in racing, depending on your point of view.

Managing a large stable of horses responsibly requires some economies of scale, referred to as "herd management." A racing barn is treated as a "herd," with a baseline of care given to the entire stable. It is absolutely critical to give some drugs, like dewormers, to the whole herd to keep the barn safe. Other treatments, like anti-ulcer medications, are given to all horses simply because it's easier to tell a shifting staff of grooms to give everyone GastroGard than to ensure they remember that only Horses A, C, and F get dosed.

Where the "herd management" approach gets more ambiguous is with drugs that are designed to maximize performance. Some trainers begin giving a drug as a way of keeping up with the trainer next door—and it's easier to simply put the entire barn on that drug. This doesn't just guarantee proper administration. It can be hard to explain to an owner why his horse isn't getting the go-fast juice when some other guy's horse is. Clenbuterol was one of these medications.

"If somebody's going to—you have to do it," Baffert said of clenbuterol, which he said he "didn't like giving" and eventually stopped using. "If you got to give it to one horse, you got to give it to all of them."

"It's a pain in the ass," he added. "You forget who you give it to and what if you give it to one that's too close to [race day]." It was the same with Thyro-L, he said: "It's a herd thing. . . . It's just the way it is."[21]

Baffert's blanket administration of Thyro-L was also a snapshot of another common dynamic surrounding medications in racing. Veterinarians, in theory, are supposed to act as a physician to the horse, evaluating and offering care with the best interests of the animal at heart. But it isn't the horse who signs the check. The trainer is the client and at the racetrack, it's often the trainer who tells the veterinarian what medication he wants his horse to receive. Of course, many owners, trainers, and veterinarians care deeply about the animal and put the "horse first" in these interactions. But as a structural matter, the animal has no independent advocate who does not have a financial stake in his racing career, other than whatever regulatory attention the state is able to offer.

"Thyroxine must be prescribed by a veterinarian, but as in the Baffert situation, thyroxine is often, if not usually, dispensed at the trainer's request," Arthur wrote.[22]

That relationship can lead to a two-way flow of information about hot new therapies that might help a horse win. Different trainers gravitate to different veterinarians, depending on their persuasion about the use of therapeutics. Some are simply willing to write a prescription for whatever a trainer might want. Some are actively selling a new miracle drug.

"To put every horse on [Thryo-L] was crazy," said one longtime racetrack vet whose clients operate at the top levels of the sport. "And the way some veterinarians sold it was by pulling a blood sample that had nothing to do with how you test for thyroid [levels]."

Some veterinarians, "the chemists," go further by trying to engineer new, untestable "therapies." But all operate at the discretion—or behest—of the trainer.

"Way too many [trainers] are, 'What can I do, Doc?' 'What do you got?' 'What's the new thing that you know?'" New York trainer Tony Dutrow said. "I don't understand because we're supposed to be in the best interest of the horse. I understand because you need to be competitive."

This was just horse racing. It was the accepted, unexamined status quo of how racing thought about drugs. It was a kind of thinking that, as the sport increasingly came under the microscope of the mainstream media, was beginning to come under fire. But absolutely none of it explained the deaths in Bob Baffert's barn.

The legend of Baffert and Thyro-L has persisted. More than a decade later, there are still trainers and racing administrators across the country who believe that the drug was singly to blame for the deaths. Tony Dutrow is among them. So is a top executive of one of the largest trade organizations in racing. Arthur, now retired, still thinks that the administration of Thyro-L may have played a part, but it's "a little bit simplistic of an explanation."

"I don't think it explains all the sudden deaths," he told me, sitting on his couch at home in California in 2023.

Baffert was frustrated by Arthur's inclusion of his findings about Thyro-L in the final report. He doesn't deny that he had kept horses on the medication for years, but he feels unfairly singled out for its use.[23] (Even after the report was issued, other trainers continued to use the medication. An undercover investigation by PETA in 2014 showed that perennial leading trainer Steve Asmussen routinely administered the drug to his string.)[24] And, Baffert says, he is angry that Arthur didn't warn him during the writing of the report that he thought that the drug might be contributing to the problem. In April 2013—more than a year after the final death—Baffert stopped administering Thyro-L after an internal review of his supplement program.[25]

Baffert's version of events attributes more of the deaths to rat poison and alleges that Arthur had a conflict of interest that led him to downplay Hollywood Park's culpability. (There is an equally vocal contingency that believes Arthur was covering for Baffert.) It wasn't just that all the deaths were at the one barn at Hollywood Park, Baffert and Marlow point out. They were all stabled on one side of one barn, a barn that had cement flooring. Hollywood Park was "dumping the rat poison in piles in the corners," Baffert said. Rats would eat the poison, climb into the feed bins looking for grain, and defecate. The horses would eat the poisoned rat feces along with their grain—a pretty fair explanation of how rat poison might have figured in at least the December 21 death.

Later, after the publication of the report, Baffert said, Hollywood "picked up all that rat poison" and put out a track-wide memo warning horsemen that rodenticide could cause sudden death. Baffert says he believes that there were other horses that had rat poison in their system and it either wasn't reported or wasn't found. And, he claims, there were other horses that died and whose deaths weren't reported. It is true that the number of sudden deaths in California doubled during the three-year period that Baffert's deaths occurred compared to the previous three-year period—a statistic that is included in Arthur's final report—but this didn't change the fact that an unaccountable proportion of those deaths had occurred in his barn alone. It's a defense that Baffert has returned to again and again: "There was a lot of horses that died around there, but they were just calling mine."

"I think Arthur was covering for Hollywood Park because he was getting paid by Hollywood Park," Baffert said, referring to what appears to be a mistaken understanding of the funding arrangement. Arthur's salary was paid by the California Horse Racing Board, the funding for which is drawn in part from parimutuel handle and did thus come from racetrack operators, including Hollywood Park—but that's a statutory requirement. Hollywood was hardly paying to be regulated voluntarily.

The main problem with Baffert's rodenticide explanation is that it doesn't fit with the necropsy findings. Rodenticide causes hemorrhage in the abdomen, which was only observed in the necropsy for one of the seven.

One other theory has persisted. There is little to no research into drug interactions in horses generally, much less into Thoroughbred racehorses. Some horsemen believe that in some horses, the therapeutics and supplements Baffert was giving had a fatal interaction. Baffert himself may not have known exactly what combination of substances was to blame. Rick Sams and Arthur, however, both believe this is unlikely. ("You'd have to stop the heart," something that the kinds of drugs Baffert appeared to have been administering simply don't do, said Sams, who like Arthur is still of the mind that liberal dosing of thyroxine may have played some unknown role.)

In the end, the deaths in the Baffert barn stubbornly defied explanation. The conclusion of Arthur's final report is devastatingly short.

"The cluster of seven sudden deaths of horses trained by Bob Baffert on the Hollywood Park main and stabled in Barn 61 at Hollywood Park remains unexplained," he wrote. "There is no evidence whatsoever CHRB rules or regulations have been violated or any illicit activity played a part in the 7 sudden deaths."[26]

Arthur said he still has no theories about what caused the sudden rash of deaths.

"I really don't," he said. "They're all a little different. That's the problem—when you go through them, they're all different."

He said he doesn't have any reason to believe that Baffert was doing anything against the rules of racing.

"Everybody wants to put some devious thoughts behind it, or some nefarious explanation," he said. "If it is, I can't figure it out."

Arthur said the most likely "confounder"—the thing that may have interacted with the Thyro-L to result in the death of at least some of these horses—is high-intensity exercise. Baffert is known for training his horses hard. His horses are, famously, just *fitter* than his competitors'. It's the quarter horse thing. He's not afraid to work a horse. Sitting next to him in the grandstand, you can listen to him tell his riders through the radio: *keep going on him*. If the horse is still dragging his rider ahead, he has plenty of gas left in the tank. Baffert tells the rider to push him.[27] On race day, that pays off. Officially, the jury is still out on the role exercise plays in sudden death: One 2022 study found that horses with fewer lifetime starts were more likely to die from a heart arrhythmia, and they were more likely to perish during training—not during a race, at peak exertion.[28] But researchers have good evidence that high-intensity exercise can cause arrythmias.[29] So can Thyro-L.[30] The link between the two hasn't been proven, but it's possible that the intensity of Baffert's training program may have compounded this known risk factor of the drug, Arthur said. "The concern is with high-intensity exercise plus thyroxine, you now have two initiators of arrythmias," he explained.[31]

As a reporter, this episode is the most difficult part of Baffert's story to adjudicate. There is no evidence to prove that Baffert was doing anything out of the ordinary, including with his broad administration of Thyro-L. But the number of deaths in his barn was a statistical anomaly that set him apart from other trainers. And as is often the case with Baffert, it's difficult to completely credit his version of events, because it doesn't fit the facts, or fits only some of the facts, or fits the facts if they were skewed one half degree off their axis. Baffert believes multiple horses died because they ingested rat poison, yet only one horse showed signs of having died from rodenticide. He claims that Arthur had a conflict of interest because his salary was funded by the racetracks; racetrack money supported Arthur's salary only indirectly—and as a matter of statute. It raises the question: Is he lying, or just a lazy student of the details? If he's lying, what isn't he telling us? Is it just a stubborn refusal to admit *any* mistake, no matter how benign, or is it something more sinister?

As a matter of personality, regulators, family members, and current and former employees all told me: Baffert is not a detail-oriented person. He seems to glom on to certain facts and apply them across the board in service of his own narrative. He also has an ego, and he is generally unwilling to acknowledge even little mistakes. It makes him difficult to trust, even in instances where the public record suggests his innocence. He can also be difficult to understand: he speaks in ever-expanding parentheticals, interrupting himself with new sentence fragments for listeners to collect and try to piece together when he returns to the thought later. Stories begin with "this guy" or "this horse"; it's up to the listener to figure out: *Which* guy? *Which* horse? He appears constantly distracted.

But he also speaks without a filter. There is a distinct sense, talking to Baffert, that if the thought enters his head, it comes out of his mouth. Sometimes it's the truth—the quiet part spoken aloud, handed over even when any savvy PR advisor would tell him to just keep it to himself—while sometimes you get the feeling that it's just an idea that he's trying on without stopping to think about whether it's correct or not. Baffert says he has always tried to be "transparent" and "above suspicion"; the reality may be that he talks even if he doesn't know the answer. Does that make his shotgun explanations any more credible, or, at the very least, forgivable? In racing's hall of mirrors, it's in the eye of the beholder.

Baffert's reputation never truly recovered from that season of death. There had been suspicion of him before. But the deaths were so unusual, so inexplicable, so many and so sudden, that they became proof positive that the white-haired Goliath must be doing *something*. Other trainers bring up the deaths in any conversation about Baffert and his training practices, because of course it was Baffert whose horses inexplicably began dropping like flies. It was simply too much of a coincidence. That there was no explanation—no evidence, no leads—only added to the strength of the theory. *He was combining EPO with rat poison. It was the Thyro-L. Baffert was experimenting on his horses with some new designer drug that the necropsies and the out-of-competition testing failed to find.*

The proof, for any one of those bar stool explanations, was the deaths.

"Great horseman. Does a great job. Got the best horses. He's a good, smart horse trainer. But he cheats," Tony Dutrow said, with utter conviction but without evidence beyond what he says is observable in the public record. "What do you have to say about when he had like seven horses die out there in the Thyro-L days? What do you say about that?"

CHAPTER 8

SOCIAL LICENSE TO OPERATE

Rick Dutrow was obnoxious. There was just no getting around it. Even his defenders will acknowledge that. But he had also just won the Kentucky Derby with a horse named Big Brown and, so, no matter how perilous a spokesman for the sport he might be, racing was stuck with him for now. Heavyset with an almost cherubic face, Dutrow could be charmingly irreverent; he was known for calling everyone he interacted with, men and women, "babe." He also had a rap sheet a mile long for petty paperwork infractions and minor drug overages—and a bad habit of publicly haranguing regulators over changes to the rules he considered stupid. He was always running his mouth, his brother Tony would later say.

The Dutrow boys were racetrackers to the core. The sons of a New York trainer, they had grown up at the track. Rick Dutrow left school at sixteen and worked for his father until he hung out his own shingle in 1995. Where his brother Tony was a trim, tidy man, rigidly disciplined, Rick seemed always to hover just on the lee side of disaster. Over the years, he struggled with substance abuse issues and at one point was reduced to living in the tack room of his barn at Aqueduct. The mother of his daughter was killed in a 1997 drug break-in. But he was a smart horse trainer and an instinctual horseman, almost unaccountably talented, and by 2008, he had successfully graduated from claiming horses to become one of New York's leading stakes trainers.

Dutrow's tale of redemption should have made for great television. Instead, Dutrow made headlines when he acknowledged on national television that he routinely treated Big Brown with the anabolic steroid Winstrol. It was 2008, and Winstrol was legal at the time in 28 out of 38 racing jurisdictions. But Dutrow had chosen to open his mouth not only in the wake of professional baseball's reckoning with muscle-building drugs, but also at a moment when racing was already engulfed in controversy over its treatment of its equine athletes. Two weeks earlier, the second-largest crowd in Derby history, which included Chelsea Clinton, the daughter of presidential hopeful Senator Hillary Clinton, had come to watch a filly called Eight Belles try to become the first female since Winning Colors in 1988 to win racing's most cherished prize. A filly so densely gray she was almost black, Eight Belles's fairy-tale story had captured national attention. It ended in tragedy: she crossed the finish line second behind Dutrow's Big Brown, then seconds later crumpled over herself, as if some invisible giant hand had wadded her up and tossed her aside. As she galloped out past the wire, Eight Belles had shattered both front ankles. The break was so severe that bone broke through skin. She floundered in a black heap on the track, panicked and desperate to stand, her destroyed ankles bent forward grotesquely. Churchill Downs outriders in red coats swarmed around the filly to keep her down until the attending veterinarian could arrive to euthanize her. The national news had talked of little else since.

Making matters worse, Dutrow appeared not to know why he was treating Big Brown with Winstrol.

"I wouldn't even know what Winstrol does with a horse," he told NBC Sports' Bob Costas. "One of my vets talked me into it five, six years ago.

"I can't say it helps. I know it doesn't hurt," he said.

Horse racing had faced outside scrutiny before. There had always been breakdowns that were amplified by the national press. (W. C. Heinz wrote "Death of a Racehorse" in 1949.) And there had been, at least since the 1990s, a growing sense both within racing and outside of it that the cocktail of medication these animals received could be contributing to the number of horses breaking down and dying on the track.[1]

Racing had largely been able to ignore the fact that it had a real public perception problem. Even as other animal entertainments like the circus, whale shows, and dog racing were facing existential crises, racing had been largely insulated. It helped to have politically connected patrons. Racing also generates an enormous number of agricultural jobs and other economic benefits in states where it operates. The hay man, the farriers, the feed production company, the shipping transport companies, and the many other ancillary support roles beyond the trainers, owners, and jockeys, all pay taxes. In Kentucky, the industry generates more than $100 million in tax revenue each year; according to statistics cited by Churchill Downs, racing generates $517 million in direct impact to Kentucky's economy.[2] (The Kentucky Derby and Oaks days, combined, create upwards of $217 million, according to the track.) At the time, there was also no federal regulation of racing, so reform efforts had for years been disjointed and ineffective.

Internally, racing had brushed aside animal welfare concerns as uneducated hot takes from animal rights wingnuts. The coverage of breakdowns by mainstream press is inevitably replete with the minute errors of vocabulary and expertise made by journalists and advocates with no horse experience, errors that tend to enrage racing professionals. Media outlets would write erroneously that Eight Belles had fractured her "feet."[3] PETA would frustrate racing professionals by arguing that the filly was "doubtlessly injured before the finish" and that the jockey should be suspended[4]—a baseless assertion belied by the fact that the filly was galloping seamlessly right up until the moment that she wasn't. The industry remained smug and cosseted in the comforting notion that outsiders "just don't understand" horse racing. What racing folks believed they didn't understand was twofold: that these horses were treated exceptionally well, and that breakdowns were an inescapable fact of life at the track. Nothing to be done.

This difference of viewpoints reflects the gulf between how average Americans see horses—essentially as pets—and how racing people see them, which is a sort of amalgam of livestock, financial asset, and anthropomorphized athlete. Neither is quite right. Horses certainly aren't pets, and the way the racing industry sees them is unsettled and ill-defined. Cattle farmers typically don't become attached to individual cattle the way horsemen might to an individual horse, yet both cattlemen and horsemen have to consider expenses and revenue if they want to make a living. Horse people both make their living on the backs of these animals and interact with them in a day-to-day way that can feel intensely personal. Most Americans today, by contrast, have little to no exposure to working animals. They have no frame of reference for the endless challenges of maintaining a performance animal, much less for the difficult practical decisions that must be made if bills are to be paid. (Is it worth doing a costly colic surgery on an older, lower-level horse that likely will never return to the races and be able to pay for its keep, for example?)

Eight Belles changed everything. It was a watershed moment, the beginning of the end of the old retreat into "business as usual." Her death had been so horrific, so gruesome, so glaringly *public*. The uproar was compounded by the fact that only two years before, the Kentucky Derby winner Barbaro had been injured during the Preakness Stakes and was eventually eutha-nized. Racing was forced to account for itself publicly. The rippling effect of that pressure would ultimately change the business in ways that would have a profound impact on some of the sport's top trainers: Rick Dutrow and, later, Bob Baffert.

In the wake of Eight Belles's death, another debate began to emerge in the mainstream press as critics spread the blame beyond the drugs used at the racetrack. People both inside and outside the industry began to point at the very start of the process: the gene pool. They asked: Had Eight Belles been doomed to death from the moment she was conceived?

Thoroughbred horses are bred all over the country—in Virginia, New York, Florida, California, and beyond. But the counties surrounding Lexington, Kentucky, are the birthplace of most of the Thoroughbreds that run in the United States. It's here that most of the sport's top stallions "stand at stud," available for the owners of top mares to pay fees that range into the hundreds of thousands of dollars to breed their mare and own the resultant offspring. That fee earns you a live foal that stands and nurses, begat the old-fashioned way. An industrialized approach to equine fertility tracking that makes *The Handmaid's Tale* look quaint by comparison has grown in response. Mares are palpated daily to judge the size of their follicle, because to miss their fertility window is to miss an entire cycle. That could cost you money down the line when the resultant foal is younger and therefore less physically mature than its peers at the sale. And because all Thoroughbreds officially turn a year older on January 1, no matter their real birth date, a May foal running in the Kentucky Derby may be at a disadvantage against a January foal. If you even get that far: if the foal drops dead two days after it's born, the mare owner must still pay the stallion owner the full amount of the stud fee.

Kentucky is also the home of most of the major commercial nurseries, where young horses are "prepped" for public auction to be sold as year-lings, or sometimes as weanlings (after they have been weaned from the mare but before January 1 of their first year). A series of top sales for horses of different ages—Keeneland September and Fasig-Tipton July for year-lings, Keeneland November and January for weanlings and so-called short yearlings—punctuate the year with buying and selling opportunities. (The entire circus moves north to Saratoga Springs, New York, in August for a glamorous nighttime Fasig-Tipton sale for yearlings.)

Kentucky is known for its racetracks. But as Robert Sangster showed the world in the 1980s, the breeding shed and the sales grounds are where the real money is made.

The problem, some trainers, bloodstock experts, and longtime racing pundits argued, was that beginning in the late 1970s and 1980s, more money than ever poured into the racing industry, with Irish and Arab money especially sparking a feeding frenzy in central Kentucky. As a result, so the argument goes, horsemen began to breed their horses for public auction instead of for the racetrack. They began to select matings that produced a more aesthetically pleasing but fragile animal. Perfect legs, more muscular bodies, and brilliant early speed brought a bigger price tag in the sales ring, these critics argued. These animals *looked* like Olympic athletes as immature yearlings. But were they too mature at too young an age? Were they being bred to be so naturally fast early in their careers that their legs couldn't stand up to the demands of racing and training over the long run?

The same change that had turned horse ownership into a commercial venture rather than a sporting one—the seismic shift that had indirectly allowed trainers like Wayne Lukas and Bob Baffert to become rich—was responsible for the damage done to the horse itself, argued training legend John Nerud. Bill Nack pinned Eight Belles's death on her pedigree and emphasized his long-standing contention that the drugs in racing were a mere symptom of a weakening breed.[5] Ellen Parker, a Thoroughbred breeding consultant, said that the animal rights picketers who came to the Preakness that year should instead have camped out in front of Robert Clay's Three Chimneys Farm in Midway, Kentucky, which bred Eight Belles and then sold her at auction for $375,000.[6] The view was calcifying: Eight Belles had been a victim of a sport that had become too greedy, had lost its nobility, its gentility, its sporting soul in the thicket of Arab money and cowboy hats signing checks for oil barons and car salesmen.

"Horses are being over-bred and over-raced, until their bodies cannot support their own ambitions, or those of the humans who race them," wrote the *Washington Post*'s Sally Jenkins. Eight Belles, she said, "ran with the heart of a locomotive, on champagne-glass ankles."

It's a pretty story, albeit one almost impossible to prove with data.

Horses today race comparatively less than they did in the 1970s and before. The average number of starts per year of a Thoroughbred racehorse was 6.2 in 2008 and 10.23 in 1975,[7] a statistic that is frequently cited by those who believe the breed is less durable than it was in those fabled days, when Secretariat was shattering course records.* Of course, there are any number of reasons beyond soundness why a horse might be removed from the racing pool—including the simple fact that it's worth more in the breeding shed than on the track†—or why it might compete in fewer races while still remaining in training. Several horsemen remarked to me that as "win percentages" became an increasingly important part of a trainer's advertisement to potential owners, there was an incentive to run a horse only when it could win, rather than follow the more old-school model of running in races as a routine part of fitness development and sporting enjoyment. Critically in 2008, the percentage of the racing population that is five years or older had remained remarkably stable going back to the 1950s, according to data presented at the annual Jockey Club forum that August.[8]

"If older horses are productive, they are racing as long as they ever have," Dr. Larry Bramlage, one of the industry's foremost experts on equine soundness, told me. "There is no indication the breed is any less durable than it ever has been. Horses train more and race less, but they last just as long."

This isn't an entirely satisfying answer, because it does little to account for the number of older hands-on horsemen who say definitively that they are dealing with a more fragile animal than they had in the barn decades ago. Baffert, known for working his horses hard, told me that if he trained any of his horses the way that Secretariat was trained in 1973, "I would have never won a Triple Crown. I'd cook 'em—there would have been nothing left of them." Two of central Kentucky's most respected horsemen, Seth Hancock and John Williams, both told me that the majority of horses they see today are "light-boned," literally a reference to thinner bones in

---

* Secretariat's autopsy famously revealed a twenty-two-pound heart, almost twice the size of a normal horse. Discussing this standing by a sales barn at Keeneland, one longtime bloodstock agent slyly remarked to me: *Of course, we know steroids can cause hypertrophy.* (Steroids were legal at the time and in use in both racing and human sports.) In 2024, former football player and sports pundit Jason Kelce made a similar suggestion to his brother, Travis Kelce, on their podcast, *New Heights*; horse racing professionals, journalists, and pundits reacted as if Kelce had come into their home, kicked their dog, and spat on their mother. Within a day, Kelce had issued a public apology for heresy. Rick Sams and others have a subtly different take: Secretariat, like many other top horses at the time, probably *was* running on steroids. Assuming that was the case, all those horses would likely have had enlarged hearts. But even in that context, Secretariat's heart was still abnormally, heroically, huge. https://www.horseracingnation.com/news/The_Tremendous _Size_of_Secretariat_s_Heart_123; https://www.today.com/popculture/jason-kelce-apology -secretariat-steroids-rcna151657.

† A relatively small proportion of the racing population fits this description, however.

the lower leg, visible to the eye. Both blame the commercial sales industry, which they say has both neglected durability in favor of speed and bulk—a recipe for a big price tag now and broken bones later—and created a market incentive to raise horses like hothouse flowers, keeping them blemish-free by restricting them from all the running and roughhousing that young animals need to build durable bones. Some trainers also point to other sales preparation practices, like so-called corrective surgery commonly done to straighten crooked legs, as a potential contributor to unsoundness. At best, you're perpetuating the flaw in the gene pool; blood will out, and that horse is still going to breed crooked horses. At worst, you might be inadvertently messing around with the horse's natural gait, something that could be damaging in ways we don't understand. There is, of course, little to no research on the impact of so-called corrective surgeries,[9] because it would require sales consignors to disclose when they have been done, something that is currently not required.

This part of the industry has virtually no regulation. Auction houses provide some light oversight—some drug testing is done as part of sales for two-year-olds in training, for example—and they nominally restrict some common therapeutics up to ninety days out from a sale. Buyers can also elect to have postsale testing done for anabolic steroids and bisphosphonates, which are approved for use in older horses to treat bone disease but if given to young horses can predispose them to injury by disrupting the natural rebuilding process that makes bones stronger as they age. There are indications that some consignors were giving them to yearlings to mask radiographic evidence of bone abnormalities that could have dented their sales price.[10] Steroids, of course, would bulk up a yearling to give him the impression of being physically mature and thus worthy of a big price.

There are yearling consignors who raise a horse like a horse, who are known for letting them run and kick in the paddock, eschewing any kind of drug use. These consignors keep "prep" exercise light so their yearlings go to the sales ring looking like the teenagers they are, not body builders. But because there is no independent oversight of sales beyond the rules put in place by the auction houses—which make their money on a percentage of each horse sold, and thus themselves benefit from higher prices—horses in this part of the business are entirely at the mercy of the profit incentive. Although in many states there are mandated records of what medications and treatments a horse receives once it arrives at the racetrack, what happens to a horse *before* that is a black box.

The maelstrom churning in the national press in 2008 largely fixated on the question of *breeding* for the sales ring, rather than management practices. But the two are connected, and in recent years, as national scrutiny of the racetrack has come to a head, racetrackers have increasingly begun to point out the double standard: *Why are we subject to all this regulation and criticism, while the Kentucky breeders are given the benefit of the doubt?* It would quickly become part of the simmering social tensions within racing.

Things were bad enough for horse racing in the spring of 2008. Then Rick Dutrow had to open his big mouth about Big Brown. Racing now had to contend with two damaging public narratives. It wasn't just that horses like Eight Belles were the product of irresponsible breeding. They were also running pumped up on drugs that were endangering their lives and weakening the breed.

Another thing to understand right away: with what we know now, it is incredibly difficult to definitively link the general use of drugs, legal or illegal, with breakdowns. It's common sense that a horse whose pain is masked by a drug might injure itself running, but there are drugs in use beyond painkillers and an even broader set of potential conditions that may contribute to a horse's death. Track conditions, the pace of high-intensity exercise, and any number of other factors, singly or in combination, could result in a catastrophic breakdown. The buzzword in the industry is that breakdowns are "multifactorial." It is impossible to diagnose precisely why any individual horse breaks down, because there is usually no *one* reason. It's maddening to people inside racing and outside of it, and it is one of the most fiercely debated questions in the sport: What, exactly, causes catastrophic injury?

Not all drugs are created equal. In some cases, there is clear and compelling research to show that repeated use of a particular "therapeutic" increases the odds of a breakdown. Corticosteroid joint injections—powerful anti-inflammatories, of which there are many variations on the market*—have been linked to catastrophic ankle injuries like the one Eight Belles suffered. But even here, the research is complicated. There is no simple conclusion that corticosteroids cause breakdowns. How they are used—which drug, at what dosage, in what combination related to exercise or rest—seems to

---

* Not to be confused with anabolic steroids, which help build muscle and increase body mass by acting like testosterone, a naturally occurring hormone in both males and females.

have a tremendous impact on whether the drug is helpful or harmful to the horse. Some prominent veterinarians believe that using lower-dose, shorter-acting corticosteroids to reduce joint inflammation within a week of a timed workout, for example, is a "medically sound" approach to help avoid long-term damage to the cartilage.[11] Of course, not every trainer and veterinarian hits that sweet spot. The rules have tightened in recent years, but there is evidence that some trainers used to have no problem injecting multiple joints the week before a race.* Because trainers keep their pre-race routines a secret, it's impossible to know what these trainers—and their veterinarians—were thinking. "You can't legislate good judgment," California regulator Greg Ferraro said.[12] "Corticosteroids in the hands of a wise, experienced equine veterinarian, you could probably do fine with it. But . . . good judgment is not something that's always [used on the] backside."

With other drugs, there's little to no peer-reviewed evidence to link their use to soundness. Lasix, for example, the drug that gets by far the most attention both inside the industry and whenever the issue of horse drugs comes up in Congress, is sometimes accused of negatively impacting bone health. But that idea comes from human research in older patients taking the drug far more regularly than racehorses, and it's probably spotty science to extrapolate the results to horses.[13]

Complicating the issue is the fact that research on the pharmacokinetics of different drugs for use in racehorses is, generally speaking, quite limited. Many studies are small, perhaps a dozen horses or fewer, and those horses are typically not young Thoroughbreds in heavy work. They might be draft horses or Standardbreds—an entirely different breed—whose only exercise is walking from one side of the pasture to the other. Their metabolism, among other factors, may be completely different and not relevant to testing Thoroughbreds.

Because of the prohibitive expense of doing this kind of research, there is also little useful information on drug interactions in racehorses. Researchers might be able to confidently say how Lasix affects a horse's body, but what about a combination of Lasix, Thyro-L, bute, and a dietary supplement?

"There's a great world of unknown out there," said Dr. Mary Scollay, the former top executive at the Racing Medication and Testing Consortium, a

---

* Almighty Silver, who suffered a catastrophic injury and died in his forty-fourth start in 2012, had received "four IA injections . . . five days prior to the race" that were "not reported to the Stewards," according to a New York State report. https://coap.gaming.ny.gov/pdf/NY%20Task%20 Force%20on%20Racehorse%20Health%20and%20Safety.pdf, 30.

research body that sets recommended guidelines for prohibited substances and therapeutic medications. "People get unhappy when we say, 'This study addressed a specific drug administered, alone, by this route of administration and at this dose.' That's not real-world. We can't replicate the real world. We don't have enough money to contemplate all the variables that go into that."[14]

In other words, when it comes to drugs and breakdowns, most horsemen are in the dark. But inside the industry, there is a growing sense that the overuse of therapeutic medication is replacing good horsemanship, by allowing bad horsemen to patch up a damaged horse that shouldn't be running and send him onto the track to make money.

"If a horse requires those medications in proximity to a race, we should be asking: Why is that horse entered to race? He's physically compromised in some capacity," Scollay said.

A prominent stakes-level trainer I spoke to put it flatly: "Not all horses are bred to race. Not all horses should stay in training."

Critics also argued that an increase in the use of medication had a darker consequence as well. Arthur Hancock, Seth's brother and another respected breeder in central Kentucky, told Congress in 2008 that "the breed is becoming softer and weaker."[15] Horses like Big Brown that needed steroids to perform were going to stud, leading to horses like Eight Belles who were breaking down at the wire. And it was happening more and more.

Steroids in particular were "used as a crutch," Seth Hancock told me. "What they did was make a weaker horse stronger, and maybe they made a weaker horse strong enough to win a Grade I, and now that horse has won a Grade I, so he goes to stud some place."

Arthur Hancock told Congress: "It's a vicious cycle. Chemical horses produce chemical babies."[16]

It's another incredibly appealing narrative: As drug use has proliferated across the backstretch, breakdowns have increased. By this logic, if only you did away with the drugs, you would do away with the breakdowns.

But once again, there's little to no data to prove the assertion. As horsemen from Tom Smith to Dr. Harthill have shown, drugs have been around since the dawn of racing. Medication use might have been much more sparing in 2008—or at the very least, on par with previous years—because of the improvements in testing sensitivity. In fact, there's anecdotal evidence that it was.

"Everything went through a transition period of being detected," Harthill told a racing reporter about practicing veterinary medicine on the racetrack in the 1960s. "The thing everyone wanted to find out was what didn't show at the time. It was just part of the game, ever since I can remember. Everybody was looking for an edge. A trainer would say, 'Don't get me caught, but keep me worried.'"[17]

An answer to the question of whether breakdowns have increased dramatically since the 1980s and the dawn of the commercial breeding industry is also, probably, lost to time. Horse racing didn't start keeping reliable figures on race-day breakdowns until 2009, the year after Eight Belles died. (The Jockey Club took up the project.) Trying to make such a comparison anecdotally—did more horses break down in the 1960s and '70s than the 2000s?—isn't a reliable gauge. Because cultural attitudes surrounding the horse have changed so drastically, with the life of an individual animal valued more highly today than in past decades, it seems reasonable to posit that most people simply paid less attention to the death of a racehorse in that era and thus do not remember the relative prevalence of breakdowns. We know they happened: in 1975, a match race between one of the most brilliant fillies of all time, Ruffian, and the Kentucky Derby–winning colt Foolish Pleasure ended when Ruffian shattered both ankles, in front of an audience of fifty thousand.[18]

But by the time Rick Dutrow talked openly about drug use in racing on national television, it had become obvious to some racing leaders—the Jockey Club in particular—that it didn't matter whether there was a defensible reason to use therapeutic medication on racehorses. It was irrelevant whether drug use and breakdowns at the track were greater in 2008 than they were in 1980. What mattered was that they were too high to be considered socially acceptable *outside* of racing *today*. Racing needs fans—specifically, bettors. If bettors believed racehorses were being doped until they dropped, they would take their wagering dollars elsewhere. If the sport wanted to survive, it had to give up the needle.

Big Brown went on to crush his rivals in the Preakness. Before the Belmont, Dutrow announced that the horse had received his final Winstrol injection on April 15 and would not be receiving another prior to the Belmont. The horse was eased in the far turn and crossed the finish line in last place. It was a huge defeat that escalated the scandal. It left the impression that Big Brown couldn't run without steroids.

By the first day of 2009, New York and all other major racing jurisdictions had banned the use of steroids. Congress, not for the last time, threatened to intervene by developing a central governing authority for the sport if horses continued to die on the track.

Then a rash of breakdowns beginning in 2011 occurred at Aqueduct, with twenty-one horses dying in the space of three and a half months. A state report found no single cause for the breakdowns but was heavily critical of both the use of corticosteroid joint injections and an increase in purse money for claiming races that incentivized trainers to run horses that perhaps weren't up to the task. The episode drew particular scrutiny to the use of a high-dose corticosteroid known as Depo-Medrol, among other perfectly legal drugs.*

Doing away with therapeutic drug use at the racetrack posed a practical difficulty. Even at the top level with good stock, "You can't *not* medicate an athlete. It's not realistic to think you can't," the stakes trainer—the one who emphasized that not all horses should race—told me. At the lower levels of the sport, not medicating an animal may be the difference between making rent and an eviction notice. In other words, to say that some horses should not race because they can't do so without drugs might mean telling that horse's trainer that they can't afford payroll this month. Then there's the practical and ethical question of who will—or can—pay to care for the animal if it's not earning money.

Even steroids had their defenders on the backstretch, especially among working trainers who said that they promoted appetite and helped horses recover from races. One California racing executive recalled trainers protesting the ban, arguing that horses wouldn't be able to run as often and the track wouldn't be able to fill races. The drugs had been legal for such a long time that many trainers had never trained horses without at least the option of using them. A 2003 study in Pennsylvania showed that in that state alone, 60 percent of racehorses had been administered one steroid, if not more.[19] It's also possible those drugs had enabled some of the greats of the 1960s and '70s—a time when anabolic steroids were also widely popular in human sports—to run as often and as hard as they did. Most of the major track records across North America today date from that period.[20]

---

* "Based upon the fact that no illicit or non-therapeutic drugs were detected in any post-race samples subjected to the full complement of drug screening during the period of investigation, and based upon further information that the Task Force was able to review, the Task Force has no reason to believe that any of the fatally injured horses was administered an illicit or non-therapeutic drug," a New York State report carefully mentioned. https://coap.gaming.ny.gov/pdf/NY%20 Task%20Force%20on%20Racehorse%20Health%20and%20Safety.pdf, 61.

The drug issue hadn't gotten worse. The individual drugs themselves had changed over the years, testing had evolved, and veterinary medicine had grown more sophisticated. But the use of *drugs* was so deeply intertwined with the history and business of Thoroughbred racing that it had become impossible to disentangle them—to know what was good, responsible management of an athlete and what was taking an edge. To know what was causing harm and what was patching over harm. To know what could be abandoned and what was needed. What had changed wasn't the drugs. It was America's view of the horse and its sense of how it should be treated. In 2008, that was beginning to become clear.

Some horsemen recognized that earlier than others. Arthur Hancock had been advocating publicly to do away with the use of medication in racing since the early 1990s. He gave a somewhat unpopular speech in 1991 decrying the "drugs and thugs" in the sport. This wasn't just the ideological proclamation of one of the scions of Thoroughbred breeding; it was also a matter of commercial interest. Arthur Hancock had bred the 1989 Kentucky Derby winner, Sunday Silence. Seth Hancock had syndicated Secretariat for a record $6 million in the 1970s. Both men made their living at the breeding of horses. But both worried about the long-term viability of the industry. Horse racing, Hancock said in 1991, could not compete with football, baseball, and other sports "if we are perceived by the masses of fans and potential fans as being dishonest and riddled by drugs and thugs."

"Something has to be done and done quickly or racing as it was meant to be and life as we have known it is over," he said. "We are riding a runaway train." He told an audience of horsemen that the industry was "dying of a disease, corruption, and the high fever is caused by greed."

He made an explicitly commercial appeal: "The way to help the little man or any owner is for breeders to breed them good, rugged, healthy, sound horses, and to do that we have to assess the true merit of horses without their performance having been enhanced by drugs. When we breeders sell someone something, we had better try our best to make sure that they have a chance to make money or they'll be gone forever."[21]

It was a powerful speech, but it didn't work. By the time Eight Belles died, the Hancocks were still fighting the same fight. In 2012, Arthur and his wife, Staci, and others launched an organization dedicated to creating a single national regulatory body and tightening the rules surrounding medication use.[22] Other elites in racing also tried to mobilize against medication. Stuart S. Janney III, then the chair of the Jockey Club's safety committee, announced in August 2012 that the breed registry was declaring its opposition to Lasix. These were some of the oldest and most influential voices in Thoroughbred racing. Yet none of their efforts gained any real traction—"because the rules are made on a state-by-state basis, and pro-medication horsemen have more clout on the state level than do the nation's elite owners and breeders," wrote Andrew Beyer, the *Washington Post*'s preeminent racing scribe.[23] Their efforts split in the industry, between working-level trainers and veterinarians across the country on one side, and the Jockey Club and a handful of prominent breeders on the other.

But even at the working level, racetrackers recognized that the sport had a serious perception problem. It had to do *something*. Rick Dutrow became perhaps the first trainer to experience the fallout when the world he had always known began to change under his feet.

Dutrow had always pissed off the wrong people in New York, his brother Tony told me. He routinely popped positives for therapeutic medications, he lacked deference to regulators, and he was widely suspected of doping—a suspicion, as always at the racetrack, based more on his strike rate than any real evidence that he used illegal drugs. He had more than a dozen positive drug tests to his name over the years, and an even longer list of citations for paperwork errors that broke the rules of racing, like a failure to have a horse in the paddock on time or have the right identification papers on file with the racing office. Penny-ante shit, but it added up.

In November 2010, officials from the regulatory body then called the New York State Racing and Wagering Board* entered Dutrow's barn at Aqueduct for an inspection. Dutrow was out of town. In a drawer in his desk, investigators say they found a box with three unlabeled syringes containing the common sedative xylazine. It was illegal in New York for nonveterinarians to possess hypodermic needles or injectable medications. Then, weeks later, a Dutrow-trained horse tested positive for an overage of butorphanol, a regulated sedative and opioid pain reliever. A little under a year later, the Racing and Wagering Board voted unanimously to suspend Dutrow for ten years and fine him $50,000. Because state racing commissions typically

---

* The New York State Racing and Wagering Board and the Division of the Lottery became, in 2012, the New York State Gaming Commission.

reciprocate suspensions handed out by other states, the ban meant Dutrow was done in racing for a decade.

The penalty was astonishing in historical terms, and deeply controversial. Some trainers in 2012 had received similar bans for the use of dermorphin—frog juice—but a ten-year ban for a regulated drug that normally would have only sparked a penalty of perhaps a month?[24] "Even Patrick Biancone, who had cobra venom discovered in his barn, was only suspended for a year by the Kentucky Horse Racing Commission," noted the Paulick Report.[25] The state's top regulator said that Dutrow's "repeated violations and disregard of the rules of racing has eroded confidence in the betting public and caused an embarrassment throughout the industry"; his brother and other allies would come to believe that Dutrow had been drummed out of the sport because New York regulators simply didn't like him.

Then, in 2020, a retired racing official wrote a letter to the New York State Gaming Commission alleging that one of the stewards of the New York Racing Association had told him "on numerous occasions" that the syringes found in Dutrow's tack room had been planted there.[26] It wasn't a new allegation: an investigator had reportedly been in Dutrow's barn unaccompanied for forty minutes prior to the search itself. Once the search began, it took only ten minutes to uncover the syringes. State regulators have denied the allegation, but Tony Dutrow, among others, still believes it.

"My brother upset the wrong people," Tony told me. "More than once or twice or three times. So they finally planted needles in his barn to get rid of him.

"Did he need to go away? Yes, he did. He did not represent horse racing well. He needed to be sanctioned. But for him to get the rap of drugging and ten years I thought was both criminal and abusive," Tony continued.

Regulators unquestionably made a judgment call in the penalty they chose to mete out to Dutrow. The ten-year ban exposed the fragmented way that racing polices its participants: sometimes not at all, and sometimes violently if that person is deemed to be "detrimental" to the sport. But the definition of what is "detrimental" to racing seems to be a matter of personal opinion. The system allows opportunities for discretion at its best, but also favoritism or a vendetta at its worst. Even among participants who understand the nuances of different drug policies and testing procedures, it has very little credibility. Many racetrackers simply don't trust that penalties are handed out fairly. How, then, are most people to tell which sins are venial and which are mortal, if venial sins are sometimes punished as mortal sins and mortal sins sometimes paid for with little more than a slap on the wrist? How do you square the nine-year delta between Patrick Biancone's and Rick Dutrow's punishments? And without trust in a clear architecture for accountability, how can you change a culture that has built up around years of permissibility, confusion, and irregularity? Little evidence exists that banning Rick Dutrow for ten years did anything to dissuade veterinarians from prescribing butorphanol or trainers from keeping illegal syringes around the barn.

But in some ways, the ten-year ban that New York handed down to Dutrow was good PR. New York "will not permit individuals who cheat," the Racing and Wagering Board chairman said in a statement at the time. With one sweep of the hand, the state could be seen to be *doing something*— whether or not that something had much of an effect on the backside. That Rick Dutrow was also a particularly acute pain in their ass was, perhaps, just a happy coincidence.

For ten years, Rick Dutrow did very little, his brother said. He sat at home and watched racing. He found no other occupation. Like most racetrackers, he couldn't exist outside the racetrack. He bided his time and waited for 2023, when he could return to the track.

"He was foolish," Tony said. "Wouldn't listen to me, wouldn't listen to nobody, having too much fun. And getting away with his world—until his world came to an end."

CHAPTER 9

THE RACING BUSINESS

Baffert was trying to give racing some badly needed good PR. Santa Anita was in crisis—and so far, it didn't have anything to do with him. Twenty-one horses had broken down and been euthanized during racing or training in the three months since the race meet had begun on December 26, 2018. The news media had noticed. The local TV stations were in Burbank, just a few minutes up the road from the racetrack, so every time there was a fatality, the satellite trucks would whisk over to the track. That morning, March 14, 2019, Baffert was being interviewed by the local Fox affiliate in Los Angeles. He was trying to explain the sport of racing—its risks, yes, but also the care that trainers took with their equine athletes—when the sirens blared, warning riders on the track of a loose horse.

Few things are more chilling than the cry of "loose horse!" at a race-track. Somewhere, a panicked one-thousand-pound animal is hurtling like a frictionless ball bearing amid the crowded warren of barns or caroming between high-strung horses out on the track. Your best hope is to stay out of the way, avoid collision, hope that the fractious filly you are holding barely on the edge of calm never glimpses the rolling eye of a loose horse. Baffert stopped talking to Fox 11 and picked up his radio to make sure his riders heard the siren: "Hey, hold up, boys, hold up, boys."[1]

Almost immediately, he saw her.

On the track in front of the grandstand where he was standing with the TV crew, three-year-old filly Princess Lili B looked as if she were standing downhill. She had lost her rider, triggering the sirens, but she wasn't a runaway. Her front ankles had shattered, her feet attached to her body by nothing but tendon and skin. Someone stood on the ground, holding her, wrapping the filly's head around him and into his chest. Within moments, two giant green tarps were brought out to shield Princess Lili B from the cameras. She was euthanized immediately. It was the only humane thing to do.

Having a horse break down is heartbreaking for horsemen. There is the stomach-churning agony of bearing witness to the confusion, fear, and pain that a horse, an innocent whose well-being rests in your care, must feel in its final moments of life. And there is the emotional reaction to the death of an animal that you care for—the sense of loss. It can be like losing a family member, trainer Jena Antonucci told the racing press the day after a particularly high-profile breakdown in a Grade I at Saratoga in 2023: "When your life revolves around another being—whether it's an animal or whatever—and that part is then gone, I can't give you words because the feeling that you have, gutted doesn't even do it. It stays for life. I can tell you every horse that I have lost."[2]

Many trainers, Baffert among them, are deeply insulted by the notion that they don't care for the horses that break down in their barn. Most horsemen share a very real feeling that there is a certain inevitability about breakdowns: Thoroughbreds just "take a wrong step," and there is nothing that even the most careful of trainers can do to avoid it. Antonucci likened it to walking out of your front door and getting hit by a car. Always, there has been a sense that anything can happen on the racetrack, that tragedy can lurk unseen on the far turn. As veterinary science has improved—and as breakdown statistics have become more comprehensive—there is a growing awareness that this long-held perception might not be true. But breakdowns have a randomness about them that makes it difficult for many horsemen to stomach the criticism that they somehow could have known or prevented any individual disaster. Worse is the suggestion that they are callous to it.

"You can villainize us and villainize this industry," Antonucci said, "but you cannot fathom the failure you feel as a human that we are doing everything we can to steward the best for our horses and then something freaky happens.

"I am very aware that the general public views this sport with a terrible light," she continued. "There is not a single human that puts a horse on a racetrack with the intent to harm, ever. Even nefarious people."[3]

Antonucci can make the point that even "nefarious people" do not knowingly send a horse to the track when it might break down because beyond the emotional impact, breakdowns come with stiff financial implications.

A beloved horse is still a financial asset. Particularly at the middle and lower levels of racing—the strata of the sport that often gets the worst publicity for allegedly providing substandard care to its equine athletes—a breakdown is an empty stall and the loss of potential purse earnings. At that level, there is no economic incentive to casually risk a catastrophic injury, even as there is a conflicting incentive to run horses as often as possible.

"You depend on them to support you and your family," explained one California trainer. "You walk around the barns many times during the day and you become friendly with them. But at the same time on race day, you're putting them in the gate. And if that guy [the jockey] has to hit that horse twenty times to get you to the winner's circle, you don't really lose any sleep over it. So exactly what are they? They're not your pets."*

Ironically, the incentives to treat a horse as expendable can sometimes be higher at the top levels of the sport, where successful trainers can always fill a stall with another million-dollar colt. Trainers like Bob Baffert,[4] Wayne Lukas,[5] and Todd Pletcher[6] sometimes get a reputation for a high rate of attrition. If a horse can't stand up to a rigorous training regimen—well, there's always another one. The ones that make it are going to win a Grade I.[†]

Horsemen in recent years have also become keenly aware of what a PR disaster breakdowns are. The entire racetrack experiences a collective wince. As the tarps went up around Princess Lili B, the vans from Burbank turned on the road toward Santa Anita, and racing, once again, was faced with explaining to outsiders why it was killing horses.

By the morning of Princess Lili B's death, Santa Anita was a hotbed of pointing fingers and dread. The California trainer described it as "soul-destroying." It felt like trench warfare: barns were just waiting for the next shell to hit and hoping it didn't land on them. And it was very much like

---

* Whip rules have been tightened in recent years, limiting jockeys to six strikes on the horse's hindquarters with no more than two more in a row without giving a horse a chance to respond. Racing "sticks," as they are called in the sport, are now padded and largely designed to produce sound rather than pain. While they are used to encourage horses to run faster in the final stretch of a race, they can also be crucial for safety during a race to, for example, encourage a horse that might be risking collision by leaning in on another horse to move back into his own lane. https://www.govinfo.gov/content/pkg/FR-2024-04-08/pdf/2024-06911.pdf, 24597.

† Not all horses whose racing careers end because they aren't sound enough to train on die; many experience soft-tissue injuries and are retired to the breeding shed or other careers. Those are still considered "attrition."

being hit with an artillery shell. Almost all the deaths had been the result of shattered sesamoids, the injury Princess Lili B had sustained. Racing calls broken bones that result in euthanasia "catastrophic breakdowns" because in many instances, the fragile ball of the animal's ankle virtually explodes. Necropsies performed after the fact have shown that most fatal breakdowns—as high as 90 percent[7]—show signs of preexisting damage at the site of the injury. But how to catch or diagnose that subtle pathology in real time? Trainers frequently report that the horse wasn't showing any physical signs of discomfort or underlying injury.

One thing everyone at the track knew was that California had received an enormous amount of rain in early 2019. A megadrought that began in 2011 had finally ended and the skies had bucketed more than a foot of water on Southern California in just two months. When the final accounting was done, 39 percent of the fatalities during the 2019 season occurred on racing surfaces that had been affected by wet weather.[8]

Maintaining a dirt racetrack is part engineering, part high-dollar landscaping, part art. A consistent racing surface is safest—and the biggest factor impacting surface consistency is the amount of moisture in the track. Racetracks across the country employ a "track man" whose job is to direct a fleet of tractors, harrows, and heavy rollers to groom the track between races. Weather stations monitor rainfall, wind speed, and sunlight, any of which can dramatically impact the racing surface from one race to the next.

Most dirt surfaces are variations on a theme: a densely packed subbase with some form of drainage system running through it, a compacted layer of granite or other drainage stone, topped by six to ten inches of some mixture of sand, silt, and clay. The exact composition of the surface layer varies based on what materials are locally available and the prevailing weather conditions where the track is located. When needed, engineers employ X-ray diffraction equipment typically used in oil exploration to analyze the mineral makeup of a racetrack and laser diffraction to scatter light across the top layer to assess how large the sand particles are. They use lasers to check the gradation of a track. There is even a machine that replicates the front leg of a Thoroughbred as it strikes the racecourse—known as a "portable biomechanical surface tester"—to test the load distribution on a galloping horse.[9]

When it rains, the track man will "seal" a racetrack by running heavy rollers or plates over the loam. The idea is to remove all the air pockets from the surface layer so that water will run horizontally off the track into drainage ditches. In theory, a sealed track is perfectly safe. No good data exists to prove a direct correlation between catastrophic breakdowns and a wet track.[10] The danger comes when a sealed track starts to dry out, creating a hard ceramic top layer, according to Mick Peterson, a consultant and widely known expert in racing surfaces. At such moments, you can hear the percussive hammer of horses' hooves like they are running on tarmac.

The methodology for what to do when it rains, and when it starts to dry out, varies from track to track, and is mostly determined through trial and error. Even the speed of the harrow can matter. Good track men are made through an informal apprenticeship process, and often only one man at the racetrack knows what to do when it rains.

At Santa Anita, that man was Dennis Moore. But Moore had retired—some sources say he was forced out by track management, which 1/ST denies—just before the crisis.

"They raced when they shouldn't have raced. They had a bad track," said Rick Arthur, medical director for CHRB at the time.[11]

It is widely accepted within racing that breakdowns tend to happen in clusters because "there's something wrong with the track," as it's said. In 2023, another cluster of fatalities at Churchill Downs leading up to the Kentucky Derby drew national attention. Some horsemen blamed the deaths on too many rocks in the top layer and a surface that had been manipulated to produce faster times.* Clusters of fatalities at Laurel Park in Maryland and Saratoga that same year drew similar explanations. Yet, in the final analysis, there usually isn't one single diagnosis of "a bad track."

During the crisis at Santa Anita, Dennis Moore was brought back on to assess the track. According to Peterson, "his immediate response was, 'Ah, this isn't that different. In '73, we had exactly the same situation.'" Moore spent two weeks in the chute leading onto the track, testing out different

---

* Both have been consistent criticisms of Churchill for years; it's not clear Churchill's track man had maintained the track any differently in the run-up to the Derby than at any other time of year. Churchill added more material to the dirt track surface and began using new harrows after the episode and the track saw no fatalities during Kentucky Derby week of the following year. But the track alone was unlikely to be the sole culprit: an after-action report found multiple risk factors for the fatalities but no single cause, and it's important to note that some of the fatalities were paddock accidents and sudden death, rather than musculoskeletal injuries. "Equine Safety a Highlight of Kentucky Derby Week," TrueNicks, accessed September 22, 2024, https://www.truenicks.com/articles/276804/equine-safety-a-highlight-of-kentucky-derby-week.

combinations of rakes, harrows, and rollers to find just the right formula to ensure a consistent surface. Peterson conducted his high-tech testing of the track too, and in late February he declared that it was "100 percent ready" for racing. The problem was supposed to be solved.

Three more horses died over the next two weeks. Princess Lili B was the third.

Belinda Stronach, the president of the Canadian conglomerate that owns Santa Anita and major racetracks in Florida and Maryland, breathes rarefied air. Immaculately presented, with shoulder-length blond hair and eyes that narrow into mascara-lined slits when she smiles, Stronach is both a product of privilege and a woman not to be trifled with. She runs in powerful circles. Longtime rumor—never substantiated and consistently denied by both parties—even had it that she engaged in an affair with former president Bill Clinton.[12]

The Stronach Group represents the racing empire of Belinda's father, an Austrian-born billionaire named Frank Stronach, who has been on and off the list of Canada's wealthiest men for decades thanks to an international auto parts business he founded in the late 1960s. He's a self-made man who had long been known as a notorious skirt chaser*—even before Canadian authorities arrested him on sexual assault charges dating back to the 1980s.[13] (Stronach has denied the charges.)[14] He's the type of guy who, in 2012, launched his own political party in Austria, Team Stronach, dedicated in large part to doing away with the euro. To achieve that goal, Stronach handed the reins of his Thoroughbred empire to Belinda: two large breeding operations in the US and Canada; Santa Anita; Gulfstream Park; and until recently, Pimlico, the home of the Preakness, in Baltimore; a company that builds and operates tote boards; and other myriad racing assets. When his political ambitions fizzled out and he wanted to resume control of the business, Belinda wasn't keen to let it go. By 2019, the Stronach family was in an extremely public feud in court. Frank had accused Belinda of mismanaging the family fortune and orchestrating what amounted to a family coup; Belinda had countersued, accusing her father

---

* Disclosure: In 2011, when I was in my early twenties, I had an encounter with Stronach that I initially believed was an informal job interview but during which it became clear to me from Stronach's conduct that his interest in me was personal. I declined an offer of "walking around" money from him and canceled the rest of our engagements.

of frittering away their millions on fanciful pet projects. The case was eventually settled in 2020, with the family fortune split. Belinda retained control of the racing and gaming operations, while Frank assumed control of the breeding operation.

In 2019, under Belinda, the Stronach Group was making a very public effort to boost field size at Santa Anita—and by extension, make the racetrack more profitable. The company had named two key executives over the past six years: Tim Ritvo, a racing executive at Gulfstream in Florida, had become the CEO of Santa Anita in 2017, and P. J. Campo, a former racing secretary in New York, had been made the vice president of racing in 2013.

Racetrack operators' basic product is competitive races on which gamblers can wager. To help promote full fields that make for a better betting product, racetracks offer free stabling to trainers, with the understanding that they will run their horses in races at that facility. Trainers who don't help fill races can lose their stall allocations. Of course, racetracks also offer incentives for horsemen to run—competitive purse money—and they write races with certain "conditions" that fit the horse population stabled at their facility. On any given day at Santa Anita, the racing secretary is working to fill specific races carved up by distance, racing surface, and the gender and relative track record of possible entrants. Some of the races are more competitive betting products than others, and for these there may be relatively fewer trainers and owners with horses that fit the model—and vice versa. But the real leverage over trainers that the racing office has at its disposal is stalls.

"We need to correct the guys who are here and not running and just using the place as a training track," Ritvo told the *Los Angeles Times* shortly after arriving at Santa Anita in 2017. "We need to replace them."[15]

Some trainers who were stabled at Santa Anita in 2019 have said that Ritvo, Campo, and other racing officials put pressure on them to run their horses even when the trainers considered the track surface unsafe or the horse in question unprepared to run. The message of "run or lose your stalls" was delivered informally, people told me, but unambiguously. (1/ST called the allegation that it pressured trainers "industry gossip which has never been substantiated.")[16]

It was "absolutely true" that the racing office under Campo put pressure on trainers to run, said Rick Arthur. "And the smaller the trainer, the more pressure they were under."

Five weeks into the meet, a young trainer named Shelbe Ruis had entered an unraced three-year-old named C Falls on the main track. It had rained, again, and the track had been sealed. At the time, a dozen horses had already died since December 26, and Ruis felt she had no choice but to "scratch" C Falls from the race.

When she made Santa Anita aware of her desire to remove the horse from the field, the then racing secretary, Steve Lym, called her to persuade her to run the horse anyway. This isn't unusual: it's up to the racetrack and the regulatory stewards to approve a scratch, and it's in the racetrack's interest to avoid them to protect the betting product. Turf writer T. D. Thornton in his chronicle of life at a hard-luck track in Massachusetts wrote about a trainer who wanted to scratch a horse, Glockenspiel, with a nagging injury; the track refused because "the field would be reduced to only four horses, resulting in a loss of revenue for Suffolk Downs because certain bets, such as the trifecta, would not be allowed with so few wagering interests. Despite the pleas from [the assistant trainer] that not scratching Glockenspiel could be dangerous to both horse and rider, the stewards refuse[d] to allow him out of the race, insisting that the animal's problematic tendon chance the unsteady footing.

"Upon hearing the news . . . the incensed [trainer] has three brief emphatic words. . . . 'Eat the fine.'" The trainer refused to move the horse from his stall, accepting a mandatory penalty, "opting to protect his Thoroughbred rather than risk running—and ruining—the colt," Thornton wrote.[17] (It is one of a million small acts of welfare at the racetrack that challenges the prevailing image of horsemen as heartless butchers.)

Immediately after her call with the Santa Anita racing secretary, Ruis took to social media to complain that Lym had "bullied" her: "I was harassed from the new racing secretary for scratching my horse for unsafe conditions. They don't care about horse safety at Santa Anita."[18]

Lym later told the racing trade publication *BloodHorse* that he was "trying to hold a card together" and that everyone who tried to scratch a horse that day had received a phone call. He denied that he had threatened to take away Ruis's stalls. (She had more than one for her string.) But he also acknowledged that there was no guarantee that she would continue to receive the same stall allocation that she had in the past.

"She felt I was threatening with stalls, " Lym said at the time. "The year is still young. I can't tell you what kind of stalls she's going to get this year. I'm not threatening anything. If you perform, you'll get stalls. If you don't, you won't get stalls. That's the same with everyone."

DEATH OF A RACEHORSE

Tim Ritvo had made a similar call to another trainer who wanted to scratch two horses that day, Jeff Mullins. Mullins told *BloodHorse* that Ritvo had merely encouraged him to remove the horses from contention sooner rather than later to protect a complicated multi-race betting product.

"I told him, 'I'd love you to run, but the horses come first,'" Ritvo said. Ritvo also pushed back forcefully against the suggestion that there was anything wrong with Santa Anita's track.

"I don't want to hear the track is unsafe, because that's untrue. We wouldn't run if the track was unsafe," he said. "The track isn't unsafe just because it's muddy. Tracks are muddy all around the country. . . . Some horses run better in the mud."[19]

Public statements from these early weeks of the crisis make clear that Santa Anita was still thinking about its primary constituents as bettors. Its goal was to preserve the betting product. Indeed, it had hired Campo for that very purpose—even though Campo had some history that raised questions about whether he had prioritized the economic needs of the racetrack over the welfare of the horse. He had served, under the auspices of the New York Racing Association, as racing secretary at Aqueduct during the 2011 cluster of breakdowns, when twenty-one horses died during a three-month period. The investigatory report ordered by then-governor Andrew Cuomo ran to two hundred pages and found no single root cause for the fatalities, pinning the blame on a combination of track surface management, overuse of joint injections, and increased purses in claiming races. But the report also found an "inappropriate dynamic" in how scratches were handled under Campo: track veterinarians, who reported to the racing office, sometimes wanted to scratch a horse for safety reasons but were overruled, the report found. The report also learned of a trainer who, "dissatisfied with a [New York Racing Association] veterinarian's assessment of his horse, arranged through the Racing Office for the veterinarian in question to no longer perform pre-race exams on his horses." It found other examples in which track veterinarians "were instructed to re-evaluate horses having been recommended for a scratch."[20] Even the basic structure of the office, with track vets responsible for ensuring horses were sound enough to run reporting to an office whose main purpose was to maximize field size, raised a troubling conflict of interest, the report found. (A model Campo only operated within and did not invent, of course.)

The state report made the connection very clearly: "Racetrack management has a vested interest in maximizing field size," they wrote. "Conversely, field size, or the economic impact of a scratch, must never be a consideration when an examining veterinarian assesses a horse's suitability to race."[21]

Campo's hiring by the Stronach Group came about a year after the Cuomo report was issued. Five years later, in 2018, he was placed in the racing office.

By the time Princess Lili B died, the Stronach Group seemed to have recognized that it had a bigger problem: the perception that Santa Anita was killing horses in service of its betting product. On the afternoon of the horse's death, Belinda Stronach issued an "open letter" to the industry that appeared to identify a new culprit for the deaths: drugs.

She announced that Santa Anita would adopt a policy of "zero tolerance for race day medication," including banning the use of Lasix and increasing the restrictions on joint injections of corticosteroids. She declared it "a watershed moment."

Although it never addresses horsemen directly, the letter carried the unmistakable suggestion that if it weren't for trainers pumping their horses full of unnecessary, injury-masking drugs, the crisis would never have happened. "There are some who will take a stand and tell us that it cannot be done," Stronach declared. "To them we say 'the health and welfare of the horses will always come first.'" By the time Stronach got around to writing that the company "recognize(s) the owners and trainers of these horses have the final responsibility to assess their fitness for racing and training," it sounded more like an indictment than a concession.[22]

Stronach made transformative changes to medication policy. Within a few years, Santa Anita became one of the safest racetracks in the country, with some of the tightest rules for race-day medication. It also became a leader for veterinary oversight and transparency.

Arguably the most impactful change that Stronach made was a new thirty-day stand-down for corticosteroid use, mandating rest for an animal that was given a joint injection. A seventy-six-page after-action report from the California Horse Racing Board found that some trainers appeared to be overusing the treatment, raising serious questions about the level of horsemanship being practiced on the backstretch. "One horse was being treated by two veterinarians without communication or even an awareness that the other was similarly treating the horse," the report found. "In one case two veterinarians injected the same joint within five days of each other. In that case, it was the major weight-bearing bone in the joint that ultimately failed in the race."[23]

Several prominent vets now attribute a dramatic drop-off across California in shattered ankles—the injury that made up all but three of the deaths at Santa Anita—to restrictions on joint injections. The Stronach Group policy became statewide in October 2021 and the results were immediate: in the 20 months leading up to that shift, there were 83 deaths from shattered ankles; in the 19 months after, there were 24.[24] The policy, proponents say, made it impossible for bad horsemen to misuse the therapy.

But Stronach's letter was also a brilliant public relations move that managed to elide the racetrack's responsibility for either the track surface or the conduct of its racing office. The villain was the drugs.

The problem is that alone, the injection practices that Stronach ultimately restricted do not explain the number of deaths in 2019. For one thing, corticosteroid use wasn't new. Plus, only eleven of the horses that died in 2019 had received intra-articular injections, and not always in the joint that ultimately failed.

The other major change Stronach implemented—the Lasix ban—also likely didn't have much impact on stopping the deaths. There is little to no evidence that the drug, which prevents hemorrhage in the lungs, has any connection to broken bones.

Indeed, Stronach's new policies did not immediately end the crisis. Racing had been canceled indefinitely on March 5, 2019, although horses had continued to train on the racetrack. (The alternative would have been to keep the animals confined to their stalls, which carries its own health and welfare risks.) Racing resumed on March 29, two weeks after Princess Lili B's death. There was no rain and no fatalities for the next six weeks. But in mid-May, it rained eight times in a twelve-day period and six horses died within three weeks.

The breakdowns continued up until virtually the end of the race meet on June 23. Governor Gavin Newsom directed the California Horse Racing Board to form a safety panel to review the fitness of every horse entered to race. The panel, headed by Rick Arthur, started work on June 14, with just two weeks left in the race meet. The thirtieth and final horse perished during a morning workout during that time. California's elite racing population moved south to the resort town of Del Mar, near San Diego, for a summer race meet there. The deaths stopped as mysteriously as they had begun.*

Disentangling the threads of what caused the cluster—and why it stopped—is impossible. Many things had to go wrong at once for thirty horses to die within such a short period. Few horsemen doubt that the impact of historic rain on the racing surface was partly to blame, and few, now, would argue against the new medication restrictions put in place by the Stronach Group.

Many of the changes to drug and medication policy appear to have made Santa Anita safer. In 2022, there were zero fatalities during racing on the main dirt track. (Twelve horses died during training, on the turf course, or from sudden death.)[25] But the exact impact of these new protocols—including increased veterinary oversight of horses prior to racing and breezing—is hard to assess. Officials also implemented continuing education requirements for trainers on the backstretch, a possibly critical element to resolving the more systemic problem that not all trainers are good horsemen. But poor horsemanship is also nothing new and alone doesn't explain why, suddenly, thirty horses perished in six months at the same track.

Some trainers at Santa Anita felt scapegoated on the medication issue. The drugs Stronach's letter seemed to suggest had led to the death of so many horses weren't illegal performance enhancers. They were perfectly permissible under California's rules and, when used responsibly, were arguably a legitimate part of keeping horses in training, healthy and sound. A subsequent investigation by the Los Angeles County district attorney found no evidence of "criminal animal cruelty or unlawful conduct relating to the equine fatalities at Santa Anita Park."[26]

What Stronach had successfully done was make the most immediate custodians of the horse—the trainers—solely responsible for the events of 2019. Undoubtedly the intersection of training and medication practices played some role. But by publicly placing the onus entirely inside individual barns, Stronach managed to escape any reckoning with the role that the economic model of racing, and her racetrack, had played.

---

* Other horses would suffer catastrophic injuries at Santa Anita when racing resumed later in 2019, including one high-profile breakdown during the Breeders' Cup in November. According to the Los Angeles County district attorney, the final count for the calendar year of 2019 was forty-two horses. Los Angeles County District Attorney's Office, "Santa Anita Task Force Report of Investigation," December 2019, https://da.lacounty.gov/sites/default/files/press/121919-District-Attorney-Jackie-Lacey-Issues-Report-on-Horse-Deaths-at-Santa-Anita-Racetrack.pdf.

"I do think the medication was definitely an important factor in improving the situation," said one former racing official with firsthand knowledge of the episode. "I don't think the racetrack surface and the pressure from the racing office ever got the public attention that it deserved."

From a business perspective, the basic imperative of Thoroughbred racing is that horses run. If horses don't run in races, gamblers don't have anything to bet on and the track loses. Racetracks are best understood as gambling houses with little intrinsic link to the horse itself. Their primary clients are gamblers: the two-dollar bettor riding the A train from Queens to Aqueduct who hands crumpled dollar bills to the teller at the window, and the titanically wealthy anonymous gambler whose volume of play is so huge that the racetrack will negotiate private terms with them.[27] Racetrack executives are businesspeople, not horsemen. (The CEO of Churchill Downs, for example, came from General Electric, not a barn; the company recorded a net revenue of $2.5 billion in 2023.)[28]

The "horse" side of the industry also depends entirely on horses running: If horses do not run in races, they neither cover the cost of their upkeep nor establish commercial value for the breeding shed—and so the owners, the breeders, and the bloodstock agents all lose. The real money in racing is made in the breeding shed and the sales ring, yes, but the core product that props up the big races that establish value in the sales ring is still a card full of competitive Thoroughbred races for gamblers to bet on. It is the engine that powers the entire industry.

In the middle of the crisis, Ritvo appeared to acknowledge as much. In an interview with the *New York Times* in April 2019, he said, "Maybe we are where we are because racing has become too much of a business and [is] not enough of a sport."

But, he told the *Times*, "We got to keep our doors open."[29]

Money, as it so often does, dictates the fates of horses. The crisis was an admonition, a stark warning of how vulnerable the horse is to the brute demands of the business. But that warning was mostly ignored in favor of an easier, siloed response that could be implemented without *too* much disruption: just fix the drugs.

CHAPTER 10

"EYES AND GUT"

n August 2018, the California Horse Racing Board held an unusual closed-door meeting. Four months before, Bob Baffert's brilliant chestnut colt Justify had won the Grade I Santa Anita Derby. He had tested positive for a prohibited substance known as scopolamine. Under California's rules as they were written at the time, Justify should have been disqualified, which would have rendered him unable to run at Churchill Downs in the Kentucky Derby the following month.

California's regulators did not immediately act. The lab notified the CHRB of the positive test about two and a half weeks before the Kentucky Derby. But the board did not notify Baffert until eight days later, just as he was about to ship Justify to Louisville. A split sample was not sent out to be tested until four days before the Derby.[1] Baffert went to Kentucky with the secret of the positive test hanging over his head. He was planning on fighting the results. Yet weeks passed and he heard nothing from the CHRB. Justify won the Derby, then he won the Preakness. And then, in June, he did the impossible: he won the Triple Crown. Still, the CHRB stayed silent.

It was otherwise a very good time to be Bob Baffert. Just three years before, in 2015, he had won the Triple Crown with a horse named American Pharoah. Now he had done it again with Justify. This wasn't just horse training—this was the stuff of legends. Moments before Baffert broke a thirty-seven-year drought with American Pharoah, he saw Penny Chenery, the Virginian owner of Secretariat, in the clubhouse at Belmont. The grande dame beckoned him to bend down to hear her: *This is the one*, she told him.[2]

The two Triple Crown victories had made Baffert one of the sport's most important spokesmen. He was one of the few horse trainers—if not the only one—that the American public recognized. American Pharoah had helped bring some badly needed positive attention to a sport that had been struggling with what academic researchers call its "social license to operate." The constant churn of suspicion around Baffert had lulled, although he had continued to receive the occasional positive test. He had two "high butes" in 2016 and 2017 that had received little notice—"high butes" are a fairly routine occurrence at the racetrack—and before that, he hadn't gotten a positive since 2010.[3]

The split test confirming Justify's positive came back on May 8, after the Kentucky Derby had already been run but before the Preakness. Rick Baedeker, the CHRB executive director, informed board members of the positive that day and, in an email, said that "the CHRB investigations unit will issue a complaint and a hearing will be scheduled."[4]

Yet neither of those things happened. It wasn't until four months later that the CHRB finally met to vote on how to handle the positive test, which still had not been made public. Justify had already been retired from racing. His breeding rights had been sold to an Irish breeding conglomerate for $60 million, with the pending positive test result written into the contract.[5] Without telling Baffert or anyone else, the CHRB voted unanimously not to bring a complaint against Baffert.

Rick Arthur thought it was a little insane that the CHRB thought it could keep the positive test a secret. He had recommended that the board dismiss the matter without charges, but he also knew how information flows at a racetrack. Too many people, including the owners and jockeys involved in the race, knew about it. But the chairman of the CHRB at the time, Chuck Winner, "was a PR guy," Arthur recalled. He didn't want the bad press. Plus, California law at the time prohibited the CHRB from releasing the results of a test that it had declined to penalize.[6]

So it wasn't until over a year later that the story appeared in the pages of the *New York Times*. In a September 2019 article by Joe Drape, the paper argued that California had broken its own rules by declining to penalize Baffert. It pointed out that Chuck Winner had a small financial interest in some horses trained by Baffert. And it quoted Rick Sams, the lab director who had run the testing lab used by the Kentucky Horse Racing Commission from 2011 until 2018, as stating that the amount of scopolamine found in Justify's system was high enough that it suggested it had been administered intentionally to enhance the horse's performance.

The story was a bombshell. It revived an old criticism of Baffert: that he was treated with kid gloves by California regulators and California racetracks.

It's a common allegation on the backstretch of racetracks across the country: big trainers are given a pass for cheating because they have a large stable and the racetrack needs them to fill races. The state commissions, of course, do not directly financially benefit from Baffert's contributions to the horse population at Santa Anita in the same way the racetrack does, but in California, commissioners are permitted to participate in the sport they regulate by owning horses. It's a shocking conflict of interest, an echo of the days when the Jockey Club—whose members are owners and breeders—regulated the sport of racing at the turn of the century. Baffert might believe he is singled out for harsher scrutiny by California regulators; outside California, many horsemen believe the opposite is true.

The revelation of the positive also ignited a host of legal problems for Baffert's team. The trainer of the horse that finished second in the Santa Anita Derby sued, arguing that his horse had rightfully won the race under California's rules at the time. He would ultimately prevail, in 2024, and the purse money and the official victory for the race would go to his horse.[7]

The saga exposed the specter of an entire parallel universe. It's possible that even had the CHRB moved more swiftly, the split sample would not have been returned before the Derby and the horse might have been allowed to run anyway. But *had* Justify been disqualified immediately after the Santa Anita Derby, he would have been unable to run in the Kentucky Derby. Baffert would not have won a second Triple Crown. And Justify would almost certainly not have been worth the $60 million that the stud farm paid for him. It all hinged on murky science—and whether you believed Bob Baffert.

Scopolamine can be manufactured in a lab and is the active ingredient both in an anti-nausea drug and medication that dilates pupils in humans. But it is also a naturally occurring chemical contained in jimsonweed, a flowering green plant that grows liberally in parts of California where hay and straw are farmed. Although it was categorized as a banned substance in California, trainers in the past had successfully argued that their horses had tested positive for scopolamine because they had consumed contaminated feed or stall bedding.

The problem is that scopolamine is closely related to atropine, a bronchodilator, and there is evidence that at some unknown concentration, it could act as a performance enhancer. But there isn't much data on what that concentration would be. In California, horses were allowed to have

60 nanograms per milliliter of scopolamine in their system without triggering a penalty, "and I don't want to say [it was] pulled out of the air, but there wasn't a lot of research as to what level was right," Rick Arthur said.

Scopolamine, like so many other so-called environmental contaminants, is the subject of fierce debate within the industry. Are scurrilous trainers giving a synthetic form of the drug to boost performance by getting more oxygen into their horse's lungs? Or are horses simply eating hay harvested from a field where jimsonweed grew wild? Justify's sample showed 300 nanograms per milliliter—an amount that Sams called "achievable by ingestion of plants, but highly unusual"[8] and Arthur said was commensurate with other positive tests for the substance that he believed were the result of contaminated feed.

There is one clue that can help indicate whether a scopolamine positive has come from jimsonweed or synthetic administration. Typically, if a scopolamine positive has arisen from jimsonweed, a small amount of atropine is also detected in the sample. Atropine was *not* found in Justify's sample, according to Arthur. That could suggest that Justify had been intentionally administered scopolamine. But both Arthur and Sams said that isn't solid proof either: if lab testing wasn't sufficiently sensitive, it "would only mean that atropine was not detected above" the so-called limit of detection.[9] Labs typically don't publicize their limits of detection, and the CHRB declined to provide it in this case. It's possible the initial screening done on Justify's urine sample simply wasn't sensitive enough to pick up what would have been good evidence that the horse had consumed jimsonweed rather than been exposed to a synthetic drug.

As usual, the limitations of drug testing—and the gaps in research in horses—had made what was meant to be the impassive arbiter of guilt or innocence into an exercise in personal judgment.

After Justify's split sample came back positive, the CHRB launched its investigation. It conducted a testing survey at Santa Anita, looking at already-cleared samples for traces of atropine and scopolamine at any level. Investigators found scopolamine in a total of seven horses with four different trainers, Arthur said—and atropine in several.[10] The scopolamine findings were all below the 60-nanograms-per-milliliter threshold, but the sheer number of horses with scopolamine in their system convinced him that Justify had probably consumed jimsonweed.

Still, as a technical matter, California's regulations at the time classified scopolamine as a drug that in any amount over the threshold should result in disqualification. That was the argument of Mick Ruis, the trainer whose horse had finished second to Justify—and the eventual judgment of a Los Angeles County Superior Court judge.[11]

But at the time, the board had a tricky decision to make. When Justify ran in the Santa Anita Derby, the CHRB was in the process of updating its rules for scopolamine, as well as other drugs, to bring itself in line with model guidelines released in 2016 by the trade association for racing commissions. Although the rules on the books at the time Justify ran stated that the drug should have sparked an immediate disqualification, under the new rules, the commission would have the discretion to set a lower penalty in the event of a positive test. The idea was to account for the possibility of accidental exposure. In the closed-door August meeting, Arthur argued that the commission should handle Baffert's case under the pending new rules.[12] (California in October 2018 formally updated the rules; in the fall of 2019, the state recorded three scopolamine positives that it determined to have arisen from contamination and issued the trainers only a warning.)[13]

Members of the California Horse Racing Board are political appointees. The decision they made was inherently political, but not unreasonable. The rules were poised to change. And there is little hard evidence that scopolamine is used as a performance enhancer on the backstretch (although it's possible that some trainers have tried it). Scopolamine is one of the few drugs that even those who are broadly skeptical of claims of "environmental contamination" say is credibly the result of accidental ingestion. The six other horses who also tested positive around the same time support that conclusion.

In the end, Arthur believed, the facts of the case weren't the only reason board commissioners upheld Justify's victory in the Santa Anita Derby. It was because he was a Triple Crown winner, in a sport struggling for good-news stories.

"My impression was that the people who made the decision, that it was out of respect for the horse," Arthur said. "Why would you want to detract from a Triple Crown winner?"

It's a strange defense, since the board didn't move to investigate and adjudicate the positive test result until after the Kentucky Derby. He was the favorite for the Derby, but there was no way they could have known for certain that he was going to win. This is horse racing; there are no sure things. Why, then, did the board not move more swiftly? In an interview with the *New York Times*, Rick Baedeker said that the panel simply didn't have enough time to adequately investigate the issue prior to the running of the Derby, suggesting that by then it was too late to penalize the horse.[14] In fact, the CHRB treated the case as unusual from the start. According to documents obtained by the *Times*, before notifying Baffert or the rest of the board of the positive test result, Arthur emailed Baedeker and a small group of other board staff. He said that the case would be "handled differently than usual" and called for additional testing—presumably the survey testing that revealed the other scopolamine positives.

None of it was necessarily unscrupulous. But once again, testing had failed to provide clarity, and the overwhelming amount of discretion with which different state racing regulators operated had created a big fat mess.

There was one other wrinkle to the Justify saga. Joe Drape, according to Arthur, had been told about the other horses whose samples showed findings of scopolamine at Santa Anita. That detail is alluded to only obliquely, relatively deep in a story that heavily suggests that Baffert was improperly let off the hook because he trained a horse partially owned by Chuck Winner. Drape had also been told of the details about the pending rule changes, Arthur said, context that is presented lower down in the article. For Arthur—and certainly for Baffert—the Justify article was proof that Drape had it in for Baffert. Drape pointed out to me that he was unable to obtain documentation of the other seven horses at the time. (CHRB provided me an anonymized record that was consistent with Arthur's description of the findings.) But for Baffert, it became a grievance that compounded his sense that he was, for reasons he couldn't understand, treated differently than other top trainers. This sense of grievance was becoming the organizing principle by which he viewed the sport. It persisted even in a situation in which California regulators had moved to quietly exonerate him.

"[Drape] knew the circumstances, about the other horses testing positive, the whole process," Arthur said. "He really does not like Bob."*

There's an organized chaos to every Thoroughbred operation. The very nature of the business—built on the backs of individual, living animals— is unpredictable. A horse that should have breezed that morning stays in

---

* Drape, in an email to me, said that he had "nothing against Bob . . . I have written fairly and accurately about him. As I have told him . . . repeatedly, it is my job to break and cover news. He has a long history of drug positives including a six-month suspension in the opening months of his career, which he wrote about in his autobiography. The list of Bob's failed drug tests is lengthy and in recent years came in bunches in some of the biggest races in the sports. In other words, it is news."

his stall with a fever. A chill in the air makes a two-year-old feel especially fractious and dump his rider at the gap.

Bob Baffert's barn could be particularly chaotic. Baffert was notoriously scatterbrained, a big picture guy who was a savant when it came to looking at the horse in front of him but a little fuzzy on the details. Baffert's genius as a trainer had always been his eye. Sure, he trained his horses a little harder, got them that much fitter than the competition. But his real power was that he could see what lesser horsemen could not. Early on, he fitted a two-way radio on his exercise riders so that he could manage a horse's workout in live time. Still, there wasn't a system. He didn't look at every horse in the barn at the end of every day the way some trainers did. His foreman, Pascual Rivera, was his "eyes and ears," he told me.[15] It wasn't that Baffert didn't put his eyes on his horses. He just looked at a horse when he was thinking of it. He might ask the assistant to bring out this horse or that horse, just to get a look at him.[16] Was he getting light? Or too heavy? "It's Bob," Mike Marlow said. "It's eyes and gut."

That mad-professor approach also trickled down to the way he ran his operation. It shocked Marlow when he first became aware of Baffert, years before, when Marlow was working for D. Wayne Lukas's stable. Lukas ran his barn with an almost fanatical devotion to organization and cleanliness. At one point in the 1980s and '90s in Baffert's barn, grooms ground up bute pills and slung them into a horse's feed bin at night, something that would never have been allowed in Lukas's barn.* Many stables have a standing prohibition against grooms handling medication to ensure there are no slip-ups that will result in a positive test. And just putting bute in the feed—rather than administering it in a single dose as an oral paste or an injection—ran the risk that a horse that didn't finish his feed until the morning would be that many hours behind in metabolizing the drug. That too risked a high bute. It was little stuff, but it could have big consequences.

In 2019, the CHRB searched Baffert's barn and found an unlocked medication cabinet, twenty-five improperly labeled medications, and the

---

* Lukas also at one point didn't allow women or radios in his barn either. (It's a particular more of racetrack sexism, the basic faulty premise for which appears akin to the old seafaring superstition about women on boats.) It didn't protect him from catastrophe: In 1993, a tough-minded colt named Tabasco Cat got loose in the barn. Lukas's son Jeff was his top assistant trainer at the time. He stepped in front of the horse, a move that will often compel a runaway to stop short. Tabasco Cat ran him over, flipping him like a rag doll into the air and fracturing his skull. He lived, but with severe cognitive and physical disabilities for the rest of his life.

presence of unsecured bute—all at least nominally against state regulations.[17] Baffert had just received another two penalties for high butes in horses that had run at Del Mar that year, paying a $500 fine for the first positive and $1,500 for the second.[18]

By that point, Baffert had long stopped giving bute in the feed. In both instances, he told CHRB investigators that a vet had injected the horses with bute forty-eight hours out from the race, in accordance with California rules.[19] (He also told California investigators that "he thinks someone is intentionally giving Bute to his horses and mentioned that he would be offering a reward to help solve the case.")[20] But privately, it appears Baffert has offered a different account of what happened. He told me that the positives arose from "mistakes" by the veterinarians—the kind of mistake that he feels generally should result in penalties for the vet, not the trainer. With one of the two horses, Baffert said, "I was out of town and it turned out that the vet, they get to bullshitting and they treat the horse twice."[21]

In 2021, he offered another explanation to a former steward in the state of New York, Steve Lewandowski.* Lewandowski said he didn't know Baffert. But that year, he would testify on his behalf at a hearing in Manhattan.

Lewandowski told me that at the hearing, he leaned forward and tapped the trainer on the shoulder.

"Bob," he said. "Don't pre-race no more." Lewandowski was referring to the standard practice of giving certain medications—in Baffert's case, bute—to all his runners before they ran.

Baffert protested. It was the vet who should have been punished, Lewandowski told me Baffert said to him, because he was late getting to the barn to administer bute on at least one of the occasions. It hadn't metabolized and was still present in the horse's system at the time of the race. (Baffert suggested a variation of this explanation to me, also.)

"I said, 'Bob, you gotta scratch the fucking horse! It's that simple!'" Lewandowski said.

"That barn has tightened up a lot over the years," Marlow told me. "But I think it used to be a little bit of a loose ship."

There was an arrogance to the way Baffert ran his barn, but there was a certain innocence about it too. In the way of a child who assumes his mother will clean up behind him, Baffert seems to have left to other people

---

* Lewandowski was the same official who had alleged being told that the syringes found in Rick Dutrow's barn had been planted there.

the details of running a racing barn that he didn't care to think about. Other people would surely tend to the boring bits, like paperwork, so that he could do what he did best: look at horses. "I think Bob just takes too much for granted," Arthur said. "He lets other people deal with . . . what other trainers would be worrying about—withdrawal times, that kind of stuff."[22] He trusted his people to take care of him.

Perhaps the person Baffert trusted the most was Jimmy Barnes, his primary assistant trainer and the man who traveled with all of Baffert's big runners to races across the country. It's a grueling job. Everyone at the racetrack could attest to the fact that Barnes worked like a yeoman. Baffert trusted Vince Baker, his longtime vet. Baker's father had worked for Baffert when he still had quarter horses, and now Baker cared for his Thoroughbreds. He trusted Marlow. He trusted his foreman, Pascual Rivera, who had worked for Baffert since he hired him from the Lukas barn decades before.

By all accounts, Baffert's team reciprocated that trust. It was something that federal and private investigators tasked with looking into Baffert would learn later, when they were unable to find even former employees who had anything bad to say about working for Baffert—at least nothing that proved he broke any rules.

When the Covid-19 pandemic hit, there was no possibility of remote work at the racetrack, where horses needed to be fed, cared for, and exercised. Tracks imposed safety precautions, like mask requirements that were especially cumbersome for exercise riders. Race meets were postponed and rescheduled with empty stands. (The Kentucky Derby was run in September in 2020; Baffert won with a horse named Authentic.) But in most ways, business continued as usual. Except that in the Baffert barn—especially as his big horses traveled to other tracks—the wheels seemed suddenly to come off.

In May 2020, Baffert sent a handful of runners to Arkansas for some prep races for the rescheduled Kentucky Derby and the Kentucky Oaks. Gamine, a filly, and Charlatan, a colt, both won their respective races that day. Both tested positive for lidocaine, a painkiller that is most commonly used in racing as a nerve block to diagnose which part of a horse's foot or leg is injured.

In July, another Baffert runner, Merneith, tested positive for dextromethorphan, the cough syrup ingredient.

Then, in September, the filly Gamine tested positive again in the Grade I Kentucky Oaks, this time for betamethasone. This was the same substance that would eventually appear in Medina Spirit's urine sample in the Kentucky Derby the following year.

All three were against racing's rules, for different reasons. Betamethasone, as a corticosteroid that has the potential to blunt pain, was tightly regulated. Lidocaine was quite literally a numbing agent. The metabolized version of dextromethorphan found in testing, meanwhile, requires extra steps for labs to distinguish from a morphine analogue known as levorphanol, and some lab directors feel it should be reported as a positive just to avoid the possibility that a horse has been given the performance enhancer.[23]

In every instance, Baffert had a different explanation. Merneith, he claimed, had ingested dextromethorphan after a groom taking DayQuil and NyQuil for a case of Covid had urinated in the stall and the horse had eaten the fouled hay. (Both drugs contain dextromethorphan.) The groom, William Alonzo, testified to peeing in the hay at the CHRB hearing. Baffert paid his $2,500 fine and that was that.*

But according to a CHRB report, Alonzo had initially denied urinating in the stall when asked by Baffert. Later, when New York racing authorities were examining Baffert's record of positives, officials wrote that Baffert's explanation "lacks credibility, especially given that the groom initially stated that he had not urinated on hay in Merneith's stall, but later changed his story, telling the CHRB that he had been scared of being fired by Baffert."[24] It's plausible, of course, that Alonzo lied when first asked by Baffert simply because he feared being fired for peeing in the stall, but the fact that he changed his story was enough to cast doubt on Baffert's version of events.

In the case of Gamine's second positive, Baffert did not dispute that the filly had received hock injections of betamethasone. But, he said, the injections had been given eighteen days before the race—well outside the recommended fourteen-day withdrawal guidelines. He had "followed every rule and guideline," he complained in a text to chief Kentucky Horse Racing Commission steward Barbara Borden.

"When did threshold change and what were they before?" he asked.

Borden told Baffert that although betamethasone used to carry a threshold of 10 picograms per milliliter, the state had changed its rules to zero tolerance for betamethasone the month before.

---

* This is a common explanation for positives at the racetrack; depending on the drug in question, according to Rick Sams, it's credible that a positive could result if a human ingests a substance and excretes it and then the horse ingests some of the fouled hay. A dextromethorphan positive in particular could plausibly arise this way, he said.

Baffert considered the whole affair "ridiculous." But even if the original threshold had remained in place, Gamine still tested for more than twice the old allowable amount. And the guidelines for withdrawal times are based on injecting a single joint. Gamine had both hocks done, meaning she received twice the load of betamethasone on which the fourteen-day stand-down guidelines were based.[25] Under racing's ultimate-insurer rule, that was on Baffert. He ultimately paid the $2,500 fine.

The two lidocaine positives, in Arkansas, were the most hotly debated. (Tim Yakteen, Baffert's former assistant, would get into a scuffle over the situation with another trainer at Santa Anita who needled him that "your boy got away with it again," a reference to Baffert.)[26] At first Baffert claimed that the positives were yet another case of "environmental contamination": Barnes, his longtime assistant, had allegedly been wearing a Salonpas pain patch for an old back injury. The patches contain lidocaine, and Baffert and his team argued that Barnes had accidentally transferred lidocaine to the horse's system when he reached into their mouths to put on a tongue tie, a strip of cloth that helps keep a horse's tongue out of its airway while it's racing.

Baffert chose to fight the positives, and during the discovery process, his legal team uncovered several things that raised questions about how, exactly, a metabolite of lidocaine had appeared in the blood samples for Gamine and Charlatan.

Almost immediately, they learned that the chain of custody had been broken when the sample was sent to the laboratory.

Typically, when blood and urine samples are taken in the test barn, those samples are sealed with a numerical tag and put in a cooler, which is also marked when it's sealed. But when the cooler with Charlatan's and Gamine's samples arrived at the lab, the original cooler tag had been broken and a new tag, with a different number, had been applied. The samples were apparently undisturbed, but somewhere along the way, the cooler appeared to have been opened.

Then they realized that the lab report for Charlatan listed the horse as a gelding. A colt accidentally analyzed as a gelding should have showed off-the-charts testosterone levels. Yet the report marked nothing unusual in his hormone levels. That too was suspicious.

Finally, and perhaps most crucially, Baffert's team said during an April hearing on the matter, they learned the horse that finished second to Char-latan had also been found to have lidocaine in his system. It didn't meet the threshold, so it wasn't flagged as a positive test, but it was there. According to testimony from the state commission's veterinarian, "substantive conversations" with the lab in question "indicates, yes, there were samples that were below the threshold."[27] That raised the possibility that multiple horses had somehow been exposed to lidocaine in the test barn, rather than by a member of Baffert's staff.

Arkansas ultimately permitted both horses to keep their respective wins. They fined Baffert $10,000 but did not suspend him, allowing him to keep running not only in Arkansas but in California.[28] (It has long been racing commission practice across the country to reciprocate suspensions meted out in other jurisdictions, so that a penalty can't be avoided by simply running horses in another state.) Public statements from Arkansas commissioners suggest that they were persuaded both that the amount of lidocaine found in the two horses could not have impacted their performance, and that there had been no intentional administration of the drug to either horse.[29]

It's difficult to credit the notion that Baffert would intentionally administer lidocaine, a serious drug that is routinely screened for, to numb a horse to pain and then send him to the post. That's "something desperate people do at desperate times," said one US-based trainer with experience in Baffert's barn. "There's no way Bob would do it, because he knows it's not going to pass the vet." Unless you believed Baffert was both a butcher *and* utterly reckless about getting caught, it just didn't make sense.

But the Arkansas commission's decision was still controversial. Although hearing testimony had suggested it was possible that the positive had come from outside his barn—what Baffert appears to believe today—his own lawyers had argued the positive likely originated with Barnes's back patch. (Sams also characterized this as the far more likely scenario.) If a member of his own staff was the source, even inadvertently, that was Baffert's responsibility.

Once again, Baffert was fighting the cardinal rule of enforcement in Thoroughbred racing: the trainer is the absolute insurer of the animal's care and welfare. Baffert had a case to make that the lidocaine positives may have come from outside his barn, but the other two positives—as well as the two high butes from the summer before at Del Mar—were indisputably the responsibility of the trainer, even if they weren't a deliberate effort to flout the rules or gain an advantage on the racetrack.

Baffert seemed incapable of accepting that premise. "The big knock on me has always been, 'well, he won't own up to his things,'" he said. "Own up to *what*?"[30] Gamine's betamethasone overage was because the rules were changed. Merneith was the sick groom's fault. The lidocaines, at least initially, were because Jimmy Barnes had foolishly worn a medicated back patch. The two high butes were the fault of the vet.[31] It didn't matter that other trainers seemed to have been able to put better controls in place, to better educate their staff on the risk of accidental exposure, to manage which horses were receiving bute and when more carefully. In Baffert's world, he had done all he could. He trusted other people to manage this sort of thing for him—and because other people were taking care of it, any mistakes couldn't possibly be his responsibility.

"A lot of them are just ticky-tack little violations. And a lot of it is sloppiness," he said. "When I get a high bute . . . it's embarrassing. . . . I get mad, like, *what happened*?"[32]

Eventually, he appeared to make some adjustments to his medication practices. He had already stopped allowing grooms to give bute to his horses in the feed and instead had a vet administer it. It can be difficult to pin down Baffert on a precise order of events—in many ways, he seems to live entirely in the present—but he also at some point had signs printed to clearly designate which horses were entered in a race that day and to whom special notice should be given to avoid accidental contamination. He issued an employee handbook emphasizing the importance of not urinating in the stall. In court testimony later, he said he ordered Baker never to administer betamethasone to any of his horses ever again.[33] And he announced in a public statement that he would be retaining a prominent Lexington vet, Dr. Michael Hore, to advise him on medication compliance.

Baffert's statement said all the right things. He said he was disappointed by the positives, vowing to "do better" and "ensure I receive no further medication complaints." He would, he said, be "personally increasing my oversight and commitment to running a tight ship."[34]

In his heart, Baffert felt that his portion of the blame was being blown out of proportion. These kinds of understandable slipups happened to everyone at the racetrack. As always, he believed he was being singled out.

"It happens every day, but you don't hear about it," he said to me, when I pressed him on the root of the problem. "When it happens to me, it's big."[35]

He had a case to make that this was true.

Baffert didn't know it at the time, but that string of positives was only the beginning. Within a year, he would receive yet another positive. The test was for betamethasone, the same drug he insisted that he had told Baker he wanted out of his barn. This time, it was found in a horse competing on racing's most important stage: the Kentucky Derby. Dr. Hore had never gone to work for him after all, and betamethasone, it appeared, was still being administered in the Baffert barn. With that positive test would come a volley of judgment so intense that it would ultimately lead to calls for ousting Baffert from the sport itself.

Several years before, before all the positives, before the pandemic, before the Santa Anita deaths in 2019, the Jockey Club had set something in motion. It was 2015, and Baffert had just won the Triple Crown with American Pharoah, and racing was riding a wave of public goodwill. That fall, the chairman of the Jockey Club had quietly hired a private intelligence firm to root out cheaters and dopers at the racetrack. Unbeknownst to almost anyone in racing, an investigation was unfurling, curling blind vines and tentacles into the barns of leading trainers.

The Jockey Club had given the PIs only one instruction: *I want you to catch big fish.*

PART II

THE BACKSTRETCH

◆

"A Thoroughbred is not a natural phenomenon. His mommy and daddy didn't fall in love, get married, and decide to have a baby. None of these horses would be here if they weren't meant to race and win. The breeder is their God and the racetrack is their destiny and running is their work, and any other way of looking at it is getting things mixed up, if you ask me. The last thing I want to do is get things mixed up, because, as fucked as I am now, I'd be really fucked then, because I wouldn't know what I was doing."

—Jane Smiley, *Horse Heaven*

CHAPTER 11

STUART JANNEY'S QUEST

One Saturday during the fall meet at Belmont, when the air cools and the ivy growing on the old brick grandstand turns red and yellow and brilliant orange, Stuart Janney III found himself hiding in the men's room. Lurking in the bathroom was the last place you might expect to find a man of Stuart Janney's stature, especially given that Belmont Park was considered Janney's home turf.

Stuart Janney III oozed old money. Not just old money, but old mid-Atlantic money, which is to say he wore his wealth lightly but with absolute assurance. He wore the understated uniform of the country club: khakis and loafers, a blue blazer, or perhaps a soft three-quarter pullover—nothing gauche, nothing to broadcast wealth. His manners were impeccable, but he wasn't stuffy. His father had been a gentleman daredevil, riding to hounds in Maryland and galloping steeplechasers over five-foot timber fences. Janney had no such ambitions: he stopped riding as a boy and preferred golf to the ringing cry of fox hounds on a winter morning. At sixty-seven, with blond hair that had gone gray, and small, blue eyes, Janney was a man concerned with the affairs of industry, not of the barn. He had a sense of humor and an absolute conviction in his own integrity. He was right in all matters.

Janney was the scion of a racing dynasty that spanned generations and multiple states, but he hadn't necessarily intended to follow in his father's footsteps as a breeder and owner of Thoroughbred racehorses, at least not right away. His grandmother, Gladys Mills Phipps, owned Wheatley Stable in New York with her brother, Ogden Mills, and was one of the country's preeminent breeders for decades. His father, Stuart Janney Jr., had bred Ruffian, the coal-black miss who passed into racing legend in 1975 when she shattered her ankles in a match race against the colt Foolish Pleasure. Together the Phippses and the Janneys represented the epitome of the old way of doing things. They were sportsmen, breeding for the pleasure of it—and probably a tax write-off, of course.* They maintained private stables, employing trainers who worked for them alone. But Stuart Janney III didn't pursue horse racing until he inherited the family stable following his parents' death in the late 1980s.

The animals weren't what most interested Janney. It was the management of the sport. In 1994 he had become the chairman of Bessemer Trust, a New York wealth management company founded by his great-grandfather in 1907. (Janney took over the role from his cousin, another financier and giant of the turf, Ogden Mills Phipps, known to all as Dinny. Their great-grandfather, Henry W. Phipps Jr., was a partner of steel magnate Andrew Carnegie. Janney was the product of a male line that had married into the Phipps family, [1] something one older New York insider once whispered to me sotto voce in the dining room at Saratoga as if it were a secret of great significance.) In his younger years, he practiced law as a partner at a firm in Baltimore, worked as a senator's aide on Capitol Hill, and had been a special assistant to US secretary of state Henry Kissinger.[2] What became of interest to him was not just the business of running a stable of racing and breeding prospects, but the larger, structural problems confronting an archaic sport trying to survive in the modern world.

Almost as a matter of birthright, Janney held prominent leadership positions in nearly every elite hub of power in racing: the New York Racing Association, the Keeneland Association, and, most importantly, the Jockey Club. It's difficult to overstate the authority and the influence of the Jockey Club in horse racing. As the breed registry for the Thoroughbred racehorse, in a very literal sense it controls eligibility to race. Even the names of Thoroughbreds—eighteen characters, no more—must be approved by the Jockey Club. It also maintains vast repositories of racing data. Although it ceded its regulatory authority over racing to state commissions beginning

---

* Up until 1986, investing in racehorses was a way for wealthy people—taxed at as high as 70 and, during World War II, 94 percent—to write off significant losses. But tax cuts for the wealthy signed into law by President Ronald Reagan that year made that a less attractive financial strategy and did away with what one senior sales executive characterized at the time as the number one reason people bought racehorses: the tax benefits. https://www.latimes.com/archives/la-xpm-1990-08-07 -sp-132-story.html; https://www.urban.org/sites/default/files/publication/59856/1000459-A-Brief -History-of-the-Top-Tax-Rate.PDF.

in 1951, the opinions of the men of the Jockey Club remain a powerful behind-the-scenes driver of racing policy. It is the oldest and most powerful racing institution.

The Jockey Club was also synonymous with New York, with moneyed authority—and with the Phipps family. For the better part of fifty years, descendants of Henry Phipps had held the reins at the Jockey Club. Dinny's father, Ogden, was chairman from 1964 to 1974.[3] Dinny Phipps served as chairman from 1983 until 2015, the longest tenure of any other chairman in the organization's 130-year history. Then, when he finally retired, through an opaque and closed-door succession process,[4] Janney was elected to take over from his cousin.[5] He was one of the single most important and well-connected people in Thoroughbred racing. While many people in horse racing have a lot of money, Janney is the sort of person who can pick up the phone and call the chairman of the Joint Chiefs of Staff—and use his first name.

And here he was, hiding in the bathroom at Belmont Park.

It had all started with a couple of unsolicited opinions, from two different people Janney trusted. One of them was his trainer, Claude "Shug" McGaughey III. The other was Seth Hancock, one of the two brothers descended from Kentucky's most legendary breeding dynasty.

Hancock had called Janney one Monday morning after a weekend of racing.

"Stuart," Hancock said. "Did you see the winner of the feature?"

Janney said he had.

"Did you see the winner of the other stake?"

Janney had. He asked Hancock to get to the point.

"Well, I'm just telling you that I've been back through those pedigrees every which way, and there isn't one horse in either of those pedigrees that ever accomplished anything more than maybe winning at six furlongs. They never went seven furlongs, and here's a horse that just won at a mile and an eighth in far better company."

Hancock continued, "I'm not saying it can't happen. But that trainer is having it happen all the time."

Around the same time, Janney ran a nice horse at Saratoga. The horse ran second or third, and afterward Janney called Shug McGaughey. He and McGaughey had known each other a long time. McGaughey had been the Phipps family's private trainer since the 1980s. He was an old hardboot, steeped in horseflesh; small-mouthed, tough, but companionable as long as you didn't get on his bad side.

The trainer told Janney that he knew the race was lost before it even began. The owners of the horse that eventually won were a couple of New York wiseguys McGaughey was familiar with, and he had watched the two men closely as the horses were saddled. These were the kinds of guys who were in on everything you *shouldn't* be in on, McGaughey told him.

"I just watched them," McGaughey told Janney. "They knew they had already won the race. It was just a matter of having the race run and then going to the winner's circle. They weren't nervous."

Janney began to understand something about his sport. It came to him in stages, this understanding. He had to be tenderized to the idea. But once he knew what he knew, he was possessed of the absolute conviction of the righteous. Racing was rotten with cheating. He didn't have any proof yet, but he knew it.

That was how he found himself ducking into the men's room at Belmont Park that fall Saturday in 2015. He was in the Trustees Room, the exclusive sanctuary of NYRA executives, carpeted in rich greens, where a coat and tie were required, and winning connections were invited to toast with champagne. (It's "where everybody who is anybody wants to be at Belmont," one NYRA employee said.) Coming straight at him was the owner of a winning horse that Janney believed in his bones had been doped. If the two men continued on their current course, Janney would have to congratulate him. He just couldn't stomach it. It was infuriating to be beat by cheaters. But it was also infuriating to feel obliged to congratulate people he didn't believe deserved their trip to the winner's circle. There was something small and indecent about it. It would make him a hypocrite, party to the whole sordid business. And so he detoured casually to the right and slipped into the bathroom like a mink into water.

Janney, and the Jockey Club, had long been outspoken against Lasix and the permissibility of other legal therapeutics. But Lasix wasn't why Janney was hiding in the bathroom. That was because of *dope*.

He had no evidence, only circumstance. People and horses who had no business winning races were winning races. Trainers at competitive racetracks were suddenly boasting strike rates of 30 percent or higher. That was the evidence, as it existed, and it was enough for Janney. But it wasn't enough to bring these guys down. It wasn't even enough to know for sure who was using drugs and who wasn't.

Janney walked out of Belmont Park holding a burning coal of anger in his closed fist. He was angry enough to do something drastic. He made a call on Monday morning to the executive director of the Jockey Club. He had just one question: What are we going to do about all the cheaters?

The idea of "the good old days," when horses ran pure and unsullied by drugs, is a myth. The term *doping* actually originated in horse racing around the turn of the twentieth century and was used to refer to both speeding up and slowing down horses to create more lucrative betting opportunities, by artificially inflating a horse's odds. Some news coverage from the time suggests that speeding horses up wasn't seen as much of a crime, initially— just as, in human sports, the use of strychnine and other stimulants was at one time seen as a valiant commitment on the part of the athlete.[6] A 1901 *New York Times* article reported that "shrewd turfmen" were using drugs to "get more speed out of certain horses," a practice that few believed "was either discreditable or dishonest," according to the paper.[7] Doping a horse to make it run slower than bettors and bookies expected was different: that was such a serious offense that in 1894, San Francisco's *Morning Call* newspaper reported that a British trainer named Dan Danson was executed for it.[8] When the Jockey Club moved to create rules around drugs in the late 1800s, it was taking aim at both practices.[9]

The Jockey Club was about to get back into the antidoping business in a big way. By the time it was all over, it had spent close to $5 million trying to root out cheaters, according to a source close to the organization. Multiple trainers would be jailed for doping. New laws would be passed in Washington that would change the regulation of Thoroughbred horse racing in ways that would split the industry in two. And Janney, the man who had engineered it all, would become, to some, the most hated man in Thoroughbred racing. He would be accused of being an out-of-touch elite who targeted only certain people in the sport, determined to regulate the blue-collar backbone out of existence. He would face accusations of siccing private eyes on his competition to keep them from beating his own horses. Janney's crusade against doping became the catalyst for outright class warfare in Thoroughbred horse racing. It would, in the end, expose how deeply entrenched the use of drugs was in the sport—and raise questions about whether it could ever be fixed.

From the start, the Jockey Club had the same problem that has dogged every authority that has ever tried to pin down cheaters in any sport: it was next to impossible to catch them. Sure, Seth Hancock could observe that cheap horses with bad pedigrees were winning too many races to be credible, but that was circumstantial evidence at best. It had ever been thus at the racetrack. If a trainer becomes known for "moving them up off of the claim"—claiming horses that go on to perform at a much higher level—or goes from winning 15 percent of his races to winning 30 percent, that's all the proof most racetrackers need that he's doping. But there was rarely any real proof, and regulators can't penalize a trainer just because they think he's winning too much.

There are also clear limitations to modern-day lab testing. It's incredibly sensitive and can pick up the presence of a foreign substance in a horse's system down to the level of one-trillionth of a gram—but only if lab operators know what they're looking for. How effective testing is at catching cheaters depends on what kind of test is being run.

For a long time, labs relied heavily on a screening method called an ELISA (enzyme-linked immunosorbent assay) test, which looked for specific substances, like bute or morphine. It was fast and cheap. But horsemen quickly learned which drugs different states tested for and adjusted their medication or doping practices accordingly.

In the late 1980s and 1990s, the technology evolved, and many labs began to do what's known as mass spectrometry analysis, which determines the mass of a molecule and then runs it against a database of known molecules of that weight. This sophisticated method made it "possible to detect several hundred different substances in a single analysis, as opposed to one or three or four by an ELISA test," explained Rick Sams, the former Kentucky lab director.

To do mass spectral analysis in "full scan mode," where lab technicians attempt to identify every substance they can find in a sample, is extremely expensive and time-consuming. State racing budgets generally aren't huge and, as a result, most labs run targeted analyses to look for known molecules. That means that even today, most testing is targeting only certain drugs, even if the list is longer than it used to be. If the lab doesn't know what it's looking for, it isn't going to find anything. And up until 2023, different states tested for different drugs at different sensitivity levels, allowing cheaters to play the system by using anything that wasn't on the list of what's tested in their state—or play the edge on withdrawal times for therapeutics in states where the lab's instruments or methods weren't detecting low concentrations of certain drugs. As creative performance-enhancing drugs proliferated, regulators struggled to identify and develop tests for them, another expensive and time-consuming endeavor that most states didn't have the budget for. The advantage was, and still is, to the cheater.

What labs are able to identify also depends on whether they are testing a urine sample or a blood sample. As Baffert's legal team had pointed out with Nautical Look, urine samples show what the body has already metabolized and excreted—perhaps offering clues about what an animal had ingested or been administered in the *past*—while blood samples show what is *actively* circulating in a horse's system and may have a pharmacological impact. Some drugs are more amenable to identification in blood, others in urine, and while racetracks typically draw both samples from every horse, they don't always test both to stretch the budget. It's not an omniscient system, although in the best-case scenario, findings in the urine sample can trigger targeted testing of the blood sample that can help labs gain greater insight into the potential significance of a positive.[10]

Most racetracks employ private investigators who, in theory, are supposed to root out evidence of cheating by developing informants and running surveillance around the barns. This intel can help point labs in the right direction. The better investigators have been able to find substantial evidence that *somebody* was doping. One prominent racetrack investigator told me that he knew he had trainers at his racetrack who were using erythropoietin because he found vials of an iron supplement that trainers were instructed to give in conjunction with the EPO. Occasionally, investigators get a hot tip. The same investigator once received an anonymous phone call alerting him that at a certain time, one of the trainers at his track would be giving a horse a cocktail of sodium bicarbonate—milkshaking—to minimize muscle fatigue by counteracting lactic acid buildup. The investigator surveilled the horse's stall and caught the trainer in the act.

But for the most part, allegations of doping were the stuff of innuendo and rumor. These are especially difficult for a regulator to sort through because, thanks in part to the peculiar internal politics of the racetrack, there is on any given day at every track across the country someone who feels that he has been dealt a grave injustice by either mankind or the cosmos. In other words, there's a lot of sore losers and petty gossip. It is simultaneously true that everyone on the backstretch knows everything that is going on and also that at least half of what you hear is a lie.

Complicating matters even more is the very real cultural appreciation for the sly bravado of the scamps and cheats and ne'er-do-wells of the race-track—especially at the blue-collar tracks. Here the racetrack is a world of chance and nerve. It's a hustler's paradise. You can come from nowhere and make it big. This is the world of Damon Runyon, and of Frank Sinatra, the neighborhood boy from Hoboken who became a star and ran with the mob. "The sport is like Ivory Soap: It's 99 and 44/100 percent pure," wrote T. D. Thornton, one of racing's greatest modern scribes. "If one sticks around horse racing long enough, the realization eventually settles in that if that 56/100 touch of larceny didn't exist, the game wouldn't be nearly as much fun."[11] The racing community—the trainers, grooms, hot-walkers, exercise riders, outriders, and assorted other working men and women who should never be confused with the big-money breeders and soft-handed bloodstock agents who populated Stuart Janney's world—lived by the track code of omertà.

Antidoping efforts in human sports have always carried with them a whiff of classism. The French aristocrat Pierre de Coubertin, the father of the modern Olympic Games, enforced the mandatory amateur status of the Olympic athlete because it was "a form of social protection, a relic of the class system," he wrote in 1925.[12] Amateur sports as an ideal of moral and social purity was an almost religious dogma for Coubertin that allowed the founding members of the committee to preserve the social order of the day—one in which the working classes and laborers were excluded from the sporting club. "Allowing pros to play next to amateurs would be tantamount to allowing the land-tilling peasant to join the estate-owning baron at the dinner table—a disruption of the social order," sports journalist Mark Johnson wrote in a history of doping in sports.[13] But even as the ideal of amateurism eventually died out in the face of its obvious unworkability for most athletes at the Games, Johnson and other sports scholars have argued that Coubertin's chivalric code of purity and "chaste fair play" lived on in antidoping regulations. Coubertin, Johnson wrote, "left a legacy that persists today as anti-doping missionaries strive to revive a contrived state of purity that never existed, most especially in pro sports."[14]

The first thing the Jockey Club needed to do, Janney decided, was to understand, with real facts and evidence, how prevalent doping actually was. The group solicited proposals for how this could be done from several companies, including Kroll, a risk-advisory firm that performs business intelligence investigations. The results were underwhelming, made by companies that clearly did not understand the alternate universe that exists behind the gates of every backstretch in America. One firm proposed placing an attractive Latina in the seamy bar just beyond the gates of a prominent racetrack to try to lure grooms and exercise riders into talking—low-level and often transient employees who would have little to no real insight into a trainer's secretive doping program. It was eye-rolling stuff—not to mention racist—almost too amateur to be believed.

Then Travis Tygart, CEO of the US Anti-Doping Agency (USADA), suggested that the Jockey Club reach out to David Tinsley. Janney trusted Tygart. The Jockey Club had initiated some discussions with USADA back in 2012, when Janney, Arthur Hancock, and other racing elites were in the midst of one of their periodic mobilizations against drugs and medication in racing.

Tygart warned the Jockey Club: Tinsley is a little *different*. But in early 2015, the World Anti-Doping Agency had hired Tinsley's company, 5 Stones Intelligence, to look into allegations of Russian doping in top-level soccer[15]—the swirling controversy surrounding FIFA, the international soccer regulator, that was dominating headlines at the time—and he did a good job. The FBI's Eurasian organized-crime unit in New York had ultimately investigated, and the case had resulted in prosecutions that year.[16] Check him out, Tygart advised.

The proposal that 5 Stones made was different. Janney was struck by the group's proposed investigative techniques, which were heavy on cyber-sleuthing and navigating the dark web. He wasn't totally sure how that was going to translate to catching cheaters, but it certainly smacked of more professionalism than hoping an attractive woman was going to convince a hot-walker to squeal on Bob Baffert or whomever.

He also wasn't entirely sure how whatever investigation 5 Stones did was going to result in any enforcement, since at the time the only real authority in horse racing was administrative regulation done by the state racing commissions. The US Food and Drug Administration (FDA) had some jurisdiction, and regulators had in the past tried to refer illegally compounded products being administered to horses to the agency; no one had ever been able to get officials to take much interest, according to one longtime regulator. But 5 Stones was made up of a bunch of ex–law enforcement types—Tinsley himself had worked for the US Drug Enforcement Administration—and so Janney knew they knew the right people in government to hand whatever they found.

The Jockey Club inked the contract with 5 Stones in December 2015. Janney had just one directive for Tinsley—an instruction that, when it became public, would become infamous within horse racing. It would become all the proof that Janney's critics needed that he was using his wealth and influence to play God in racing, picking favorites and putting a fat target on the back of anyone he didn't like. (It was widely perceived that chief among those he didn't like, of course, was Bob Baffert—but there were others.)

Janney told Tinsley he didn't want hot-walkers, grooms, and exercise boys. He wanted big names—what Janney called "big fish." To Janney's critics, that meant he had provided a list of specific people.

The way Dave Tinsley tells it, he's led the most interesting life imaginable. He talks of killing two people at close range in the line of duty, being an exceptional fighter, and having once put a pistol in the mouth of the man who was abusing his sister—in his words, bouncing Campbell's Soup cans off her skull. He's a man who insists he wants no credit for all his accomplishments, including the many multimillion-dollar federal contracts that he is quick to tell you his company has received over the years. The credit, he says, belongs to God. Five Stones Intelligence proclaims itself to be the first Judeo-Christian intelligence company in the world. Tinsley, thick around the middle in middle age but robust in the way well-fed old cops can be, weaves God and money together seamlessly in the telling of his own story. Observers who had contact with him during his work on the racetrack described him variously; some as colorful self-promoter, but effective; others, as a carnival barker loyal only to himself, at times known to overpromise and underdeliver.

Tinsley had an eventful career at the DEA. He was fired by the agency amid swirling allegations that he might have been involved in a payoff scheme run by an informant with CIA ties.[17] He had supervised what began as a $5.8 million money-laundering sting but grew into a sprawling anti-cartel operation that led to over 200 arrests and the seizure of more than 30,000 pounds of drugs. The informant, a photographer in Miami Beach's trendy South Beach who helped enable the arrest of more than one hundred drug suspects, took between $6 million and $100 million from some of them in exchange for what he promised would be favorable deals with a US prosecutor. Although repeated DEA reviews found no evidence that the scheme was real or that Tinsley had participated, he was dismissed for violating expense rules and other clerical infractions amid the uproar.[18] An administrative judge ultimately ordered his reinstatement in 2004, characterizing his mistakes as "very minor" and "the result of an excess of zeal."[19]

Over the years, Tinsley would engage in some apparent dramatizing when asked how many staff he put on the Jockey Club investigation. He would have you believe he had investigators swarming the backstretch of every racetrack up and down the East Coast, multiple people who had spoken to him over the years told me. But in fact it appears it was never more than a dozen or so at any given moment. And in the beginning, it was mainly one man: an old New York cop named Tim Harrington.

Harrington had spent fourteen years with the New York City Police Department, rising to the rank of detective.[20] His main problem now was that he knew absolutely nothing about Thoroughbred horse racing. He was an experienced investigator, but if you had dropped him on the Af-Pak border and told him to figure out where the Taliban were, he would have had a better idea of where to start than he did on the backstretch of a racetrack.

But Harrington got lucky. He teamed up with Brice Cote, another former cop. Cote had been with the New Jersey State Police as a detective and a trooper until he went to work for Jeff Gural, a New York real estate developer who ran the Meadowlands Racetrack, just north of Newark. Gural and Cote were both single-mindedly obsessed with catching cheaters. Cote had been part of a struggling racetrack unit when he was on the police force and had been collecting intelligence on suspected and known dopers for decades. Now he was sort of a lone vigilante who spent his existence in a state of constant frustration that he couldn't get the right authorities to support his mission to eradicate drugs. Gural shared his passion and was known to gleefully throw trainers off his racetrack on the mere suspicion of doping.* (Gural could bypass regulators entirely based on the simple fact that the track was his private property and he could kick anyone off that he wanted.) Now, Gural had teamed up with the Jockey Club and was contributing some money to the 5 Stones contract. Most importantly, he was contributing the services of Brice Cote.

Cote became Harrington's sherpa in the racing world. Five Stones, for Cote, was a godsend. He had spent years trying to track down and eject cheaters from the sport with evangelical zeal. Finally, someone else cared.

Cote educated Harrington on the finer points of performance-enhancing drugs (PEDs). He shared years' worth of reports from his own informants on different trainers and what drugs he believed they were using. Harrington, meanwhile, dove headfirst into the byzantine stockpiles of racing-related

---

* They had had some real success too: in 2017, Gural and Cote had instituted a widespread out-of-competition testing program that had caught trainers using cobalt, believed to boost performance by enhancing red blood cell production.

data held by the Jockey Club. He studied past performances and the success rates of different trainers over time. He dug into social media accounts and real estate records. He began to build what is known in the law enforcement world as an i2 chart—a web of different names and how they connect to one another, a digital version of the map of red yarn snaking between photographs tacked to the office wall.

In the beginning, they found little that would meet Stuart Janney's instruction to catch big fish. The Meadowlands held some Thoroughbred races but ran mostly harness racing. Trotters are a different sport than the Thoroughbreds entirely. Rather than gallop, they trot or pace pulling a little cart carrying a driver. The Standardbred horses used in harness racing are a different breed and are often derided by the Thoroughbred people as "jugheads." The participants of the two worlds do not intermingle; most Thoroughbred people would struggle to name even the top trotting trainers. It's a smaller, poorer sport. It's also under even less regulatory scrutiny than Thoroughbred racing and infamously rife with drugs. It took some time, but studying drugs in harness racing would ultimately lead Harrington and Cote to the Thoroughbreds.

The first link they found was Chris Oakes, a harness trainer who looked more like a bouncer than a horseman. On May 18, 2017, Harrington filed his first report on a Florida-based Thoroughbred trainer named Jorge Navarro:

Source reports Thoroughbred trainer NAVARRO is working with standardbred trainer OAKES. Source says trainer named NAVARRO winning a lot of races over the last couple of years and NAVARRO supplying OAKES with unknown drugs.

It wasn't much, hearsay mostly. But it was enough to get started.

CHAPTER 12

THE COPS

Panama-born Jorge Navarro got his start at the racetrack at the bottom of the ladder, grooming horses in his stepfather's stable. The year he launched his own career training Thoroughbreds, in Florida in 2008, he won just one race. The next year, he won only ten.

But five years later, thirty-eight-year-old Navarro was dominating in mid- and lower-tier races up and down the East Coast. Horses under his care won an astronomical 35 percent of the races he entered in 2013, bringing home more than $2 million in purses. His owners, of course, claimed most of the winning money, with Navarro taking home a 10 percent cut. But the more money a trainer's clients make, the more likely they are to send him more and better horses. Navarro, an immigrant who had once had to sleep over barns and on the backstretch, was on his way up.

When Tim Harrington started looking into him, Navarro was at the height of his career. His horses amassed more than $6 million in earnings that year, meaning that Navarro probably received about $600,000 in revenue. Sporting a thick gold chain and unshaven stubble, Navarro seemed to fit the caricature of a hustler, cocky and swollen with self-regard. In on-camera interviews with racing journalists, he affected a moue of earnest humility and tentative optimism, and a heartfelt love of his horses—but among those who raced against him, there was no question that he did whatever it took to win races. According to Harrington and Cote's confidential sources, Navarro was supplying two harness trainers with drugs. It was the bridge that the investigators hoped would lead them into the Thoroughbred world.

It wasn't difficult to piece together Navarro's connections to the two men. Harrington could look at Equibase—the Jockey Club–owned data repository that tracks most of racing's data—and see that Oakes owned some

Thoroughbreds and Navarro trained them. The same went for Nick Surick, a young and slickly good-looking trainer who was tough to miss. By early 2018, 5 Stones investigators were able to build evidence of the intertwined relationship between the three men by photographing Navarro and Oakes together in the paddock at Gulfstream, where Navarro was based. Social media posts from around the same time showed Surick hanging around down at the Florida track.

Oakes was the first connection to Navarro, and the Thoroughbred world, that Harrington had found. The case would ultimately turn on Surick, even if Harrington and Cote didn't know it at the time.

Besides Navarro, 5 Stones had identified another "big fish."

Seth Fishman was a dumpy, almost cherubic veterinarian in his late forties based out of Highland Beach, Florida, about halfway between West Palm Beach and Fort Lauderdale. Fishman was also a hustler, a health-and-fitness freak with two American Express Black cards in his wallet and his hands in a lot of different schemes. Outside of his veterinary business, Equestology, he also ran a Bangkok fight promotion company under the name Elite Boxing and littered his Facebook page with grainy photos of himself pressed against bikini-clad fight girls who stood a head taller than him. He seemed to believe, with absolute conviction, that he was the smartest person in the room, and he took pleasure in delivering patronizing explanations of The Way the World Works.

Fishman could be generous, but he also had a ballistic temper. "He could be your best friend and your worst enemy," according to one person who knew him. He would turn scarlet while screaming at a business associate on the phone or threatening to sue his next-door neighbor, this person said. Being around Seth Fishman was like standing next to someone holding a grenade: you never knew when he was going to pull the pin out.

A long list of investigators had looked into Fishman over the years. In 2014, the US Anti-Doping Agency got a tip from an informant that a veterinarian was supplying drugs to an antiaging clinic in Florida frequented by professional cyclists. USADA tried to investigate and even took the tip to the DEA, but nothing ever came of it. When 5 Stones took the Jockey Club contract, USADA passed along what it knew about Seth Fishman to see if they could do anything with it. Brice Cote was also intimately familiar with Seth Fishman. He had heard rumors about the vet's drugmaking enterprise for years. In 2011 he had provided information to Delaware state investigators who were looking into a horse that had died after being administered one of Fishman's products, according to a source familiar with the matter.

Fishman didn't treat racehorses. Instead he developed his own drug formulations. He would create a formula, procure the ingredients, then send them to a chemist to manufacture his bespoke solutions. The end products were sometimes labeled with nothing more than color-coded bottle caps. Others had apparently homemade labels featuring galloping horses, manes whipped by the wind. None were FDA-approved. The website for his company, Equestology, was branded "the science of performance horses"—and required a user login.[1] There was little public evidence that he was doing anything illegal or even against the rules of racing.

Sources had told Harrington and Cote that Fishman made two powerful products: an untestable blood builder that acted exactly like EPO and a pain-blocking shot. The pain blocker might mask injury and coax a horse to run himself into a broken leg. Like other opiates given to horses, it also acted like an electric cattle prod if administered at the right dosage.[2]

Within a month, 5 Stones had gone back to the Jockey Club with Fishman's name and website. This guy, they said, was central.

Stuart Janney wasn't so sure. It all seemed too easy. How had 5 Stones, in just a few weeks, already turned up some kind of doping kingpin? Wasn't it more likely that they had found an easy target, someone who might lead them to a few harness trainers or cheap claiming trainers, but wouldn't implicate the big fish? Fishman was almost too colorful to credit, the kind of sleazy issue of the two-bit tracks who lacked the sophistication to ply his trade at the top levels of the sport.

Janney was entirely and stunningly wrong.

Tim Harrington was flying. But his boss, Tinsley, had a problem. He hadn't been able to sell his racehorse project to federal law enforcement. The Jockey Club wanted results, and the kind of results that 5 Stones was supposed to deliver was some kind of prosecution. All Harrington had produced so far was an i2 map of the guys he and Cote thought were the big players in a network of dopers, drawn from a mix of publicly available information and source interviews—a map that included both Navarro and Fishman.

Tinsley had shopped the package around, including to the DEA, but nobody bit. Finally, in late 2017, he took what he had to the New York field office of the FBI. Based there was a storied unit that focused on

Russian organized crime—the same unit that 5 Stones had provided some information to as part of the ultimate racketeering and corruption charges against FIFA. One agent in that unit was particularly experienced: Naushaun "Shaun" Richards. Now in his late forties, he was nearing his twenty-year mark at the bureau and his ego matched his competence. Richards was intense, with neat gray hair and inscrutable eyes. He sat down with Tinsley and Harrington in the FBI offices at 26 Federal Plaza, and looked at the snarled i2 chart full of names drawn from a world so obscure that it is nearly irrelevant to mainstream America. He looked with curiosity and recognition.

Shaun Richards was almost killed by a Thoroughbred when he was about thirteen years old, and the first thing his old man had to say after it happened was to watch his mouth.

The day it happened, Richards was wearing a helmet for the first time in his life that he can recall. His father trained Standardbreds and a handful of Thoroughbreds as a backyard hobby—a family legacy dating back generations, or so he told Richards. Two thousand miles from Nogales, Arizona, and more than a decade after Bob Baffert was getting dumped off the Chief's young horses, Richards grew up breaking his father's yearlings. He got paid five dollars a head to gallop them around a homemade Thoroughbred track that his father had cut himself around the outside of a local harness training track.

Richards's father was not the Chief and the boy did not hero-worship him. Even now, they "fight like cats and dogs," Richards told me. But he did make a horseman out of his son. One of the first things the elder Richards taught him was how to do an emergency dismount. Richards was about eleven and riding a bad little pony named Bobo. His father put a big pile of fill dirt in the ring at the farm as cushion and schooled his son in how to ride the pony past at speed—and then bail out. It was a rough sort of lesson for an eleven-year-old boy, but it was the kind of horsemanship that stuck with you.

The elder Richards was on his second marriage, to a woman under whose name the family horses all raced. That day, his stepmother had given Richards the helmet, blue and silver, still vivid in his memory. He was supposed to breeze the horse he was riding a half mile—something he was doing with a stopwatch wrapped in his palm with the reins like the old Standardbred drivers used to do, so that he could mark the time at every panel. He was too country to know that Thoroughbred exercise boys keep the clock in their head. He ticked through the first couple of panels. As he came around the bend into the stretch, he felt a sickening wobble. The saddle was slipping.

This, to anyone going close to 40 miles an hour with nothing for brakes but a slim metal bar set in the tender mouth of a runaway animal, is disaster.

There was no way he could stop the horse. So Richards made a quick determination to use what his father had taught him. He kicked his feet out of the irons and made to bail. The maneuver did not go as planned: He got tangled up and the force of his efforts whipped his thirteen-year-old body around the front of the horse. Boy and horse rolled.

The fall knocked the wind out of him. He lay in the dirt, making the terrifying sucking sound of a calf pulling its foot out of the mud, hot pain flooding his mouth from biting his tongue. There is always a horrible moment when you believe your wind will never come back to you, that you will suffocate surrounded by oxygen—a drowning man just feet from shore.

Eventually, his wind rushed back in.

"What happened?" his father asked.

"The fucking saddle slipped," Richards gasped.

"Watch your mouth," his father retorted. Richards was flabbergasted. His father swore like a sailor. *Really? Right now?*

Richards, annoyed, knew exactly what had happened. His father had tacked up the horse for him, and he'd got to running his mouth and not paying attention to what he was doing. (This is somewhat of an ironic annoyance, since as an adult, Richards too has a well-evolved talent for gab.)

It was exactly the kind of half-assery that defined his father, Richards thought. When the two-hundred-year-old family barn burned down, his father bought a bunch of out-of-use school buses, chopped the cab off the frame, and used the hollowed-out yellow shells as weather shelter for the horses. But he didn't bother to shore up the flooring, and eventually the floor rotted and one of the Thoroughbred fillies put her foot through it and into the metal undercarriage of the bus. She was never sound again.

Still, a father's hobby became the backdrop to Richards's boyhood. The harness circuit in the Northeast Corridor was a lively scene in those days, with racetracks dotting the region from Massachusetts to Maryland. It was a mom-and-pop kind of business where everyone knew one another. Richards's father became friendly with Hall of Fame driver Warren Cameron and in 1985, when Liberty Bell Park in Philadelphia went under, Richards and Cameron bought the surface materials. Richards borrowed some earth movers from his brother, piled up the stone dust, and for two years used a dump truck to run loads to the family farm to build a half-mile racetrack there. The old railing from the Liberty Bell Thoroughbred oval is there too, now grown over with weeds.

In 2000, when he was about thirty years old, Richards joined the FBI. He spent the last six months before he joined the bureau breaking in young horses for his dad—better stock that his old man had gone to Kentucky to buy, but still nothing he was going to win any big purses with. His sister eventually took over the remnants of the family stable from his aging father. For ten or fifteen years after that, Richards didn't mess with a racehorse.

But horses have a way of staying with you, especially racehorses. They capture the imagination of humans in a way few other animals do, and it is difficult, when presented with an opportunity to once more enter their mysterious world, to decline. Two weeks after his fall, thirteen-year-old Richards was at the farm, ready to get back in the saddle. Now, decades later, he looked at the thin makings of a doping investigation at the racetrack and thought: *I can do this*. In fact, he might have been the only person in the whole of the US government who could. He had the investigative skills and the legal authority necessary. He had the institutional clout to make the Federal Bureau of Investigation care about racehorse doping. And, most importantly, he knew horse racing.

The first thing Richards did was run the names that 5 Stones had brought him through the bureau's various databases. Very quickly, several of them popped. In a twist of racing fate, Fishman had once cooperated with the feds, during the 2010 criminal prosecution of a former military contractor named David Brooks. Fishman had done some work for Brooks's racing stable, and he testified that Brooks repeatedly pressured him to create a memory-erasing pill to give to the former chief financial officer of his company.[3] What was even more remarkable was that when he was interviewed in that case, Fishman had described his doping activities. He told FBI agent Angela Jett that he provided EPO to Brooks to give to his horses in advance of a race. "Brooks's horses do not test positive because they do not test for the right drugs," Jett recorded in notes documenting one of her interviews with Fishman.[4]

But to get permission to proceed with the case, Richards had to find a connection with Russian organized crime. This proved surprisingly simple. A video circulating on social media at the time showed Navarro celebrating in the Monmouth Park track bar with owner Randal Gindi as they watched a horse trained by Navarro's brother, Marcial, win a race at Gulfstream Park.[5]

"The Juice Man!" Gindi whoops, pumping a fist. "That's the juice! That's the vegetable juice!"

"That's the way we do it," Navarro crows. "We fuck everyone!"

"We fuck everyone, and I line my pockets with the bookie with another twenty thousand," said Gindi. "Oh, yeah! Life is great."*

What was interesting to Richards was not Navarro's shameless and public boasting about doping his horses. It was Randal Gindi.

According to a source familiar with the investigation, Gindi had placed some bets with an illegal Russian gambling and money-laundering operation run out of unit 63A in Trump Tower in New York, three floors beneath Donald Trump's penthouse, which Richards's unit had investigated back in 2013.[6] The architect of the ring, Vadim Trincher, ultimately pleaded guilty in Manhattan federal court to participating in a racketeering conspiracy.[7] Gindi had never been a subject of the investigation, but when the FBI ran his name through its systems, it returned a hit, according to the source. (Gindi told me that he recalled using a local bookie to bet sports around that time, and although he didn't know who was ultimately taking the bets, he acknowledged it was possible some of the wagers had passed through Trincher's operation.)[8]

That simple connection gave Richards the chit he needed to tie racehorse doping to his unit's mandate, Russian organized crime. He knew now that he could sell this investigation internally.

It was still early days. Richards had a lot of work left to do. He didn't even know what charges they were going to try to get these guys on. Sitting at his desk on the twenty-third floor at 26 Fed, he heard Special Agent Robert Hanratty start laughing.

"What the fuck are you laughing at?" Richards asked. Hanratty had worked a recent Russian gangster case with him and they knew each other well.

"These guys have no idea what's coming for them," Hanratty chuckled.

---

* Gindi would later claim that he was trying to needle a horseplayer in the bar who had previously accused him of doping his horses. "So what I did was really a show to get back at that guy. I didn't even have a dollar on the horse. I've been in the game as an owner for two years, but I still feel like a horseplayer where you can scream those things. You can have fun like that as a horseplayer," Gindi said at the time. "I was trying to get a rise out of the guy." https://www.bloodhorse.com/horse-racing/articles/223520/monmouth-stewards-urge-large-fines-for-gindi-navarro.

CHAPTER 13

"NOBODY GOES TO JAIL FOR AN EPOGEN POSITIVE"

In the little windowless cubicle in the paddock at the Meadowlands that served as his office, Brice Cote sat across from a Standardbred vet who he had caught using EPO on some horses that he also trained.* If this goes public, Cote had intimated to him, you're done. Gural—the track owner—and the state will throw you off the track and you'll never race here again.

But maybe they could cut a deal. Behind the scenes, the FBI had quietly reached an arrangement with the New Jersey Racing Commission. If the veterinarian would cooperate with the investigation, the commission would let his positive slide for now.

The vet slid a clear glass bottle with a top no bigger than a quarter onto the desk. At the bottom was a fine dusting of white powder.

"This is Seth Fishman's pain medication," he said. "It's worth a lot of money. And if you use it right, you're going to win."

It was early 2018, and the FBI and 5 Stones had by that point settled into a battle rhythm at the Meadowlands. Both organizations were relying on Brice Cote, and his mental file cabinet of rumors and leads. Richards had immediately come to trust the former state trooper. They had a history in common: Cote's father had been a harness trainer who was friendly with Warren Cameron, the same driver Richards's father had teamed up with to buy the old Liberty Bell track surface. The relationship appealed to the image Richards had of himself as a kind of Forrest Gump figure, subtly but defiantly present at the great moments of history, connected to everyone.[1]

---

* My sources declined to identify this cooperator and others to protect their identity.

Cote gave Richards the inside track he needed to the seedy underbelly of harness racing.

Meanwhile, 5 Stones was trying to show the Jockey Club that they provided a value beyond just getting the FBI involved. They were determined to generate original reporting that would be of use to the FBI. Harrington passed along tips and rumors by phone to Richards, sometimes two or three times a week. Some of them were good; others, Richards didn't want to touch. But he kept working with 5 Stones, treating them in the same way he would treat a source. Five Stones wasn't a partner in the investigation—the FBI didn't pay them and especially later, some officials would become privately derisive of the group's work—but it was sometimes useful to have a middleman communicate with sources on the backstretch to keep the FBI's presence a secret. Harrington and Cote had initially interviewed the vet with the EPO positive together, before passing the relationship on to the FBI.

The FBI had also begun conducting clandestine out-of-competition testing at the Meadowlands. Richards had an agreement with the New Jersey Racing Commission and Gural that when he wanted to test,* he would notify the track authorities that day, and then, without identifying himself, he would go with Cote to draw blood and urine from a list of horses that they had chosen together. They intentionally gathered samples from Gural's horses: Gural was paying for the testing, not the FBI, and Richards wanted to be sure that he wasn't getting played by the canny old track operator.

The first night that they went to draw samples, in early February 2018, Cote said, "You know, Richards, they're picking off three seconds with the stuff they're using."

Richards didn't *disbelieve* Cote, but it was a big claim. Three seconds was an enormous improvement. He filed it away.

Two of the horses that they tested that night were of particular interest. One was trained by the vet who had been caught using EPO and was now cooperating with the FBI. The other was trained by Rick Dane, a target of the investigation. The vet had worn a wire for the bureau, known as "consensual monitoring," to discuss a pain shot he had purchased from Dane.

---

* The New Jersey Racing Commission declined to comment on reporting that it declined to pursue citation against an FBI cooperator. When asked about the broader agreement with the FBI that permitted the bureau to perform clandestine testing on horses at New Jersey tracks, a spokesman said that the commission "has no information to suggest such an agreement existed with the FBI regarding the testing of horses." The spokesman declined to say if she was denying such an agreement existed.

Richards had already confiscated the pain shot, but he had the source call up Dane and pretend that he had used it to dope his horse.

"I'm worried," the source said. "They tested my horse. Am I going to get caught?"

"Ah, fuck 'em, you're fine," Dane said. He rattled off the cocktail of substances he had given his own horse that night—one of the horses that the FBI had tested. If he wasn't going to get caught, then the vet certainly wasn't going to either. Besides, Dane said, the race was only a cheap claimer worth $12,500. State commissions would sometimes draw samples but not test them to stretch the budget. Who the hell was going to pay to test horses in a twelve-five claimer?

Sleet sheeted from the black winter sky as the horses came onto a track heavy with rain and ice. Dane was sending out an older animal called Glass Prince with more than a half a million dollars to his name—a good horse, but the kind that because of his age had likely already demonstrated the limit of what he was capable of. That night, on a sloppy track in terrible conditions, Glass Prince blew past the competition, peeling more than a second off his best race time of the previous year. His test sample came back positive for an illegal painkiller, according to two sources familiar with the testing.

From that moment on, Richards knew he was on to the right target. This was clear evidence of fraud: money was changing hands on a product that had been surreptitiously altered. The victims were both the bettors and the competition who were none the wiser. More importantly from the FBI's perspective, because of simulcast wagering, some of the money spent on that fraudulent product had come from across state lines. Interstate commerce was the FBI's jurisdiction. Now Richards just had to build out the case, and see how far it would reach.

In particular, he wanted to identify some of the *untestable* substances, the drugs trainers were giving that they knew wouldn't show up on traditional drug screening. With the vial of Fishman's pain medication in hand, he could do that.

Using Gural's credit card, Cote packed up and mailed the little glass vial of unlabeled white powder to Hong Kong, where the booming financial hub had its own Jockey Club—a holdover from its days as a British colony—a thriving racing industry, and a testing lab that is widely credited as among the best in the world. When the lab analyzed the sample, they found it to be a novel drug[2]—one that had never before been identified, meaning it would be invisible to even the mass spectrometry analysis done by racing commissions in the United States. According to the source who had provided the drug, a trainer was supposed to dissolve the powder in sterile water shortly before the race and then administer it to the horse by injection either in the muscle or in a vein in the neck. It was incredibly potent. The new drug was part of a class of synthetic peptide-based performance enhancers that can be hundreds or even thousands of times stronger than morphine. This wasn't just a go-fast drug. This was a rocket ship.

The identification of the drug known in the scientific literature as [Dmt1]-DALDA proved something that racing regulators had long suspected. There had been tremendous research and development into the technology used for peptide synthesis over the preceding decade, developments that now made it shockingly easy for scurrilous drugmakers to insert tiny changes in the chemical structure of a known drug and create an entirely new—and therefore untestable—formula that had the same performance-enhancing capabilities as the original variant. The replacement of just a single molecule would make a drug virtually invisible. "It's the substitution of a letter in a sentence that doesn't alter the meaning of the sentence," said Sams. And thanks to improvements in the technology, you didn't have to be a genius to do it. It was like the evolution of web creation: In the 1990s, if you wanted to build a website, you had to know how to write code. By the 2000s, you could use a plug-and-play interface like WordPress without having any understanding of the underlying architecture.

These kinds of performance enhancers were known as "designer drugs," and while regulators had long assumed that they were being used, proving it had been like chasing a ghost in the engine. It was the same problem that plagued antidoping authorities in human sports.[3]

By June 2018—under instructions from Richards—Harrington had traveled to an opulent farm in central Kentucky to acquire another sealed glass vile of crystalline white powder produced by Fishman. Using a form of mass spectrometry analysis in full scan mode, the Hong Kong lab identified another designer drug, this one a mimetic for EPO. What was astonishing about Fishman's product, marketed as BB3, was that even if you knew what metabolite you were looking for in post-race testing, it would only be detectable for four hours in a horse's blood sample—the same narrow window of time that Lance Armstrong later confessed had allowed him to stay one step ahead of drug testing.[4] Although BB3 could be found for up to twenty-seven hours in a horse's urine, if the urine sample wasn't tested—which it sometimes isn't, if a horse cannot be coaxed to pee after a race—it would be invisible.

Richards and Harrington had begun to believe that trainers were timing the administration of the BB3 down to the minute by measuring how long it took to walk to the test barn after a race so that they could give the drug as close to post time as possible while staying just outside that four-hour detection window.

It was another huge breakthrough in the case, one that irrefutably showed that there was fraud being perpetrated at the racetrack. Richards had come to believe that he had enough proof of concept to escalate the investigation and bring in the prosecutors.

On a sunny day in June 2018, Richards was walking out of the Daniel Patrick Moynihan Courthouse on Pearl Street in lower Manhattan, the home of the Southern District of New York. The Justice Department had just secured a conviction in another case that Richards had investigated, this one against a brutal Russian gangster named Razhden Shulaya, known for violently beating underlings and pistol-whipping a member of his own family.[5] Richards was on a high. On his way out of the trial room, he snagged the prosecutor he had worked with to charge the case, a slim up-and-comer in his midthirties named Andrew Adams.

"Andrew," he said, "I got an idea for another case."

Richards had a problem that only Adams could solve. He had to catch these guys in the act of doing something illegal. But many of the investigative techniques that the bureau might have normally availed itself of—like traditional surveillance or the use of undercover officers—were useless in the cloistered world of horse racing. Cameras would likely be spotted, and forget getting an officer not just within eyesight of the barn but inside the stall where a horse was being doped. He would be clocked before he hit the track gate. Investigators quickly learned they couldn't trust even track security, who were known to tip trainers off that regulators were sniffing around. Meanwhile, the idea that an investigation target might discuss his doping activities with an undercover officer was laughable on several levels. Not only would a trainer never talk about even his *legal* pre-race medication regimen with an outsider—much less his illicit doping activities—but it would have taken years of intensive study to get a G-man to speak "racetrack" without giving himself away. Even the syntax of racing is unique; trainers often speak in a jumbled present tense to describe a race in the past: *She was hiding in the bushes at the quarter pole and jumped in and win by three.*

Shaun Richards might have spoken enough of the lingua franca to get along, sort of, but no one else on his team did.

The FBI needed wiretaps. They needed to hear the dopers discussing their crimes in their own words.

Adams was interested in this case. His grandfather used to take him to Fair Grounds Race Course in New Orleans when he was a kid. At Fair Grounds, true Cajun accents drift seductively out of stalls. Some of the jocks who made it big there came from the bush tracks that still run in hot, forgotten pockets of Louisiana. On summer afternoons, they would drive down from Shreveport and his grandfather would buy him the horse player's bible: the racing form, printed daily on cheap newsprint and densely jammed with the past performance statistics for every horse running that day. His grandfather would put down quarter or dollar bets for him and they would watch their horses run, horses that would invariably lose. ("It was a very unserious sort of event," Adams recalled.) Minors aren't legally allowed to bet, but there is a time-honored tradition that a father or a grandfather should take a boy to the racetrack and teach him to play the ponies.

Adams hadn't thought much about horse racing since he was a boy. He lived in New York City now, a sharp and competent prosecutor poised to make a mint when he shifted into private practice. He was handsome and well-dressed, worldly and consummately professional. He was far from the apron of the Fair Grounds, a paradise of the degenerate and the downtrodden, where losing betting slips, soggy in the humidity, scatter the concrete, a fluttering testimony to the majesty of human striving and the romantic notion that greatness may be just around the corner. In one of those unbelievable coincidences that make racetrackers believe in fate, so it was that the prosecutor Richards was most accustomed to working with was himself another person whose heart could be tugged by the gravity of the racetrack.

Richards and Adams were feeling pretty good, flush with a sense of infinite possibility: *We can really get things done together.* Adams was at a point in his career where the Justice Department trusted him to develop cases that would result in convictions, so he had some latitude.

But he would still have to convince the DOJ not only that there was sufficient probable cause to suggest a federal crime was being committed, but also that the government should use limited resources to pursue a bunch of horse dopers. There was no guarantee Adams would be successful, according to two sources familiar with the department's internal deliberations, even given his reputation.

Adams would need a clear and identifiable charge that the DOJ could pursue. The problem was that there is no federal "racehorse doping" statute. Neither could the Justice Department pursue animal cruelty charges, because most animal cruelty laws are at the state level.[6] Prosecutors wanted to get to a racketeering charge, the same sources told me, but the standards for those charges are particularly difficult to meet. The original theory of the case was primarily built on wire fraud, which meant that the Justice Department was going to have to identify interstate fraud that had been carried out over email, phone, or some other form of electronic media. Finding that documentation could be very, very hard.

Sarah Mortazavi, another prosecutor on Adams's team, had a eureka moment: she suggested that they could pursue charges of misbranding, an FDA violation that covers everything from false or misleading product labeling to selling a product that doesn't have FDA approval that it is safe and effective for its intended use. That obviously implicated Fishman's products, none of which had been granted FDA approval or even were produced at facilities that were registered with the FDA.

It was like getting Al Capone on his income taxes. Richards, Adams, and the rest of the team cared about catching dopers. But the only way they could put these guys away was on a charge that had very little to do with doping. What the FBI now had to prove was not the impact that these drugs had on the horses themselves or on the outcome of a race. What mattered legally was the FDA violations, and that the crime had involved interstate commerce. Many participants in Thoroughbred racing would never understand that distinction. Much of what the FBI learned about BB3 and Fishman's pain shot would never make it into court documents, because it wasn't relevant to the legal case the Justice Department had to prove. Years later, racetrackers would still be complaining that the FBI had accused a bunch of trainers of cheating without ever proving that they had used any real performance enhancers—just made some pettifogging clerical errors.

In the end, it all hinged on horse-sized amounts of illegally purchased Viagra.

Shaun Richards and his team were looking into several people associated with Jorge Navarro, the Thoroughbred trainer who had been seen apparently celebrating doping in the bar at Monmouth Park. Chris Oakes, the trainer who had appeared in Tim Harrington's first report, was one of them. The New Jersey Standardbred trainer Nick Surick was another. Surick, who wore his dark hair spiked with gel and had a dimpled chin that winked roguishly from under a wide grin, also owned a handful of Thoroughbreds that he kept in training with Navarro. As with 5 Stones, the FBI hoped that Oakes and Surick were going to offer the connections they could follow that would lead them out of the harness world and into the Thoroughbred world, where the real money was.

Finally, another one of the FBI's confidential informants confessed that he had been selling Surick what one source familiar with the investigation described as "an enormous quantity" of Viagra.[7]

The informant said that Surick had told him he was using Viagra as a vasodilator to improve the performance of his horses by, he thought, maximizing the amount of oxygen in their bloodstream. From there it was a relatively simple matter to get the evidence they needed to get a judge to approve a wiretap: the FBI simply had the informant call Surick and sell him scores of pills while agents listened in, sources told me.

The FBI also leaned on the veterinarian who had been caught using EPO. The vet didn't want to cooperate, but the EPO positive gave the FBI the leverage it needed to get him to engineer conversations with Surick. Richards told him to ask Surick if he could drive down to New Jersey and talk about doing some work for him. But for weeks, the vet claimed that Surick wasn't taking his calls. Richards had finally had enough, having experienced this kind of runaround before. Some sources, when cornered, will participate just enough—they think—to get the FBI off their backs. It rarely works. Richards told the vet to drive down and meet him near Monmouth Park. Three of them sat in a car: Richards, the vet, and Bruce Turpin, another FBI agent who was working the case.

"Look," Richards said to the vet. "I don't know if you understand the position you're in. You could go to jail for this. You need to make up your mind whether you're going to work with me, or we'll just go see the judge right now."

With the familiar territory of the backstretch of a racetrack just down the road, the vet scoffed.

"What, for an Epogen positive?" he said, using a brand name for EPO. "Nobody goes to jail for an Epogen positive."

"You don't know it," Richards said, "but you're the first of your kind."

Richards had the informant call Surick while they sat together in the car. Surick, unsurprisingly, answered right away. They wired up the vet and sent him into the barns to talk. While the FBI listened in, the two men "talked about doping horses and doing business," one of the sources familiar with the investigation said. "And we're off to the races."

It had to be one of the weirder Title III wiretap applications that the judge in question had ever seen. It said, in essence, *The Justice Department would like to get up on a wire because this guy is buying a bunch of Viagra to give to horses*. But, perhaps miraculously, it worked. The judge—who would have been forgiven for being just a little mystified—approved the application. Beginning in October 2018, the FBI was able to listen in on every conversation Nick Surick had. Soon they would be doing the same with trainers and veterinarians up and down the East Coast.

CHAPTER 14

THE BACKSIDE

Outside of the racetrack at four o'clock in the morning, the roads are empty except for long-haul truckers and the night shift going home, white lines Dopplering in and out of their headlights. This is the hour that belongs to stale black coffee on a Bunn burner and Hostess Honey Buns eaten out of cellophane. It's a private time of the day.

Behind the chain-link fence of the racetrack, another private world has already come alive in run-down dormitories and concrete community bathhouses with paper signs written in Spanish stuck to the stall doors: Please flush your toilet paper. While the men who own racehorses still sleep, the massive workforce required to feed, groom, walk, bandage, and care for those horses is already in the barn. They never left the racetrack.

There is an art to mucking a straw box: Start in the middle, sift through the bedding with a metal-tined pitchfork for piles of manure and matted sheets of urine-soaked straw. Mound the clean straw in the corners to save, slide the heavy soiled bedding into the aisle with quick, practiced gestures. Replenish the bedding, stabbing the dense pats of fresh straw with the metal fork and shaking vigorously to break and scatter them evenly. Rake and sweep the front of the stall so that it is clean. Empty and scrub the two water buckets. (There is always one horse that, like clockwork, likes to shit in his water bucket every night. You can either get annoyed or you can laugh at him. It won't make any difference to the horse.) This is all harder than it sounds to do right, and to do quickly.

There is an art to grooming a horse. The old-timers called it "rubbing a horse": Wash clean the white clay poultice that's applied the night before to cool sore tendons and has now dried and caked below the knee. Clip the horse to the stall wall. If you're lucky, he will lip contentedly at the snap

169

securing the lead to the little loop of baling twine on the wall while you work. That tiny string loop is all that is securing the horse, the illusion of restraint. It's intended to break if the horse startles back, because if he feels trapped, he may panic, flail, and injure himself.

Begin at the top of the neck with the hard rubber curry first, working back over the horse's body to loosen dead skin and hair—always in the direction of the hair, or you will give him a rub rash. Then perform a graceful and rhythmic two-handed dance using a stiff body brush in one hand and a softer brush in the other, alternating strokes to remove dirt and bring out the natural oils in the coat. Next, clean the manure and dirt from his hooves using a hoof pick stashed in a back pocket. Finally, rub the animal's coat nose to tail with a soft rag to make it shine. The old-school guys used burlap sacks, a vanishing art. (The old-timers also didn't believe in getting a horse wet—he should be groomed clean no matter how much manure he has managed to grind into his coat—but those days are gone.)

This must all be done with unwavering attention to the horse himself, who is young and thrumming with energy, sensitive to every flicker of cosmic energy in his world. When you rub him, he might snake around quick as lightning and close his teeth around the soft, loose skin on the back of your arm. The fillies will try to cow-kick with a back foot while you're rubbing their belly or picking their feet; the colts might try to strike you with a front foot or stand up on their hind legs. If you're not paying perfect attention to every twitch of his ear, steadying him with your voice and your hands and your quiet confidence, you're going to get your shit rocked. (You might anyway.)

It's soothing work to watch. It's husbandry, the kind of simple caretaking that must be repeated every day. And it's often the moment when a quieter, less glamorous—and purer—kind of horsemanship shines through.

Some grooms are better at their jobs than others, of course. Some are rough-handed and impatient. But there are those whose generous touch with the animal is remembered across decades.* *There was nothing he couldn't do with a horse.*

The men and women who do this work, and often their children, live on the backstretch of the racetrack. Primarily immigrants from Mexico and Central America, they are paid minimum-wage salaries, often without

---

* Eddie Sweat, Secretariat's groom, is still a household name in horse racing, as is Will Harbut, groom to Man O' War, one of the greatest racehorses of all time. But there are many other humble horsemen who are remembered the same way. I learned from Jesse Herrera, whose eye for detail and whose frank and obvious affection for the animal were unparalleled.

benefits. Labor violations are common.[1] If they are undocumented, as many are, they may not even be paid minimum wage. The expectation in many barns is that they will work seven days a week.

Some of the better racetracks, like Saratoga in New York, provide some health care options, religious support, childcare, and other services for the families living there. At cheaper tracks, these invisible communities struggle. Addiction and drugs are an unquantified but widespread problem.* Food security is a bigger one.† And even if you had food, where would you cook it? There are no hot plates allowed in the dorms.

In spite of these hardships—or perhaps because of them—the backstretch of a racetrack is a family. It's a hard world, full of people with messed-up lives. But it's not a grim, colorless world. It is a world bursting with ambition and generosity. In the track kitchen and around the dorms, where bicycles lean against the cinder-block walls and the smell of grilling goat meat fills the air, people take care of each other.

It is also, on occasion, a world pockmarked by disaster and unexpected cruelty.

When Jorge Navarro was a kid, he worked for his stepfather before school, hot-walking and grooming horses. His mother would pick him up for class and then drop him back off in the afternoon to do the 4 p.m. feeding. Jorge, as a middle schooler only recently arrived from Panama, struggled to learn English and fit in.[2] But he fit in at the racetrack. He grew up on the backstretch and he never left. He worked his way up as an assistant trainer, traveling around the country following horses, often living on the backstretch before he got settled somewhere new.

---

* Among the evidence for this is the fact that horses routinely test positive for cocaine or metham-phetamine at levels that suggest it has wound up in their system through accidental exposure—a residue of coke on a groom's fingers that is transferred when he is handling a horse before a race, for example. https://www.thoroughbreddailynews.com/morfin-meth-case-highlights-backstretch-substance-abuse-problems/.

† A spokesman for an industry aid group told a conference in 2022: "Quite regularly we receive calls for help with filling a food pantry for the backstretch workers. This assistance does not come in [the] form of a few cans of soup. We are allocating tens of thousands of dollars for food pantries. What does that tell us? That tells us that our workforce on our own backstretches are unable to satisfy this basic human need. The people who feed our precious equine athletes cannot feed themselves." https://paulickreport.com/news/ray-s-paddock/voss-equine-caretakers-shouldnt-need-a-safety-net-we-need-to-understand-why-theyre-falling-through-the-cracks.

There was little money and there were a lot of mouths to feed. At one point, Jorge lived with seven other family members in a one-bedroom apartment attached to a barn.[3] But he was the star that a large and loving family revolved around. By the time he was in his forties, he already had two grandchildren.[4] His mother, in her early sixties, had eighteen—and two great-grandchildren.[5] A bevy of nieces and nephews and friends' kids from up the block thought of him as a life-sized teddy bear, the grill master, someone who always made time for them. He was religious and seen by those who knew him best as a man of faith. He had trouble in his marriage sometimes—his wife, Jennifer, would complain that he cared more for the horses than he did for her—but "like most good families," they loved each other even in the bad times, one of his owners said.[6]

Navarro was also ambitious. As a brown man knocking around in the basement of racing's upstairs-and-downstairs divide, he was frustrated to be locked out of the glittering playground of racing's elite. He wanted to prove himself.[7] Attending a two-year-old sale in Florida not long after he started training, he asked his father-in-law, "Will they ever respect me? Will the big owners ever give me a chance?"[8]

That chance came in November 2014, when Navarro was sent a striking gray sprinter named X Y Jet to train. The colt had just won his first race for another trainer but had fallen short when sent out for a bigger purse the next time.

X Y Jet was a difficult horse. Navarro would say later that he had a connection with the animal from the day he entered the barn. He stood out in the paddock: a silver, dappled gray, the sort of horse people who don't know anything about horses love to bet on. He was "moody," the trainer would say, affectionately.[9] He had a contender's spirit. By the end of his first season in Navarro's barn, he had notched his first stakes win by a jaw-dropping 9 1/4 lengths. In 2016, when the horse was a four-year-old, Navarro took him to Dubai to try for the $2 million Golden Shaheen.

X Y Jet streaked to the front of the field and ran for his life. When the closer Muarrab came for him in the stretch, X Y Jet kept finding more, and more, and more, matching the other horse stride for stride and refusing to let him pass. Only in the final jumps before the wire did Muarrab edge his nose in front. It was a hell of a race. X Y Jet had guts.

By early 2019, X Y Jet was Navarro's most famous horse. He was a popular favorite among horse racing fans thanks to his gutsy performances and bare-knuckled style. He had gone to Dubai again in 2018 and once more run second. Some of Navarro's large and loving family had gone; one had commissioned a painting of the horse galloping on the desert oval. Now he was pointing for a third try at the race at the end of March.

He was also "loaded" with drugs.[10] And unbeknownst to Navarro, the FBI was watching.

Beginning as early as January 2017, Navarro had begun to consult Seth Fishman about drugs. It's not clear how they first became acquainted. Fishman was well-known, certainly in the Standardbred world and apparently also among a certain cohort of Thoroughbred trainers. "His reputation preceded him," one Thoroughbred trainer who purchased drugs from Fishman testified during his 2022 trial.[11] His emails and texts with Navarro from this period are matter-of-fact instructions about how to mix and administer the drugs he sold, how far out from a race to give them, and the horse's likely reaction to them. In one email, Fishman advised the trainer that a pair of his custom-made analgesics could cause the horse to hyperventilate.

"IV [intravenous injection] will hit them harder and IM [intramuscular injection] will be less consistent," he wrote. "I have never had a horse drop, but sometimes they will blow hard."[12]

In some instances, Fishman was frank that the drugs he was hawking had barely been studied. BB3—his primary blood builder—"takes two weeks to work," he told Navarro. "Typically one bottle per week for two weeks." But, he said, other "fractions" he was developing—BB1 and BB2—"in theory may move blood faster. It was studied but never brought to market or even discussed much in literature." With BB1, he advised that Navarro "wait for more feedback from people testing for me." In other words, Fishman appears to have provided, or at least offered, Navarro a drug he hadn't even fully tested *himself,* much less submitted to the FDA for approval.[13]

Navarro was hungry for knowledge while Fishman lurked in the background, a Svengali with a syringe. In March 2017, Navarro texted him: "Are you in Dubai? Need to ask you about pills, how to use them."

"I just landed in Qatar. Going through transfer," Fishman replied. "Will call you in a few minutes.

"As for the pills," he added, "since it also has anti-inflammatory I generally load them over three days for better horses."[14]

Fishman's business records show that by that time, Navarro was buying everything from blood builders to thousands of bleeder pills. He was racking up a serious bill. A record from that year suggests Navarro spent over $20,000 in a six-month period on Fishman's products,[15] including $3,000 on "an enhanced version of the naturally occurring peptide" thymosin.[16] According to Fishman's documentation, Navarro spent $2,000 on something described in the vet's spreadsheets as only "Green cap no label."[17]

Some of these products were likely useless. Peptides are nothing more than the building blocks of proteins, broken down and isolated in a lab. There is huge variation in how proteins function in the body. Some might have dramatic implications as a performance enhancer; others might have none at all. Fishman's thymosin product, branded "TB-7," probably had little to no pharmacological impact on the horse, according to Rick Sams. But Navarro kept buying them.

He seemed to sometimes fall behind. "Seth, I am going to pay you," he wrote in a text in October 2017. "I promise, just things are so crazy for me right now. I won too many races and they are trying to put me out of the game but I promise. . . . I am going to paid [sic] you boss, and I do appreciate what you have done for me."[18] Still, he kept buying more and more. In late May 2018, with more than $6,000 on his account with Equestology, he wrote Fishman: "Send me an address, Boss, so my wife can send you a check today. . . . Also send me ten BB3 and 2,000 bleeder pills."[19]

By February 2019, Navarro seemed dependent on Fishman, but the stress of maintaining his access to the drugs he felt he needed to win races and the pressure he was getting from racing authorities bubbled just below the surface. In January, Fishman called Navarro about yet another unpaid bill. Navarro at first tried to suggest he had been led to believe Fishman was out of town. Then he claimed that Fishman had never sent him an invoice. Barely restrained tension sharpened the two men's voices. Navarro asked that the vet send him some "amino acid injectable shit" for a horse that was tying up, a relatively common but mysterious condition that causes muscle cramping. Fishman asked, challengingly, in a voice that suggested Navarro ought to know the drug he wanted: "Which one?" Navarro swiftly tried to move on, insisting that he hadn't received an invoice in a long time and that Fishman should send him one. Fishman said he would, then returned to the amino acid product, wanting to know which one Navarro wanted—clearly still interested in making a sale. "I have hundreds of products," he said.

Navarro snapped: "Listen, Seth, I'm at the track right now. There's people in front of me. I'm not talking about medication in front of people, okay? They—they—they already—they already got at me, like, a monster, so please. Okay? I'll talk to you."[20]

A few weeks later, Navarro was preparing to run X Y Jet in an allowance race, set for February 13, to get the horse ready to return to Dubai for a third shot at the Golden Shaheen. But, as happens with horses, a couple of things went wrong at once.

X Y Jet was unsound. At seven years old, he'd had three separate knee surgeries. He had raced only once in 2017. Before this upcoming allowance race, Navarro wanted to give him a special pain blocker. But the twenty bottles he had ordered—it's not clear if from Fishman or someone else—hadn't arrived yet.

Fishman wasn't Navarro's only source for performance enhancers. He texted a friend, a trainer at Gulfstream named Marcos Zulueta.

"I have a problem and you need to get me out of it," Navarro told him.[21] Navarro trusted Zulueta. He felt that the other trainer had showed his loyalty by screaming his guts out for an old claimer Navarro trained that had just won a $60,000 race.[22] They sometimes helped each other out with medication, and Zulueta promised to send Navarro a bottle of the pain blocker overnight so that it would arrive in time for the race.

Then, X Y Jet tied up. The horse "never tied up in his fucking life and he ties up today," Navarro complained to Chris Oakes.[23] Navarro bounced calls to Zulueta, Oakes, and a veterinarian named Gregory Skelton, who offered a "product . . . for tie-ups" to discuss what he should give the horse.[24] He was determined that the animal should run.

At one point, Zulueta suggested: "Do not race him—do not race him, then."

Navarro brushed that idea aside.

"I started treating him right away," Navarro said, according to government prosecutors. "When he peed . . . he didn't pee too much blood or anything ugly." (When horses tie up, they can excrete damaged muscle cells that appear red in the urine. A higher concentration of red can indicate a higher risk of severe kidney damage.)

He told Zulueta he had already given X Y Jet a milkshake—baking soda—through a nasogastric tube. He also told Zulueta that he planned to dose the horse with the pain blocker they had discussed earlier.

"Let me warn you," Zulueta said. "When you get a hold of that blocker . . . don't show it to anyone."[25]

Navarro knew what he was doing was against racing's rules.[26] He often arrived at the barn in the middle of the night to administer different drugs. At least one person involved with the syndicate that owned X Y Jet knew as well. On a separate call with someone that federal officials would later identify only as "a representative of one of X Y Jet's owners," Navarro said that he intended to milkshake the horse. The syndicate representative asked if the horse would pop a positive test as a result.

"Don't worry about it," Navarro responded. "I use something that covers the baking soda."

X Y Jet wasn't the only horse Navarro was drugging. Navarro seemed to be using everything he could get his hands on to try to get his horses across the line first.[27] The government later put the total value of the drugs he purchased at $70,000.[28] He gave horses something called "red acid," advertised as an anti-inflammatory that could mask injury. He gave an EPO mimetic he referred to as "monkey." He milkshaked his horses. The different cocktails had a homemade feel. There were plastic squeeze bottles with "Blood Builder" written in Sharpie on them, little glass vials with dosing instructions printed with a label maker. None of the drugs, of course, were approved by the FDA.

Navarro knew that he was the subject of rampant backstretch suspicion for, in the words of one racing trade publication, "his ability to transform ordinary horses into stars."[29] After the infamous "Juice Man" video filmed at Monmouth Park, where he was the leading trainer at the time, Navarro and Gindi were each fined $5,000 for "conduct detrimental to racing," and Navarro apologized for his behavior. Publicly, he was defensive.

"Everyone wants to pick on Navarro when I win a race," he told the Paulick Report in August 2017, when the video was recorded by another bar patron.[30] "They call me the 'juice man,' even when my kids are around."

"When people call me 'The Juice Man' how do I handle myself?" he told *BloodHorse*. "My best answer to people calling me 'The Juice Man,' or 'The Drug Man' is to come back and hit them again; win another race."[31]

And Navarro was winning races. He was absolutely shattering records. At Monmouth in 2016, the year before the video was filmed, he set a win record for the Monmouth Park season, winning 59 races. In 2017, he won 65—an unheard-of 41 percent rate.[32] And he was doing it with horses that other trainers couldn't get run out of. In 2017, he was sent a horse named El Deal who had finished ninth at odds of 102-1 in his last start for another trainer. He immediately won three races in a row for Navarro, including an eight-length victory in a Grade I sprint race at the prestigious Saratoga meet.[33]

Navarro had some close calls. Sometime in February 2019, he got a call from Jason Servis, a Northeast trainer he was stabled next to at Monmouth and had developed a relationship with. According to Navarro, Servis told him that he had gotten a call from a friend in racetrack security who warned him that a track official was going to search Navarro's barn.

"Jason Servis called me yesterday to let me know," Navarro told Michael Tannuzzo, a New York–based trainer with whom he was close friends. "Yea fuckin' . . . if he showed up at 5, he would of caught our asses fuckin' pumpin' and pumping and fuming every fucking horse runs today."

Everyone at the racetrack knew Jorge Navarro was up to no good—racetrack rumor can also be as reliable as an affidavit—but no one, it seemed, could catch him. On February 13, X Y Jet entered the starting gate for his prep race for Dubai. He won by almost eight lengths.

Navarro's family knew he was under pressure. His mother and his grandmother, who had raised Navarro for a time in Panama, talked about it at family gatherings. He had separated from Jennifer.[34] There was a sense that he was unraveling a little bit. He was drinking too much. The wins were never enough. His owners, he felt, were constantly demanding more, more, *more* from him. Navarro confided to Tannuzzo that he was going to call his bookie and settle up, close his account, stop gambling. He owed the bookie $24,000 on football. He couldn't keep betting like this, Navarro told Tannuzzo: he needed a clear head. He was going to stop gambling *today.*[35]

He had never been more successful. But the horses, and the drugs it took to keep them running, were expensive. It was as if he was on a treadmill that kept running out beneath him. Navarro was liberal with his money in other ways too. He paid his staff well and he was quick to give you a job, or a second chance. He once gave a struggling jockey $450, no questions asked.[36] The rider needed it to send home to Panama to cover his mother's rent, but Navarro didn't know that. All he had told Navarro was that he needed some money. The trainer had asked no questions. Navarro was a villain to some people in racing. But for some of the Spanish-speaking community on the backstretch, he was representation.[37] One of their own had made it to the top of the trainer leaderboards. The pressure to stay there was enormous. Navarro seemed to feel under siege.

"I got something new, big daddy," Navarro told Tannuzzo. "But I want you to . . . Mikey, you don't tell nobody, *nobody*, Mikey.

"You know what's wrong with us?" he went on. "We want to help the world. Fuck everybody."[38]

The "something new" was the pain blocker he had tried to get from Zulueta, who appeared to have come through. Navarro had paid him $3,000 for twenty bottles of the stuff and had given it to all his runners. Only one horse "ran bad," Navarro said to Tannuzzo, and that horse had gotten himself worked up beforehand and "left his race in the stall." But Navarro was getting paranoid.

"We gotta close the circle," Navarro said. "I can't feel bad for anybody."

"No, you can't, you can't, you can't," Tannuzzo said.[39]

X Y Jet took Navarro back to the deserts of Dubai, where the sand and exhaust make the hot air a hazy yellow smog. Here you sometimes see a Lamborghini flying in the wrong direction down Sheikh Zayed Road and wonder if you're on the wrong side of the road or they are.

The Meydan Racecourse is a behemoth. Its massive arced grandstand hooks out over the track like a hawk casting a shadow over the desert, its sheer glass front conveying limitless money, limitless power, limitless luxury. In the exclusive areas of the track apron, polished and well-heeled Emirati men stride about in the traditional white dishdasha. Giant gilded trophies wait like Portkeys to a better life.

Nominally, at least, the United Arab Emirates adheres to a strict policy of no race-day medication, in line with European rules. (Sheikh Moham-med bin Rashid Al Maktoum, the racing-obsessed ruler of Dubai whose pet project Meydan is, is known as an Anglophile.) Navarro had to be careful not to give X Y Jet anything that would test positive—and not to give anything in a way that would show.

When X Y Jet entered the starting gate under the floodlights at Meydan, he was doped. Navarro told Zulueta after the race that he had administered an unknown drug through "50 injections" in the horse's mouth.*

"Everything through the mouth, everything through the mouth," he said.

X Y Jet did just what he was supposed to: He took the lead from the start, gobbling up the ground in huge strides, and charged past the finish line first—despite losing a shoe midway through the race. X Y Jet's owners shrieked with excitement and mobbed Navarro with huge hugs.

Later, Seth Fishman texted Navarro to congratulate him on the $2.5 million purse. Navarro replied: Thank u boss u are a big part of it.

---

* This is likely a reference to oral administration rather than a shot, but I wasn't able to determine that.

The FBI had been listening to all of it. The Surick wiretap had yielded enough incriminating conversations that by January 2019, a judge had approved a wiretap for Navarro's cell phone. Every morning, Shaun Richards and Andrew Adams had been receiving readouts of the most interesting material.

What they heard was chilling, but also thrilling. They didn't have enough to charge yet. But they knew they had this guy dead to rights.

"You know how many f—ing horses he [Navarro] f—ing killed and broke down that I made disappear," Surick told Tannuzzo. "You know how much trouble he could get in . . . if they found out . . . the six horses we killed?"[40]

CHAPTER 15

BELONGING

The Surick wiretap had given the FBI enough evidence to get a wiretap approved for Navarro, and by early 2019, the Navarro wire had yielded enough to get an order to listen in on Seth Fishman.[1]

Richards, along with just about everybody else who knew Fishman, thought the guy was certifiable. Even Navarro called him "this crazy fuck Seth." In January 2019, he told Chris Oakes that Fishman had sent him "something with amino acid." (Oakes and Navarro, like many of the trainers who would either be indicted or testify in the case, appeared to have little grasp of what, exactly, they were giving to their horses.) Navarro had given it to a horse, he told Oakes, and "the motherfucker galloped. *Galloped.*"[2] That, combined with the sample of Fishman's pain shot that 5 Stones had helped the FBI acquire, was enough to get a judge to approve a wiretap.

They listened during the early winter months of 2019 as Fishman began to court a new client, a pretty young woman named Adrienne Hall, who was struggling along with a stable of five harness horses in the backwaters of Ohio. She came to believe, later, that Fishman saw her as a business opportunity, a way to get to one of the biggest trainers in Thoroughbred racing. But it seems obvious that he also saw in Hall's wide-eyed credulity a willing audience.

The first time she met Fishman, it was over dinner at a restaurant on Atlantic Avenue in the South Florida resort town of Delray Beach. Hall had a handful of cheap harness horses stabled near there at the time that she was trying to make a go of—unsuccessfully. She wanted his help "pre-racing" her horses, the catch-all term that refers to the standard schedule of medication, legal or illegal, that trainers give to all the horses in their barn prior to a race. At the time, Hall has insisted since, she wasn't looking for illegal performance enhancers from Fishman. But she was desperate for anything that might give her struggling stable a competitive edge.

Hall didn't have much hands-on experience with horses, but she loved them.[3] She was a horse girl, right down to her jeans and boots. She had done administrative work for a Thoroughbred breeding farm and later had worked in the office of leading Thoroughbred trainer Todd Pletcher. But when she and her husband moved to Ohio, she had to give up the job. Lost in the featureless belly of the Midwest, she missed horses so much that she started visiting the harness track near her home. It's hard to leave behind that world, where everyone from the millionaire owner to lowliest hot-walker holds no fonder ambition than to be an insider: an accepted native in an all-consuming culture built around the horse, this voiceless vessel for all their dreams. The yearning pull of *belonging* at the racetrack is as powerful as a drug. Soon Hall had claimed a few horses of her own to train. But she was losing.

She had bought some pre-race options from someone else in Ohio,[4] but it wasn't helping. There were rumors among trainers at the track that these products were not as they were labeled. "Horses were having bad reactions," she testified later in court. Other trainers suspected that "some of it . . . could have just been saline, so they were wasting money." That was how she came across Equestology.

When she first reached out to Fishman, Hall was very clear with the vet: She did not want to use EPO. She did not want to milkshake her horses. "I just really was desperate to find some help giving my horses an edge. I needed to be able to compete or I was going to lose them," she said.

As they ate, she asked Fishman who his clients were. Fishman was coy. He told her he was helping one of the leading Thoroughbred trainers in the country. He would say only that he was "a minority."

"Oh," Hall said. There was only one person who fit that description at the top of the training ranks. She knew instantly: "You're helping Navarro."[5]

After dinner, Fishman asked Hall to walk to his car, and he gave her a gift bag that had some samples in it: some syringes of a bleeder paste and some bottles of something called VO2 Max,[6] a product that was designed to maximize oxygen consumption but probably had very little actual impact on the horse.[7] Hall knew that it was against racing's rules to use, but she was desperate. She gave it to one of her horses the morning of a race.

It didn't help. Her horses were still losing. Within a few months, Hall had tried her first blood builder, from another drug provider. That too failed to make any difference.

In early March 2019 she called Fishman. He was in Thailand, and sounded a little surprised to hear from her—his voice almost suggesting to her, *Why are you calling me?*

"My stable needs your help," she said.

"What's wrong?" His voice was immediately gentle, almost fatherly.

"I don't know, my horses are falling apart," Hall said. "My one horse tied up really badly the other day. I pulled blood and that's when I saw, like the red blood cell count was bad. . . . I mean, like everything is—this blood builder doesn't do shit, obviously." She trailed off and sighed. "I don't know—I don't know what's going on."[8]

Even then, Hall now claims, she wasn't looking specifically for illegal drugs.

"I had horses who were tying up," she told the industry publication *Thoroughbred Daily News* in 2022.[9] "I had questions about how to raise red blood cell counts because my horses were borderline anemic. I really wanted help and I trusted him. I had heard really good things about him and how smart he was and that's why I wanted to utilize him. I did not specifically reach out to Dr. Fishman for performance-enhancing drugs."

But she also knew that everyone at the track was using something. It was "chemical warfare," she says now. "How was I supposed to compete against horses that don't get tired?"

Hall knew she was breaking the rules at the time—she has testified as much under oath—so it's hard to square these two viewpoints. There seems to be a delta between Hall's definition of "performance enhancers" and racetrack regulators' definition. Or perhaps the delta is between the drugs Hall considered to be an acceptable price of doing business in a corrupt industry and the drugs that were within the rules of racing. It's the frictionless slide between a human being's highest expectation of themself and their observable behavior. In between is the rationalization. The relationship with Fishman took on a life of its own.

Fishman began to provide her with his primary blood builder, BB3, and his thymosin product, the one that, according to Rick Sams, probably doesn't "do anything" to a horse.[10] He seemed eager to help Hall, and she continued to confide in him about her horses. She asked him questions, took his advice. His program could be expensive, and Hall's budget was limited. Almost immediately, he offered her ways to pay for the drugs through referral fees. He educated her about what other, less scrupulous trainers were up to. He talked to her about the pharmacokinetics of medication, about the permeable line between testability and permissibility. He softened her to the idea of building blood *responsibly*. He was professorial, always happy to explain how things *really* worked. He flattered her at times, telling her she knew her horses better than most because she treated them as pets, not racehorses.

In retrospect, Hall would come to believe she was being used. By early April, Fishman was encouraging her to approach Tony Alagna, a harness trainer whose barn Hall had some connections in. What Fishman really seemed to want was Hall's connections to Todd Pletcher's barn.

Fishman told Hall that he was fed up with Navarro. He needed another client.

"I fucking hate him," he told Hall. "He is just a proof of concept. . . . I just want one or two good Thoroughbred trainers and I would not work for that guy anymore."

Hall told Fishman that she had texted a friend who knew Pletcher well. Her text reached the friend while he was at Keeneland, at the sales.

"If I can tell you how Navarro wins so many races, would you and Todd have any interest in knowing?" she asked him. Her friend wrote back immediately, Hall told Fishman: "Absolutely. Knowledge is power."

"I hear the guy likes Dairy Queen," he added, a reference to milkshaking a horse.

As Hall described the text exchange, Fishman saw an opportunity. "Well, if you are tight with him, just say, 'I know for a . . . undisputable fact that I know a guy that [Navarro] is working with and that he [has] actually acknowledged to that guy that he is a major part of his success," Fishman told Hall to tell her friend.

"I basically said, 'I am doing work with a vet that helps [Navarro],'" Hall told Fishman. Her friend promised that he would talk to Pletcher when he got back to New York from Keeneland, she told Fishman. "He's absolutely wanting to know what the fuck—everyone wants to know what [Navarro] is doing. I mean everyone has always talked about [it], wondering what the fuck that guy does to win so many races."[11]

Hall later testified under oath that she never spoke to Pletcher about any of this, because she knew that the top trainer would never be interested in the opinions of a former office staffer. She said that it was not clear whether her friend did either.

By this point, Hall was either enjoying being in the know, or she was putting up a good front to maintain her access to Fishman and his products.

In the same conversation, she strategized how to get Fishman's products into Tony Alagna's barn in a more confident, knowing tone. Fishman was equally direct about the quid pro quo he was offering.

"Life is about give-and-take," he said. "Let's be honest, you have two horses, if I help you with your two horses and he is going to buy for 30–40 horses I am not going to charge you.

"I'm not a dick, I'm not like these other guys," he added.

"Well, that's why I am hoping he buys 'cause that would be fabulous," Hall responded.[12]

Aside from complaining about Navarro, Fishman also told Hall about other clients. Some bought more drugs than they needed for their own horses and then resold them. He boasted about outsmarting Brice Cote, alleging that Cote had sent down an undercover cop to try to trick him into selling EPO. But in Fishman's telling, the cover story the alleged cop concocted didn't make any sense—because he didn't really understand how EPO worked. Fishman saw right through him, he told Hall, and walked away scot-free. "Wooow," Hall exclaimed.[13] (As with most of Fishman's boasts, it's unclear how much truth there was to the story, or when it took place. Cote, as private security for a racetrack, would not have had the authority to order law enforcement to do anything.)

Most tantalizingly, Fishman boasted about his clients overseas in Dubai. The blood-building program that he was helping Hall put her horses on, he told her, had been designed, for $2 million, for use in the equine hospital built by the ruler of Dubai. In addition to building the glittering racecourse where the Golden Shaheen is held, and a series of other expensive supporting equine facilities, Sheikh Mohammed is among the sport's biggest owners and breeders anywhere, with roughly one thousand horses in training worldwide, including in the United States.[14]

"This is what they do for all their horses and overall, they are very happy," Fishman claimed to Hall. "Sheikh Mohammed Maktoum had the best 3 years, you know, in the 30 years he has been racing and they are very happy."

Throughout, Hall was receptive. His stuff worked for her. In March 2019, one of her horses won a race by five lengths. "I wish you could have watched the race replay," she told Fishman. He was "a completely different animal," she enthused. "He dominated." She cried when he won, she told him. She loved this horse so much, and he had won.

"Yeah, well if you think it is a pet horse, you got to race it a few more times and then fucking find it a home," Fishman said, offhandedly. "I mean, you fall in love with these [horses] . . . why don't you be a fucking hunter/jumper trainer?"

Hall quickly pivoted, her tone shifting. She told him she had drawn and tested blood samples from another horse because he raced "like complete shit." She was hard enough for this, she seemed to be saying.[15]

But even as she was talking tough to Fishman, Hall wasn't confident she was doing the right thing. She was nervous about the blood builder that he gave her, and she didn't use all of it. The medications came in color-coded bottles with complex instructions for mixing them, and she worried she would screw something up.[16] Fishman had emphasized that she shouldn't "overdo" it, because the horse might "crash" if she got him too hopped up.

"Mother Nature's a bitch. You want to take from her, you are going to have to give back sooner or later," Fishman told her.[17]

The relationship had soured by the time summer rolled around. Hall hadn't come through on Pletcher or Alagna. She and Fishman spoke for the last time in June 2019. He told her that he regretted helping her because she had done nothing but waste his time.[18]*

That year, Hall's horses earned about $60,000 in purse money. She made no profit.[19]

"You were in it for the love of the sport, isn't that right?" she was asked during Fishman's trial.

"The love of the horse," Hall said, "yes."

Seth Fishman seemed to have been lurking, just out of the grasp of countless regulators in different states and different jurisdictions, for years. In 2011, a Delaware veterinarian named Dr. Brittany Faison received an urgent call from a harness racing barn whose horses she treated. When she arrived, she found a horse named Louisville dead in the aisleway. The horse's groom told

---

* Fishman told me in an email that he had only helped Hall as "a favor" to a friend and that he "didn't need the drama as I wasn't even sure what her real reason for calling me was." He claimed that in other conversations that were not used by the government in their prosecution, he advised Tony Alagna how to "do the right thing with young expensive horses" and advised Hall that "she can NOT do what others do especially since she wants to treat her horses like a pet." He denied needing Hall to broker contact with Pletcher: "Pletcher? Seriously? She worked in his office, and for all I know she could have been a horrible employee that was fired," he wrote. "Truth be known when you have very effective products that can be verified with basic blood analysis that are far less likely to be detected than what is commonly being used, do you need anyone to introduce or vouch for YOU?"

her that he had tried to administer a shot of pentosan, an antiarthritic, into a vein in the horse's neck. He was confident that he had found a vein, not an artery, but the horse quickly began to hyperventilate and went down. He took a few agonal breaths and died.

Faison was pretty sure that the groom had accidentally administered the shot to the horse's artery, carrying the drug straight to the horse's brain without being diluted by the heart,[20] a known risk of IV injections. But what concerned her was that she had not prescribed the pentosan. The barn had bought the drug from a woman named Lisa Giannelli, who Faison believed was selling it on behalf of Dr. Seth Fishman. She called Fishman to tell him what had happened. According to a complaint she filed with the Delaware Division of Professional Regulation, he was "surprised and expressed he had just returned state side from being out of the country (I believe he said Brazil) for an extended period of time."

"I am concerned this veterinarian is not physically examining these animals and is in this medications sales situation strictly for profit," Faison wrote in her complaint. She also raised concerns that Giannelli was "driving around this state selling medications, needles, syringes and prescription drugs without a license and no professional training in regards to the medications she is dispensing"—including, Faison believed, anabolic steroids.*

"I am concerned this is going to happen again to another innocent victim, the horse," she wrote.[21]

A lawyer for Giannelli and Fishman denied the allegations at the time, and the complaint was ultimately dismissed. Fishman, the attorney insisted, personally examined all the horses he treated.

Yet Fishman, court testimony would later reveal, did no such thing. His business, Equestology, was entirely built around the creation of bespoke drugs, novel recipes that he cooked up himself and sent to a lab to mass-produce—and then marketed to trainers around the country and across the globe. Fishman sold a dizzying array of products. A 2018 product list had some five hundred different substances on it,[22] the work of a restless mind. Some were knockoff versions of FDA-approved drugs. Others were explicit performance enhancers that Fishman had designed to be untestable by regulators. Some, based on formulas in his business records, were a combination of naturally

---

* Giannelli too would later become a focus of the federal investigation and was among the targets followed not only by the FBI but also 5 Stones. Going back as far as 2017, the PI group had sent contractors to tail her car as she made deliveries from Delaware to upstate New York.

occurring amino acids that likely would have had no pharmacological effect whatsoever on a horse, according to Rick Sams. ("But as a buyer, you don't know," he noted.) Fishman was constantly experimenting, including with an analgesic peptide derived from the venom of a South American rattlesnake.*

But the cornerstone of Fishman's business model was to tweak a molecule here or there and make an illegal product invisible. During a lunch with a small Thoroughbred trainer named Jamen Davidovich in 2017, Fishman explained over sushi how he engineered his BB3 so that it was untestable. He took a paper napkin from the table and ripped two corners off. In court, Davidovich said that according to Fishman, this "changed the molecular weight of it, and they were looking for the molecular weight of this drug, and he changed it to this."[23]

"Since the molecule is altered, the labs could never detect unless a snitch tuned [sic] a bottle in and the racing authorities decide to make a test," what appears to be a fact sheet for Fishman's sales representative, Giannelli, reports about one of the products.[24]

He had been selling these "untestable" products to harness trainers going back at least to the early 2000s. Harness trainer Ross Cohen was an Equestology client in 2001. Cohen appeared to have little compunction about cheating: Over the years, he had injected his horses with EPO and run a nasogastric tube down horses' nostrils and into their stomachs to "drench" them with everything from yogurt and Gatorade to baking soda and bleeder pills. He purchased adrenocorticotropic hormone, or ACTH, from Equestology, used for its anti-inflammatory properties and undetectable in lab testing because it's a naturally occurring substance. He bought a product called Frozen Pain. Giannelli had recommended he use Fishman's bleeder pills.[25]

Giannelli told him that there was "always a risk" that administering the drugs could result in a positive post-race test, but that at the moment, New York regulators weren't testing for any of the Equestology products she sold. Once a week, Giannelli would drop off a box with Cohen's order. Occasionally, he would send blood work results—"a CBC and chemistry, just like a person gets done of their muscle enzymes, their red blood cells, white blood cells, liver enzymes, kidney function"[26]—for underperforming horses to Fishman to get his opinion on how to tailor "the program" that Fishman has designed.

---

* Cobra venom has long been known to be used in horse racing as a powerful painkiller. US Customs and Border Protection occasionally intercepts shipments bound for the racetrack. https://www.cbp.gov/newsroom/local-media-release/cobra-scorpion-spider-venom-and-other-illicit-horse-performance.

None of it, of course, had been tested by FDA-approved labs. Fishman appears to have bought tens of thousands of dollars' worth of raw ingredients from several sources, including a Chinese company and a commercial peptide producer in Massachusetts. He sent these to a drug formulator along with a recipe. He would then design unique "programs" for individual clients. Fishman said in what appears to be a pitch letter that investigators later found among his documents that his "products have been extensively tested and researched already in a decade of performance veterinary practice." He seemed to suggest that this was a net positive that would make any efforts to make the product legal easier: "Going to an independent R&D phase for basic safety studies would be with confidence knowing that the product was proven in actual application already. Going backwards is much easier and cheaper!"[27] (It also, of course, suggests that "basic safety studies" had never been done. His clients—and their horses, nonconsenting and utterly without an advocate—were his guinea pigs.)

Some of Fishman's products were so unreliable that Fishman would ultimately discontinue them—*after* selling them to trainers for use on their horses. Cohen called Fishman to tell him that horses would run lights-out after he administered some of the bottles of Frozen Pain, but that other batches would have little impact on the animal's performance.

"I expressed some feelings that they were not consistent, and in the conversation he said it was very hard to keep stable and to have proper employees make it, and that that's why he was going to stop making it," Cohen would later testify in court.[28]

In conversations with his clients, Fishman did not hide the fact that his products constituted "doping," but he took a nuanced, almost philosophical approach to the question—a rationalization so mind-bending that it feels like stepping through Alice's looking glass. On the other side is the backstretch of the racetrack. In April 2019, Fishman took a phone call from a client who Fishman told me in an email was looking for "legal doping agents" for his endurance stable.

"But it's not doping, yeah?" the client said.

"Of course it's doping," Fishman said. "The question is, is it testable doping? Any time you give something to a horse, that's doping. Whether or not they test for it is a different story.

"Don't kid yourself," he went on. "If you're giving something to a horse to make it better and you're not supposed to do that . . . that's doping."

CHAPTER 16

THE GHOST OF ALEX HARTHILL

The wire also caught Jorge Navarro talking to another Thoroughbred trainer, a slim, neat man he knew from Monmouth Park. More than perhaps any other target of the FBI's investigation, Jason Servis would come to epitomize racing's drug culture. In his innocence and his mendacity, he was the embodiment of the way that the through-the-looking-glass nature of the sport could lead even those who believed themselves to be on the straight and narrow to lose their way in all the refractions.

Servis was born in Charles Town, West Virginia, in 1957, to a racetrack family. His dad was a jockey and later became a steward at the Charles Town Races. The track was a two-bit oval run under lights in the dark plateaus of a poor state. But the Servis boys were horsemen. John Servis, Jason's brother, would go on to be an under-the-radar trainer, winning the Kentucky Derby in 2004 with Smarty Jones. Jason Servis began his career in the saddle, first as a jockey, until his weight and height became too much, and then as an exercise rider. He was known for his quiet ability to ride rough, dangerous horses. He worked in the jock's room as a valet—pronounced on the backstretch as "VAL-et," with a hard *t*—laying out race riders' saddles and gear for each race. He was deeply steeped in the rhythms and economies of life at the racetrack.

"That's where I cut my teeth," he said, years later.[1] "No money. But they were the good old days. My dad made me. I learned the straight and narrow. Work hard. Keep your nose clean."

He didn't start training under his own name until he was forty-three. He was now in his sixties, with pale blue eyes and straw-colored hair. The wind whipping between the ears of a Thoroughbred had creased and weathered the skin on his face and made his hands hard and smooth.

Servis's training methods were old-school, a little anachronistic: he liked to give horses long, slow two-mile gallops to get them fit, preferring that rhythmic work over the frequent short bursts of speed work many trainers today drill. He thought it was easier on a horse.[2] He was small, tidy in the way of an old jock. Many people at the racetrack thought of him as a quiet, mild-mannered man. He was a soft touch. He and his family lived on a dead-end street that had an animal shelter on it; his children knew him as the father who took in strays and taught them how to quietly approach unwanted pets dropped off at the bottom of the road so that they could bring them safely to the shelter.[3]

Yet by early 2019, the FBI had built a solid case that he was buying an illegal version of clenbuterol from Jorge Navarro.

It was, in some ways, shocking company for Servis to keep. There was something refined about Servis, a man out of time, and there was nothing refined about Jorge Navarro, by then infamous for celebrating "the juice" loudly at a racetrack bar. But somehow, out of the neighborly proximity of their barns, the two men began to trade information and, eventually, clenbuterol.

Clenbuterol is a bronchodilator that is highly effective at treating lower-airway respiratory illnesses. But it also has a powerful anabolic impact on the horse when given routinely, a steroidlike effect that helps build lean muscle mass. When the FDA approved it for use in horses in 1998, racing regulators in different states set thresholds—the amount of the drug that could be detected in a horse's system on race day without triggering a positive—so that trainers could use it during training. As long as they stayed under those limits, which in some states were incredibly generous, its use was entirely permissible. Clenbuterol became so common that I can recall, when I first went to work in a racing stable in 2004, grooms walking down the aisle in different barns at the end of morning training every day, carrying the kind of long metal dosing gun used to worm cattle and administering the drug to every horse.

By the time Servis was buying clenbuterol from Navarro, regulations had tightened around the drug. Thresholds were lowered to the so-called limit of detection,[4] meaning that any trace of the drug would trigger a positive test, and many states began requiring that horses treated with clenbuterol be put on the vet's list,[5] restricting them from racing. The idea was to weed out routine administration of the drug for its anabolic impacts and limit its use to horses that needed the drug to cure a respiratory illness. It only sort of worked. Some trainers then, and now, insist that it's *necessary*, even humane, to give clenbuterol to horses asked to run on dirt tracks, where they breathe in kicked-up dirt and mud.

"I thought it was helping my horses' airways stay clean," said trainer Tony Dutrow, who used clenbuterol on every horse in the barn when it was legal. "And I guess that it had the anabolic properties that I was told—and the horses responded very well on it."

But, he added, now that New York has tightened its rules and he can no longer use it routinely, "I don't need it. I don't miss it."

Clenbuterol is perhaps the most egregious example of a drug that is classified as a "therapeutic," intended to treat a medical condition, and is instead exploited for its performance-enhancing capabilities. Although its use is tightly restricted, clenbuterol is not a banned substance. Servis's violation with the drug was not just that he was taking advantage of loopholes in the rules and gaps in enforcement to use it as part of a training program— probably not a matter of federal law per se—but that he was also buying a compounded version of the drug, made in bulk by a pharmacy with- out FDA approval. Some compounded variations of clenbuterol are more concentrated than the FDA-approved version, offering a bigger potential performance-enhancing impact, but risking overdose. Racetrackers often refer to "that Mexican clenbuterol" as being ten times more concentrated than the FDA-approved version, a reference to where at least some of the illegal variations are believed to be manufactured; Servis likely believed what he was giving was more effective at building up his horses. The compounding made it a criminal matter.

It may also have been, in part, an economic decision in line with routine racetrack practice. When every horse in the barn is on an expensive "ther- apeutic," trainers have an incentive to look for economies of scale to try to lower their costs. This is true even for drugs that are entirely legitimate and part of obvious good-faith care of the animal: virtually all racehorses are on omeprazole to treat ulcers, which can cost upwards of $40 per horse per day if you give the name brand, GastroGard. One source familiar with the FBI investigation told me that the bureau had good evidence that one prominent trainer was buying an illegally compounded version of the drug, clearly to cut costs. The Justice Department declined to prosecute, likely because omeprazole is a harmless therapeutic with no known performance- enhancing capabilities. Prosecutors may also have considered the fact that the rules surrounding compounding are also deeply confusing: there are some instances in which vets are permitted to prescribe and administer a compounded drug; several vets told me they barely understand what will and won't get them in trouble.

It was yet another way in which the entrenched culture of medication use at the racetrack had collided with the raw economy of the sport to put horses at risk. As long as the compounded clenbuterol that Servis was buying didn't have any major quality problems, like bacterial or fungal contamination—a big "if"—and as long as it wasn't so concentrated that his horses overdosed—it appears they didn't—his horses probably weren't harmed by its use. But that was the gamble that Servis, a blue-collar trainer working with mostly blue-collar horseflesh, had taken.

"You got a minute, I want to talk to you about something." Servis was on the phone with his assistant trainer, Henry Argueta. Servis needed to get a bottle of clenbuterol from Monmouth Park to Belmont, to give to a horse before it ran. But how to get it onto the track without attracting the notice of regulators?

"Okay, so listen, I got a Sprite bottle, you know, Sprite," Servis said. "What about poultice, you got poultice?" he asked, referring to the twenty-five-pound buckets of plain clay mud, often smeared on horses' knees and shins to keep them cool, that are a staple in any racing barn.

"We got it, like, um, six?" Argueta said.

"Yeah, you know what I'm thinking, if I take the lid off one new poultice . . . Stick the bottle down and then cover it over—"

"Put it inside the poultice, right?"

"Exactly," Servis said.[6]

In 2019, Servis was winning more races than he ever had—and he had the best horse he had ever trained in his barn, a colt named Maximum Security that he was pointing to the Kentucky Derby. Servis had been to the Derby the year before, with a horse named Firenze Fire, but he had finished a distant 11th. Since 2005, Servis's strike rate had nearly always been above 20 percent. But after a couple of lean years in 2014 and 2015, his luck suddenly seemed to turn. In 2018, his horses won at a 32 percent clip, bringing home more than $7.5 million in earnings. The usual racetrack chatter that he was doping his horses was in full force.

"People are talking a lot of shit," Servis said at the time, "and I'm really not happy about it."[7]

There is no suggestion that Servis was able to sneak clenbuterol past regulators on race day. Racetracks screen for clenbuterol with a well-established test as part of routine race-day procedure. But he *was* buying and using the compounded version of the drug. Separately, he was also violating the rules of racing by giving bottles of the FDA-approved version of clenbuterol from his vet using a prescription for a single horse, but then splitting the bottle across the barn. It's a common practice on the backside, but technically prohibited.

Servis knew he was skating the rules with the compounded bottles he bought from Navarro—fifteen in total—but there's some evidence that he hadn't really differentiated it in his mind from the FDA-approved version. In one conversation with Argueta, he tried to explain why what they were doing could get them in trouble. Neither of them appeared to grasp the seriousness of the crime.

"That clen is supposed to be for Sunny Ridge," Servis said.

"Yeah, but what, it's legal," Argueta said.

"I know, but . . . it's supposed to be for whatever you got the prescription for."

"It might be having a problem but it's legal. It's a fourteen-day rule," Argueta said, referencing the New York withdrawal time for clenbuterol.

"Yeah, but it's not," Servis said. "In New York it's supposed to be for a horse you have a prescription for and you have to get permission from the Gaming Commission to even get a prescription."

"Yeah, that's a little problem but the rest . . . it's little, it's not like you're doing something very illegal," Argueta said. "The only problem you get is what you don't report about it. That's it."

"Yeah, it's not reported right."

"That's it. What else can they do?" Argueta said.

"Well," Servis said. "They might do shit."

Navarro, Servis told Argueta, was giving his horses clenbuterol at midnight.[8]

Their conversations about the drug and how to sneak it past regulators is strongly reminiscent of Doc Harthill, sneaking onto the backstretch of Churchill Downs to administer Lasix to Northern Dancer. Harthill's twinkly cloak-and-dagger antics are well remembered in racetrack lore—as mischief. Servis and Argueta seemed primarily to view their own crimes as a matter of petty paperwork. At no point, at least in the conversations captured by the FBI and made public during court proceedings, do the two men appear to grapple with their use of the drug itself. Taking minor liberties with the rules and outsmarting regulators in the service of winning races—that was an intrinsic part of the culture of the racetrack. It had ever been thus.

Apart from his use of clenbuterol, Servis had also been buying, for three years, a shadowy injectable drug from another New York vet, Dr. Kristian Rhein. The drug was called SGF-1000 and was advertised as "an innovative formulation consisting of Regenerative Proteins, Cytokines . . . Peptides, potent Growth Factors and Signalling Molecules derived from Ovine Placental Extract"—sheep placenta. The marketing materials boasted that it would "increase stamina, performance, and overall health," and promised that it was "safe and legal" and "natural."[9] Rhein told clients that it was a form of cutting-edge regenerative medicine that "helped" and "healed" horses with soft-tissue injuries by promoting the body's natural recovery process.[10]

SGF-1000 was somewhat in vogue across the backstretch at the time. It was one of a few products offered by a Kentucky-based company called MediVet that Rhein had a 25 percent stake in. Rhein, a talkative, energetic entrepreneur from a part of North Carolina that had once been the home of a buoyant furniture industry and was now a hollowed-out flatland, sold the stuff for $300 a bottle on the promise that it wouldn't result in a positive test.

It's worth noting here that in most performance-horse sports, there has long been a gray area between "untestable" and "illegal." The attitude was, "If there's not a test for it, then go ahead and use it," said George Maylin, the lab director for the state of New York, with a chuckle. By September 2019, the New York State Gaming Commission and the New York Racing Association had issued a notice listing "MediVet SGF-1000" as a prohibited substance under rules that had been in force since 2012. It's not clear if there was any published guidance on SGF-1000 specifically prior to that, but it was against racing's rules to use anything that included "growth factors," naturally occurring proteins that were thought to speed recovery if given therapeutically, and which MediVet's marketing materials claimed SGF-1000 included. Yet MediVet was actively marketing the product both online and in person as within racing's guidelines. MediVet hawked the drug on Facebook and on a company website. (Prosecutors say—and the court agreed—that Servis, as a longtime horse trainer, should have known better.) Rhein was selling, he said, "assloads" of it and according to prosecutors was making millions.[11] He was part of a flourishing cottage industry of so-called all-natural products masquerading as supplements for sale to trainers; the vast majority are not FDA-approved and sometimes contained banned substances.[12]

Other trainers, large and small, used Rhein's product, including Navarro. In some quarters, it wasn't seen as problematic. Dr. Rhein was "a good vet, especially on soundness," one larger New York–based trainer told the industry trade publication *Thoroughbred Daily News*, adding, "Dr. Rhein . . . dispensed it as something that was great for recovery and wellbeing."[13] He was trusted, at least by some.

One of his Grade I horses that now stands as a stud in Kentucky was on it, the trainer said. He continued: "Dr. Rhein had a lot of clients, and everyone knew everyone else was using it. . . . No one told us it was illegal before" the state commission issued its warning that it was against the rules. "There was nothing nefarious about it."

It was also hard to know how much it helped. In general, it's impossible to determine the impact of a drug on performance. Certainly, Servis and Navarro were doing extremely well, but they were also routinely administering clenbuterol, a drug with known performance-enhancing effects. There's strong evidence that SGF-1000 was little more than snake oil. When the FBI had the Hong Kong lab test a bottle in 2019, the lab "did not detect the presence of any growth factors or growth hormones in the sample that was analyzed."[14] It did test positive for some sheep collagens, of the kind used in face creams for human beings.[15] The Jockey Club had acquired six vials of the stuff in 2014 and had it tested; they found a sample to "consist of more than 80% ovine collagen with smaller amounts of other ovine proteins."[16] Dr. Mary Scollay, one of the foremost experts on the testing of performance-enhancing drugs in Thoroughbred racing, called the manufacturing of SGF-1000 "the equivalent of bathtub gin." That, today, is basically the consensus of most veterinarians and horsemen I spoke to.

That didn't make it not a "drug" under FDA regulations, which considers any substance introduced to a horse's body that isn't food subject to its jurisdiction.* And in any case, by September 2019, it was indisputably against the rules of racing. Rhein continued to prescribe it and Jason Servis continued to give it to his horses.

---

* According to the FDA, "there is no 'dietary supplement' regulatory classification for animal food substances and products. They are considered either 'foods' or 'new animal drugs' depending on the intended use. . . . [E]xpressed or implied claims that establish the intended use of the product to cure, treat, prevent, or mitigate disease, or affect the structure or function of the body in a manner other than food (nutrition, aroma, or taste) can identify an intent to offer the product as a 'new animal drug.'" This clearly implicated SGF-1000—even if it had never been enforced before. https://www.fda.gov/animal-veterinary/animal-food-feeds/product-regulation.

◆

The roiling heat of that summer bled into the fall. Richards and Adams listened as, over and over, Fishman, Rhein, Servis, and Navarro incriminated themselves on the wire. They had already built a strong case against Nick Surick, the Standardbred trainer. One night back in December 2018, while he was at a Christmas party, one of Richards's agents had called him with news. Bruce Turpin—young, capable, and hard-charging—had heard on the wire that Nick Surick was trying to hide a horse named Northern Virgin from state regulators. Surick, it appeared, had given the horse EPO and now had reason to believe that he was about to undergo some out-of-competition testing. To get around it, he had taken the horse to a farm off the racetrack property. This was the FBI's chance to establish fraud by catching Surick with a positive test.

Sarah Mortazavi worked frantically to get an application for a search warrant written and approved in time. Brice Cote was enlisted to recruit a veterinarian to draw blood from the horse. Turpin hooked up with another one of Richards's agents, and they met at midnight at a Wawa convenience store near the farm where Surick had stashed the horse. Mortazavi came through with the warrant approval and they all drove around to the back of the property. Between them and the barn were dense, black woods.

"Are we really fucking doing this?" the other agent asked in disbelief. Turpin was pulling on Gore-Tex pants in preparation.

"Yeah," Turpin said. "We're doing this."

It was pitch-black in the woods and the vet, who was older than the two feds, fell down twice. They stumbled through the dark, crept into the barn, and drew a sample from Northern Virgin. It came back positive for EPO.

But anything that they could use to expand the case beyond the people they were already listening in on hung beyond reach, frustratingly unsaid on the hours of calls and texts. The wire was getting "stale," Richards told me. The bureau needed to do something to flush out fresh game, to try to get beyond the targets they knew to those they didn't. Fishman's client list, they felt sure, would open investigative pathways for them to follow—if only he would cooperate.

And so, in the fall of 2019, they decided to arrest him.

CHAPTER 17

THROUGH THE LOOKING GLASS

It was eleven o'clock at night. Richards sat in a windowless room with nothing on the walls in a nameless hallway in Miami International Airport. Sitting across from him, fresh off the plane from Dubai, was Seth Fishman. The vet was in his element, delivering a lecture.

He had worked with the FBI before, Fishman let it be known, in the David Brooks case, when he had been asked to make a memory-erasing pill. Everything he did was aboveboard, of course—that business in Delaware had been complete bullshit. And then, very delicately, he intimated that he had powerful friends who would never let anything happen to him. If Richards wanted to pursue this matter further, Fishman appeared to suggest, it wouldn't be very good for his career.

But Richards had an ego too. He let him talk, confident in his own ability to play the vet. Fishman wasn't under arrest, yet. Richards was trying to "flip" him. What he wanted was Fishman's client lists and the names of everyone he had worked with over the years to produce his drugs.

He had started out with the soft-pedal approach, trying to play on Fishman's delusions of grandeur and whatever loyalty to the game of horse racing he might have. Drugs were pushing out the mom-and-pop operations, Richards said. He'd grown up in that kind of grassroots family barn, he told Fishman. Help the FBI help the sport, and help the little guy.

"You could probably arrest me right now," Fishman told Richards.

"I probably could, but I don't want to get to that point," Richards said. "I'm looking for your help."

It didn't work.

"He was very cocky. He didn't believe we had anything," said one source familiar with the interview. "He just thought he was smarter and he could outtalk it and that nobody had pinned anything on him."

So the FBI put the handcuffs on him.

Fishman remained defiant that his business was not only legal but that it also operated in the best interests of the horses whose trainers he supplied. It was Thoroughbred racing's regulatory structure that was woefully outdated, he argued, in ways that allowed for both cheating and animal abuse.

Fishman's line of thinking is difficult to follow unless you abide by his definitions of "doping" and "performance-enhancing drug." In Fishman's dictionary, neither term inherently implies rule-breaking. As best as I can understand him, Fishman seems to believe that what makes the use of a PED illegal is the intent of the administrator. "When and why a drug is given is what ultimately should determine if it is a PED or not," he wrote to me in an email. In Fishman's telling, there is an innocent explanation for his answer to the client who asked, "But it's not doping, yeah?" ("Don't kid yourself.") The client was looking for "legal doping agents" that were "NOT listed as banned or prohibited," he told me.

Horse racing regulation, he said, is behind other major competitive equine sports, like show jumping, whose international competitions largely follow rules set by a body headquartered in Switzerland. He insisted that there are "several PEDs" commonly referred to as doping agents "that are actually legal because they do NOT appear on the banned or prohibited list," and that "there are 100's of PEDs that are 100% safe and legal to use in" other prominent competitive equine events outside of horse racing.

Considerations about "testability"—whether a drug will show up on an ELISA panel or in mass spectrometry analysis—are just the responsible practice of a good vet, Fishman argued to me.

"Despite the government's opinion, a performance vet is responsible to know proper withdrawal times and should understand not only the pharmacokinetics but also the pharmacodynamics of what they are using," he wrote me in an email that is typical of the dense, jargon-heavy way he speaks. "While most doctors never really need to think about this beyond safety and efficacy it is not criminal thinking as a performance veterinarian to continually be concerned and outspoken about testability and likely detection of anything they or their clients consider using!"*

---

* Here I have reproduced Fishman's email to me without editing for punctuation and clarity.

It's a reasonably cogent articulation of the old racetrack attitude: If it's not explicitly banned, then it's fair game to use.

It's hard to know how genuinely Fishman believes all this. He was, of course, also producing mimetics of explicitly banned substances, like EPO and opioids, for Navarro and others, and in those cases there should have been no question of their being "legal doping agents." Shaun Richards remains convinced that Fishman knew his conduct was both illegal and wrong. He just thought he could outsmart everyone. But it's just as possible that in Fishman's cubist worldview, his conduct isn't just rationalized but *rational*. His attorney would later disclose under oath that Fishman has "substantial" psychiatric disabilities. According to the lawyer, Fishman struggles with anxiety and depression and has been diagnosed with a bipolar disorder.[1]

"It's somewhere in the middle," said one person who worked closely with him. "I never heard him say, 'This is good for the horse.' But the way he spoke to me about it, he did believe that what he was doing was not an illegal thing."

After his arrest, Fishman tried to convince agents that he could help them clean up the sport, which he agreed was plagued by cheating. But he refused to do what Richards had in mind, which was to have the vet wear a wire.[2] The investigation had been going on for more than a year. The wires had been humming—with multiple renewals—since the beginning of 2019. Behind the scenes, the FBI was under growing pressure to wrap things up.

Andrew Adams thought he was going to throw up in the back of the taxicab.[3] It was the first Saturday in May and he was watching the Kentucky Derby on his phone while he and his wife were on their way to a birthday party. This was a catastrophe.

"What is happening?" his wife asked, alarmed. All the color had drained out of his face.

"I can't tell you," he said. *But oh my God.*

It was a dark, stormy day in Louisville. The sky was black and the track was heavy with rain. Wet manes lay stringy and limp on horses' necks. And the wrong horse had just won the Kentucky Derby.

The problem, for Adams, was that he had all but promised his boss that a horse named Maximum Security wouldn't win. The horse wasn't a total long shot—he had won an important prep race in Florida and was 10-1 on the morning line[4]—but he had an undistinguished pedigree and was trained by a man who had never won the Kentucky Derby before. He was trained by Jason Servis, who the Department of Justice knew by then was giving illegal drugs to his horses.

Their racehorse investigation had already drawn some scrutiny. A new deputy assistant attorney general down at main Justice in Washington, DC, was balking at approving wiretap extensions because she was concerned that the DOJ was willfully endangering doped horses' lives by allowing them to continue to race while the FBI built its case. And Geoffrey Berman, then the US attorney for the Southern District of New York, had made it very clear to Adams that it wouldn't look too good for the Department of Justice if it knowingly allowed a doped horse to win the most prestigious horse race in the United States, a race that was worth $3 million in purse money and on which countless Americans wagered, cumulatively, hundreds of millions of dollars each year.[5]

Now that was exactly what had happened. Adams turned off the video.

Five Stones was also under some heat by then. The Jockey Club was starting to get impatient. Now that the FBI was involved, they were getting less information out of 5 Stones, according to sources with both organizations. There were two reasons for this: One was that 5 Stones wanted to maintain the integrity of the bureau investigation. But the second and more important reason was that 5 Stones knew very little about what the FBI was up to. Harrington would try to introduce sources to the bureau and pass along tips. There was a time when he would talk to Richards multiple times a week, sometimes a couple of times a day. But he was passing along information, not receiving it. Adams, whose job it was to build the actual charges that the DOJ would bring, deliberately kept 5 Stones at a distance. Although 5 Stones—with the help of Brice Cote—had gotten the bureau started on the investigation, at some point there wasn't much more they could do. They couldn't tap phones. They didn't know what was being intercepted on those calls. They had absolutely nothing on Servis. Some of the materials from that era make it appear as if 5 Stones was scrambling for relevance. The i2 maps—the digital webs that 5 Stones put together—look convoluted and impressive. But it's not clear that 5 Stones was able to take their investigation any further: links between different people were sometimes built on little more than a Facebook connection. Some of the black lines were drawn on the claims of a single source.

Harrington tried to zero in on Chad Brown, a top New York–based trainer. Brown was a native of upstate New York who had apprenticed under Bobby Frankel before going out on his own. He was in his early forties, with a tightly shaved buzz cut and an intense, busy air about him.

Brown specialized in turf runners, often imported from Europe, public scuffles on social media, and a handful of run-ins with the law, including a domestic dispute in 2022 that had turned violent enough for the cops to get interested.[6] In 2019, a judge ordered him to pay almost $2 million in back wages and fines after a three-year investigation by the Department of Labor found that he had failed to pay overtime when employees worked more than forty hours.[7] Although there were many in the sport who considered him something of an asshole, he was a good horse trainer. There was, as there always is with successful trainers in racing, widespread suspicion that he doped his horses. The evidence cited by backstretch gossipers was that his horses "re-broke" in the stretch, meaning that they were able to suddenly accelerate just when they should be growing leg-weary and slowing down at the end of a race.[*] He had never received a drug positive for anything more serious than omeprazole.[8] He was also among the trainers who would come to believe that Stuart Janney was—personally—out to get him.

An i2 map produced by 5 Stones titled "Chad Brown career path and meteoric progress from 2008" seems less than compelling. It lays out his career trajectory, then records that a source had told investigators that veterinarian Dr. Bernard Dowd was known as "Chemist Dowd" and did some work for Brown. It also references a report written by Tim Harrington, recording that a source had told him in August 2017 that they had once seen multiple cases of 200 mg tablets of something called quinidine sulfate in Brown's barn. Quinidine sulfate is a banned substance in racing, but it is prescribed in horses to treat irregular heartbeats. Five Stones investigators came to believe that it was possible that Brown was using quinidine to help counteract the blood thickening effects of EPO by helping the heart pump more effectively—but that conclusion doesn't make any sense, according to Rick Sams, since quinidine actually *decreases* the force of contraction of the heart. It was just one more tip that 5 Stones would receive over the years it held the Jockey Club contract that investigators would use to show they were on to something, but which would turn out to be nothing.

---

[*] The notion that horses "re-break" in the stretch is routinely cited as evidence that this trainer or that trainer is cheating. It's a fallacious expression; skilled handicappers who analyze the fractional times of these races will point out that it's an optical illusion. Other horses are slowing down in the stretch while the horse who has allegedly been doped is just maintaining the same pace—giving him the appearance that he has found another gear and gunned down the front-runners. Of course, this *could* be evidence that a horse has been doped: a performance enhancer could allow a horse to stave off fatigue and continue to run at the same pace for longer, theoretically. But the suggestion that horses "re-break" is, more often than not, misleading.

Adams, sitting in the back of the cab on Derby day and feeling vaguely nauseated, was saved by an incredible quirk of racing fate. By the time he had gotten out of the cab, the stewards at Churchill Downs had moved to disqualify Maximum Security. Despite putting in a clearly winning performance, the horse drifted out in the stretch and was judged to have impeded the path of other horses making their run for the wire—a violation of racing rules. The second-place horse, Country House, was ultimately declared the winner of the Derby. Adams's despair turned to elation. He, and the investigation, were saved. For now.

"You got lucky this time," Geoffrey Berman told him. "Let's not do this again."

Meanwhile, Jason Servis was also getting nervous. One Wednesday in June 2019, a month after Maximum Security crossed the line of the Kentucky Derby first, Servis called Rhein. Regulators had just come to his barn in New Jersey to take a urine sample from Max, he said.

"You got a minute?" he asked Rhein.

On the other end of the line, Rhein stepped out of the barn where he had been working. Rhein, then in his forties, was ambitious and a bit excitable, the kind of guy who admired Elon Musk and wanted to be doing things that would put him ahead of the curve.

"Are you by yourself?" Servis asked.

"Yeah, I just walked out of the barn," Rhein assured him.

Servis explained the problem. "They've been doing some out-of-competition testing," he said, referring to state regulators who, two days before, had been by to take samples from Maximum Security. That day, Servis had given Maximum Security an injection of SGF-1000. Now the regulators had returned a second time. They were looking for something.

"Monday he got the [SGF-1000]," Servis said. "I just want to make sure we are all good with that."

Rhein told him he had nothing to worry about. SGF-1000 would never appear on a doping test. If it did, it would look like a routinely administered—and legal—therapeutic drug, an anti-inflammatory called dexamethasone that Rhein told me he would advise trainers to give concurrently with the SGF-1000 if they were worried that the horse might have a reaction to the dose.

"There's no test for it in America. There's no testing. There's nothing," Rhein reassured Servis.

"Right," Servis said.

"There's nothing you did that would test."

Behind the scenes, Rhein was scrambling. It had already come to Medi-Vet's attention that SGF-1000 was under some scrutiny from regulators, and he and the other owners of MediVet had become concerned that it could hurt their sales.

Part of the problem was MediVet's claim in its marketing materials that SGF-1000 contained "growth factors," prohibited under rules adopted by most racing jurisdictions. At that point, MediVet didn't really know *what* was in SGF-1000. It was made by an Australian company and MediVet was simply acting as the US distributor. Rhein told me that MediVet "leadership"—which included his father and brother-in-law—never felt the need to do its own testing, because the parent company had represented to them that "all samples were clean and would not swab in any testing jurisdiction." (Once again—and even now—the evident logic is that testability is the only standard by which the acceptability of a drug is judged.)

There was also some awareness within MediVet that the drug might run afoul of FDA regulations in some way.

"We gotta think of re-branding if it goes sideways," Rhein said to Michael Kegley Jr., his brother-in-law and the sales director for MediVet, about how to change the product's packaging and labeling to get around the concerns that it might require the agency's approval. "What was the fucking name that somebody told me? It was a good name. It was kinda cheesy, but shit . . . it was a one-word name . . . like Encore, something like that. . . . Repair? . . . RepairRx?

"What you do is you just say it's a preventative," he said. He and Kegley wanted SGF-1000 to be called a "dietary supplement."

"That way . . . no one even has to question if it's FDA approved or not—it's strictly a supplement," they agreed.[9] Rhein said to me that at the time, he had come to understand that there might be concerns related to the product's FDA status because of the labeling, not the contents of the product itself. "Since there was no drug in the product, it never occurred to me that it needed FDA approval. Collagen is not a drug," he said in an email. As a technical matter, he's wrong: as a nonfood substance, SGF-1000 was absolutely considered an animal drug that required a prescription to administer under FDA rules. Whether or not he—or anybody at the racetrack—understood this is unclear.

For the most part, however, everyone associated with SGF-1000 appeared entirely focused on satisfying racing regulations, rather than addressing the potential federal violation that at least MediVet was clearly aware of. Rhein, according to prosecutors, stopped storing the drug in his car, worried that racing regulators might sweep his vehicle, and he advised another vet selling the product to "lay a bit low" and avoid documenting his use of the drug for a little while. Rhein told Servis that he never put SGF-1000 on a bill. Instead, he billed the little vials as acupuncture.[10] (In Rhein's own telling, he was following a known racetrack practice to avoid angry owners calling to ask why their horse was getting such expensive veterinary treatments—one of dozens of examples of behavior that appears logical, even routine, inside racing, and totally indefensible when exposed to outside scrutiny.)

In early August, MediVet finally sent SGF-1000 off to a lab in Colorado for analysis as part of an effort to get the Racing Medication and Testing Consortium (RMTC), the national research body that most racing juris-dictions relied on to set drug rules, to issue guidance that the "supplement" was permissible. They did this through a bit of legerdemain: on August 8, the company received the results from the lab confirming that SGF-1000 was negative for growth factors. In fact, as the Jockey Club had already learned, SGF-1000 didn't appear to have much of anything in it except for sheep collagen. But it did return positive for "low levels" of a hodgepodge of other drugs, including a common narcotic, several common large-animal sedatives, and caffeine—likely evidence of contamination during the man-ufacturing process. MediVet requested that the lab split the positive and the negative findings into two separate reports and only delivered the findings that showed SGF-1000 did not contain growth factors to the RMTC.[11]

MediVet's counsel at the time was a woman named Karen Murphy, a combative lawyer who frequently represents trainers fighting drug posi-tives. She told me that MediVet only sent part of the findings because Dr. Mary Scollay, then the executive director at the RMTC, only cared about whether SGF-1000 contained growth factors.* This put MediVet in the ironic position of defending to the RMTC that its product didn't contain the very thing that its own marketing label said it did.

---

* When I initially asked Murphy about the government's allegation that MediVet had split the test results, she flatly stated that it was "completely not true," before amending to acknowledge that only the negative test results for growth factors had been sent to the RMTC.

Around the same time, Rhein had a conversation with the head of the lab used by the New York commission. The lab director, George Maylin, told him, "Either cease and desist or you're gonna go to jail. One or the other. What do you want to do? I'm saying if you want to stay out of jail, don't use it." Rhein, according to prosecutors, tried to "self-soothe" by reassuring himself of what he believed: he couldn't get caught because he didn't document his use of the drug.

"I mean it's not on any of my records, I don't write it down—I mean, I sold it but, shit, it's—it's not in my records," he said. "I don't have any positives. I don't have anything like that."[12]

Rhein, as well as two other sources familiar with the federal wiretaps, told me that Maylin also suggested to him during that conversation that he ought to burn his records related to the drug. Some officials thought it was possible he might have been kidding; others thought he was serious. ("I don't remember that, and that was not on the recorded conversation that the DOJ guys played back for me," Maylin told me.)

In August, state police approached Servis to ask him about his use of SGF-1000. He lied, telling them he had only a couple of horses in the barn on it.

"But I'll tell you I have asked [Rhein] once, I've asked him 10, 20 times, 'I don't want any problems,'" Servis told them. He said that Rhein had assured him, "This is all natural."

"What do you mean, 'No problems'?" the officer asked.

"You know, I'm using something illegal."

"Oh, okay."

Servis kept going, sounding increasingly defensive.

"I don't want no . . . I have got too much to lose. I am good. I don't need no help."

"Sure."

"Drugs or anything," Servis said. "I've got good horses. They speak for themselves."[13]

He was deeply freaked-out: "I am dying, man," he told Argueta. "Shitting. If they came to my house, I am afraid they are going to come search my house."[14] He should have asked for a lawyer, he said. Maybe a lawyer could clean things up for him.

Servis called Rhein the day after the cops came to his house, wanting to know if SGF-1000 was FDA-approved.[15] Rhein told him the truth: no, it wasn't. But, he continued to insist, incorrectly, that because SGF-1000 wasn't a "drug," it didn't have to be.

"It has no drug in it. It's literally just a purified protein from a sheep's placenta. . . . This isn't a drug, this isn't manufactured," he said. "So the Federal Drug Administration [sic], they wouldn't approve it anyways just because it's not a drug."

"Should we stop using it?" Servis asked.

"No. I mean, it's not illegal," Rhein said.[16]

Rhein was also freaked-out, he told me. But he was convinced that regulators were on a witch hunt. He had asked George Maylin, *Did I get a positive or something?* Maylin, he said, told him no. He thought, "'Well, what am I doing illegal?' And I thought, 'Oh, my God, if I stop, I look guilty.' And then I was like, they're going to come to their senses." He was convinced, then and now, that SGF-1000 was an exciting and safe new treatment for injured horses. Murphy, he said, was advising him that he was in no real legal peril.

When the New York Racing Association and the New York Gaming Commission finally issued their notice explicitly stating that SGF-1000 was banned in September, neither Servis nor Rhein stopped using it. It was as if they simply couldn't conceive that there might be consequences to their actions, that regulators were *really* going to step in and do something about their use of an unregulated, unknown drug. It's either staggering hubris or staggering naïveté—or both. It's especially bizarre given that there's little evidence that it improved Servis's horses. Servis himself, in his conversation with the police, mused: "There were days when I was like, somebody is making a lot of money for nothing."[17]

Some evidence suggests that Servis sought reassurance that his use of SGF-1000 was within racing's rules. Murphy said she had "several conversations" with him about her efforts to get the RMTC to list SGF-1000 as permissible so that New York authorities would reverse their ban, and told him that she believed "the issues concerning SGF-1000 . . . would all likely be resolved."* But whatever Servis (and Rhein) believed about the extent of

---

* The RMTC, she said, would eventually advise her in March 2020 that it believed FDA approval of the product was not required. This seems to be a bit of revisionist history: In an email to me, Scollay said she told Murphy that she "would notify NYRA that the product no longer met criteria as a Banned Substance" under racing's rules—which have nothing to do with the FDA. Still, it does seem that Scollay may have given some indication that MediVet could continue doing what it was doing: the FDA had long been "generally unresponsive to requests for help," Scollay told me, and given that, she "felt that the product was not substantially different from other non-drugs [that] have conventional use at the racetrack." Here note that even Scollay is classifying SGF-1000 as a "non-drug." Her remark about the FDA's previous lack of interest also shows why racetrackers like Rhein might come to believe that the only law they need concern themselves with is the law of the racetrack.

the federal laws they were breaking, at the time they were using SGF-1000, they absolutely knew it was not permitted by the state racing commission and the racetrack. It's a telling indictment of the culture of racing that one of the sport's top lawyers would, apparently, knowingly suggest to a business associate of her client that he could continue to flout track rules,* and that the state's lab director, who clearly grasped the federal violation, would do nothing more than advise a person over whom he had regulatory jurisdiction how to stay out of jail.

As that tense summer went on and it became obvious that MediVet's problems extended far beyond racetrack rules, Rhein and Servis continued to operate as if the only law that mattered was the law of the turf. For most racetrackers, who live their whole lives bounded by the contours of this all-consuming world, that is the only authority they know. The stewards are judge, jury, and God Almighty—and God can always be reasoned with. Everything outside of the backstretch gates feels distant and unreal.

By October 2019, the marketing descriptions of SGF-1000 had been updated to describe it as a "homeopathic placental extract." This too was probably a false assertion. According to the 2014 testing done at the behest of the Jockey Club, the collagen levels found in SGF-1000 were higher than those found in sheep placenta, meaning that was unlikely to be the origin—and leaving the question of what tissue *was* the source unanswered. This also did nothing to resolve the problem that the substance itself had never been reviewed by the FDA. MediVet went on to scrub the website of any reference to growth factors, in an apparent bid to make the problem go away.[18]

If this all sounds unnecessarily complicated, it's because it is. It's a ridiculous dance between the drugmakers and users on one side, and a poorly understood and disjointed web of state, federal, and industry regulators on the other. Murphy argued to me that Servis and Rhein were taking good-faith steps to ensure that the sale and use of a harmless therapeutic substance abided by all the necessary regulations—even though they knowingly continued to use a product that had been explicitly barred by state regulators—and that the government had been heavy-handed in its prosecution. (When it comes to SGF-1000, it is possible that the government

---

* In a conversation with me, Murphy insisted that Servis was not a client and that she did not advise him to continue using SGF-1000—she simply conveyed to him that she believed the matter would be resolved in such a way that SGF-1000 would be officially listed as permissible. Whether Servis understood that distinction is another matter.

made some misleading assertions. Prosecutors would represent in a filing to the judge that a second round of testing done by the company in October at the University of Kentucky had been "positive" for growth factors. None of the other labs that looked at the stuff had the same finding—including the Hong Kong Jockey Club—and according to Rhein and a court filing by Servis's lawyer, the result was ultimately deemed to be a false positive.)

The government, meanwhile, argued that Rhein and Servis were scurrilous deceivers, hell-bent on doping horses with growth factors—even though, as it turned out, SGF-1000 did not contain them and wiretap transcripts do show Rhein appearing to discuss the product as a healing agent.

Both narratives are wrong. Servis and Rhein weren't uniquely evil dopers, nor were they innocent businessmen unfairly targeted by government. They were two people operating by the only rules they had ever known. They were doing what countless horsemen before them had done in a chaotic, sometimes senseless world that did not question that drugs should be given to racehorses—or police it in any comprehensible way. Racetrackers could perhaps be forgiven for failing to understand FDA law, given that the agency had largely ignored them until now. For years regulators had tried and failed to get the FDA's attention, and in the meantime, scores of legally dubious products had circulated the backstretch with little to no enforcement by the feds or anyone else.[19] Not much had changed in racing since the days of Alex Harthill. The only thing that had really changed, in fact, was that the outside world had started paying attention.

So entrenched is the culture of "therapeutic drugs" at the racetrack, so wholly do horsemen believe that the giving of supplements and therapeutics is a necessary, even humane, part of racing horses, that when faced with clear regulatory scrutiny, Rhein and Servis both barreled ahead. No one associated with SGF-1000 ever seemed to pause long enough to question whether they should stop using the product. Rhein and Michael Kegley Jr., it seems, didn't even bother to establish what was *in* the drug until they realized they might lose the opportunity to sell it. That SGF-1000 was probably very expensive quackery that had very little impact on the horse hardly mattered. Because the drug *might* offer a competitive edge, it was worth money. And because it was worth money to both its producers and its purchasers, no one associated with it appeared to consider whether they *should* be giving it at all. The only question was whether they *could*. This wasn't a regulatory failing. It was a cultural one.

Rhein seemed truly to believe that he was helping the horse. There is almost an idealism to the way he describes his practice: he was helping horses heal with regenerative medicine and convincing trainers to slow down rather than pound on horses, acting as a force for good inside a broken system, a saint for lost causes. He described other trainers and vets openly boasting about testing how far within the withdrawal guidelines they could give drugs like clenbuterol. He wasn't like that, Rhein felt. He believed SGF-1000 was good medicine. But he was still operating inside the logic of the racetrack. He understood very clearly that the "help" he was providing was to get the horse back to the races. "You cannot do nothing and train horses to go fast," he said. "They just have too many bumps and bruises."

Rhein wasn't just trying to help the horses. He was also trying to help another lost cause, he told me: Jorge Navarro's friend Mike Tannuzzo. Tannuzzo, Rhein said, was struggling to make ends meet. He was living in a tack room in New York, training a few cheap horses and supporting some other family members; Rhein tried to get him to come to church with him. One of Tannuzzo's owners—a scary-looking dude who Rhein worried might be tied up with the mafia in some way—kept dropping off glass vials of illegal performance-enhancing drugs that he wanted Rhein to administer to Tannuzzo's horses. He didn't do it, Rhein said—he was still trying to be a force for good in a bad system. But he held on to them in his fridge at home, he said, out of fear of the owner and as a favor to Tannuzzo. He knew he was in a bad situation, but thought: "I'm just gonna have to play this hand out."[20] The drugs sat there in his fridge, little reminders of all the ways a person could become lost at the racetrack.

With Fishman declining to cooperate, Adams decided it was time to wrap up the case and charge what they could with what they had. He wanted to try to issue indictments by January 2020, and he and his team set to work deciding what to charge. Richards's team began trying to fill in the holes that the prosecutors needed to fill while Adams, Mortazavi, and other Justice Department officials debated whether the facts of the case supported wire fraud charges. There had been some recent wire fraud cases that had been overturned in the Southern District that led Adams's team to question whether they would be successful, or whether they would have to stick to misbranding charges.

Part of the issue was that to successfully charge wire fraud, they would have to establish that there had been clear misrepresentation: a horse was represented as running clean when in fact he was doped, in violation of accepted rules and regulations. This, for Adams's team, meant establishing exact moments in time at which a horse had run on a substance that was explicitly not permitted by racing rules. Then, that had to be coupled with documentation of money benefiting the fraudster crossing state lines. It was a difficult task, given the inexplicably arcane miasma of racing regulations. Mortazavi and Adams built a massive PDF mapping out "the PED, the way the PED violates the rule, the specific point in time that person violated that rule; and here's a check that was cut to him via interstate wire," said one person familiar with the process.

Another question was whether they could establish a *victim* for wire fraud charges. Who, exactly, had been defrauded? "Bettors" was too non-specific, and some DOJ officials were uncomfortable naming the racetracks as victims "because a lot of those tracks knew what was going on and either had willful blindness or just let it go for business," said one of the sources familiar with the investigation.

They were still debating the issue by New Year's 2019, when Adams had wanted to finish. The FBI also had to coordinate the schedules of more than one hundred agents to conduct multiple raids and arrests for dozens of defendants across the country simultaneously.

In the meantime, something happened that seemed to underscore everything that was at stake: On January 8, 2020, Jorge Navarro issued a public statement announcing that X Y Jet had died.[21]

X Y Jet had raced only once in the nine months since he had won the Golden Shaheen, a Grade III at Gulfstream in December. The old warrior had set a fast early pace, but faded to last place in the stretch, easing up under the wire twenty lengths behind the winner. After the race, Navarro said he had simply gone too fast too early and that his plan was still to get the horse back to Dubai for a fourth try at the Golden Shaheen in March.

"Twenty-one, :43, 1:08, that's it," Navarro said at the time, clicking off the fast fractions that the horse had run.[22] "I was upset going that fast, but he cooled out well and today he's perfect. We always X-ray after every race, and everything's good. That's what we needed for him."

On a Wednesday morning less than three weeks later, after a routine gallop, X Y Jet died of an apparent heart arrythmia.

X Y Jet was a mature horse by then. By racehorse standards, he was old, still racing only because as a gelding he had no value as a breeding prospect. His steel-gray coat had turned nearly white, his black mane and tail a sharp contrast when he galloped around the track. In his statement announcing the horse's death, Navarro called him "swift, moody, but noble." He said he was "part of my family, was like the older brother of my children," "a friend that I will carry forever in my heart." By all accounts, Navarro—that perfect product of the backstretch—was devastated. He wept and for two days, didn't want to leave his house.[23]

CHAPTER 18

THE RAID

Andrew Adams brought the Dunkin' the morning of the raid. He was jacked up. By 4 a.m., he'd already had his coffee and was headed to 26 Fed to meet Richards. The war room, where he and Richards would watch the raid unfold and coordinate between the various search and arrest teams and the local prosecutors, was a big, stadium-tiered space with computer screens, TV monitors, and telephones. It was March 2020—just days before the first pandemic shutdown was scheduled to begin—and the world was cold and still. This raid, like almost all raids, would go off at 6 a.m. on the dot. It was pretty tame, as raids go. There was no live news coverage and there were no helicopters with infrared up on the big screens.

Most 6 a.m. raids mean a knock on somebody's front door, finding them in their pajamas or still in bed. But these raids took place at the racetrack. At 6 a.m., everyone was already at work.

At the appointed hour, more than one hundred FBI agents poured onto the backstretch at Monmouth, Gulfstream, and Belmont Park. It was chaotic: "Backstretches were swarming with windbreaker-type people," said one source familiar with the day. The FBI arrested and charged twenty-six people that day, Servis, Navarro, Rhein, Oakes, Surick, and Giannelli among them. (Fishman had already been charged in November.) The day quickly became immortal in racetrack storytelling, as much for who wasn't arrested as who was. Multiple people told me that one prominent Florida-based trainer who was not charged was nevertheless seen "doing an approximation of a 100-yard dash to a dumpster"; no law enforcement officials saw this, according to Richards, and I found no evidence it happened. But like a lot of racetrack rumor, it would be discussed—for years—as a matter of historical record.

After the raid, they were able to seize more evidence. They found medication with homemade labels hidden in the ceiling tiles of Rhein's work trailer at Belmont Park.* Navarro, investigators found, had a pair of custom-made Crocs emblazoned with the words "Juice Man." The FBI also seized defendants' cell phones. On Nick Surick's, the bureau found an image that even years later, Richards would remember. It was a photo of a dead horse in the bucket of a backhoe.

The other thing that Richards would remember later is that no one really believed they were in trouble.

The news of the arrests rocked the sport. There was some schadenfreude among trainers and owners who had competed against Navarro and Servis and some complacency that the majority of those arrested came from harness racing. But above all, an eerie sense of exposure hung heavy over racetracks across the country. Racing people were shocked that the federal government had begun to care about their little domain that for so long had been sheltered from the universe beyond. The charges, too, were confusing. The feds referred to the case in their press releases as a doping case. But the charges were for the FDA violations of drug misbranding and adulteration.

Other fresh evidence from email accounts, barn searches, interviews, and plea deals allowed the Justice Department to broaden the charges on some of the defendants. In November 2020, prosecutors filed what's known as a superseding indictment. Rhein and Servis had originally been charged with misbranding. Now both faced charges of mail and wire fraud conspiracy. Adams's office had finally been able to locate the document they needed to prove those charges: an email from Kristian Rhein's computer showed a provably fraudulent product that was sent to a named recipient, across state lines, listed on a bill, paid for with actual money.

But the investigation was effectively over. For years, rumors continued to circulate on the backstretch that additional arrests of Thoroughbred trainers were coming. It wasn't true. What officials learned after the raid deepened their understanding of the existing defendants and allowed them to layer on additional charges, but it did not broaden their pool of targets, according to one source familiar with the investigation. There were no additional wiretaps, nor was there a situation in which investigators felt they were close

---

* Rhein says that it was a legal medication for the neurological condition EPM that he had color-coded for staff who don't read English—"a lot of the medication was given by people that are illiterate . . . and they will give the wrong thing and they will kill horses"—and that he believes his cleaning lady, frightened, must have hidden the tubes there after the arrests.

to probable cause to apply for one. There was no one that the FBI had been watching who "went underground" after the raids, the same person said.

Investigators were interested in a few other people who were not named in the original indictments, according to another source with knowledge of the investigation, but prosecutors felt they didn't have quite enough to ensure that the charges would stick. At the time, the charges that Adams and his team were bringing were novel. It wasn't a guarantee that they would be successful in front of a judge. "Collectively, we didn't know how it was going to play out," this person said. "We didn't know if people were going to think, 'Good job, FBI, DOJ,' or they were going to think, 'What are you guys doing? Why are you wasting all these resources on this?'"

Some of those people cooperated with the investigation and thus escaped indictment. Others, including a handful of trainers, "could have gotten banged up," this person said. "We had stuff that we could have possibly stretched to get in the courtroom, but they're really kind of bottom-feeders and we [didn't] have great evidence."

Then Adams and Richards retired from federal government, and the Justice Department's interest in racehorse doping waned. For the most part, when it was over, it was over.

There were also persistent rumors that Fishman had maintained a "master list" of Thoroughbred clients. It was said to have been buried, sealed, in the court record. From what I can tell, it doesn't exist—or if it does, it doesn't reflect who was actually buying his products. Fishman appears to have been trying to cultivate additional Thoroughbred business, not conceal it. He kept business records, mainly in the form of Excel spreadsheets documenting, by date, how much of each product was purchased by different clients. Those records, which were introduced in court, show "what actually went out the door," according to one of the sources familiar with the investigation. There are no Thoroughbred trainers on them whose names haven't already been publicized as Fishman clients.*

The FBI investigation was done. But 5 Stones continued its investigation, funded by the Jockey Club. It had already begun to get a little messy.

High on 5 Stones's list was Saffie Joseph Jr., a Florida-based trainer who has made his way up through the claiming ranks.† Shortly before the

---

* There are a handful of clients who are listed only by their first name; it's certainly possible some of these might be Thoroughbred trainers.

† Joseph did not reply to multiple efforts to reach him for comment.

indictments came down, Tim Harrington and two other 5 Stones investigators, Louis Sastre and Steve Diaz, were surveilling his barn on a big stakes day at Gulfstream Park. According to a 5 Stones report, they saw one of Joseph's grooms use a metal syringe to squirt liquid drawn from two buckets of ice water into the mouth of a mare running in a stakes race later that day. Suspecting that the horse had been "drenched" with some kind of water-soluble performance enhancer, they took photographs and drew samples from both water buckets that Diaz packed up and sent to the Hong Kong lab. Afterward, Joseph complained to Gulfstream Park, which had given 5 Stones permission to be on the backside. Much later, Joseph would accuse Harrington of threatening his assistant and planting drugs on him—even though, unbeknownst to Joseph, the test results of the sample the investigators had collected were clear. To 5 Stones, this only made Joseph look more suspicious.

The incident set off a firestorm inside the company that owned both Gulfstream and Pimlico, 1/ST. This was Belinda Stronach's company, the same family-run enterprise that owned Santa Anita, where Bob Baffert is based. Stronach had apparently not been informed of the 5 Stones operation and was caught by surprise when she learned of the episode at Gulfstream. She is known for hating bad press, and several sources told me that she was angry about the situation. Afterward, sources told me, 1/ST cracked down on 5 Stones's access to the backstretch. Joseph, through a lawyer, also later sent letters to the Jockey Club directly raising concerns about the group's work. (The Jockey Club, according to a source close to the organization, insisted it knew nothing about it and directed him to 5 Stones.)

In October 2020, things devolved further. Joseph was at Pimlico in Maryland on the day of the Preakness, the second jewel in the Triple Crown, which was being run in the fall that year because of the pandemic. According to a 5 Stones report, a company contractor named Dennis Turman began surveilling stall 5 in Joseph's barn beginning at about 12:30 that afternoon. Joseph, in a dark suit, with his long hair pulled back in a ponytail and the cuffs of his sleeves rolled up, was attending to Ny Traffic, a New York–bred horse that had run eighth in the Kentucky Derby.

During surveillance, Turman recorded in his report, he observed Joseph produce "a silver colored cylindrical-shaped object with a plunger" and what appeared to be a tube on the opposite end. According to the report, Joseph walked over to a bucket hanging on the fence, placed the silver object inside, pulled back the plunger, and then walked into Ny Traffic's stall. The

5 Stones contractor reported that Joseph repeated this activity several more times over the course of the afternoon.

Eventually, the contractor started videotaping what he was witnessing with his cell phone, according to several sources familiar with the episode. Joseph looked in his direction and spotted him. According to the 5 Stones report, the contractor heard Joseph say, "He's got me on video." Joseph then turned his own phone on the contractor.

Afterward, according to multiple people familiar with the situation, 5 Stones quietly declined to renew Harrington's contract at the end of the year, along with some other investigators working on the case. A 5 Stones executive insisted that this was purely a budgetary decision—the Jockey Club contract was winding down—but the limitations on their access to Gulfstream had been a setback for 5 Stones. Tinsley was convinced that the track was a hotbed of organized crime, according to sources familiar with his thinking at the time, and he was hell-bent on reaping the glory of uncovering it.

For 5 Stones investigators, the moral of the story was obvious: as far as the racetrack was concerned, catching dopers was all well and good—as long as it didn't interfere with the bottom line. The investigators believed they had credible evidence that Saffie Joseph was a cheater. But they concluded that for 1/ST, the more important thing was the full fields that made a good wagering product. Full fields meant profit. Like Baffert at Santa Anita, Saffie Joseph was a valuable commodity to Gulfstream. He ran horses in hundreds of races that year, and he helped fill the kind of workaday claimers and allowance races that for a racetrack are money in the bank.

There's a weakness with that theory. The activity that 5 Stones had observed—using a syringe to squirt water in a horse's mouth prior to racing—was a commonplace practice going back many years. Rinsing out the inside of a horse's mouth prior to putting the tongue tie on was a key part of softening the fabric of the tongue tie and making sure there was no hay or food matter inside the animal's mouth that it could choke on while running. Countless horsemen used the kind of metal plunger that the 5 Stones investigators observed Joseph using. The practice has become less common in recent years, multiple trainers told me, as race-day rules have tightened, and trainers have grown wary of exposing themselves to even the perception that they might be doping. Nowadays most trainers use a wet sponge for the purpose instead—but some trainers still use the old metal syringes. The 5 Stones interpretation of the episode raised questions about how well the Jockey Club's private investigators understood the industry they had been sent to police.

It took more than three years for all the defendants to work their way through the court system. Many cut a plea deal quickly, including Jorge Navarro, who was sentenced to five years in prison and ordered to forfeit more than $25 million. Although he was in the country legally, he is not a citizen and will almost certainly be deported to Panama when he is released, according to his lawyer. For Jorge Navarro, the American dream is over—an infinitely harsher punishment than his white codefendants, born in the United States, will face.

On the stand, faced with the full measure of the US Justice Department, few of the defendants came off as criminal masterminds. Most of them were hardly the "big fish" the Jockey Club had said it wanted. Living in his tack room and limping along with his tiny stable, Tannuzzo would likely have earned about $60,000 in 2019—before expenses. He was sentenced to more than two years. Rick Dane, one of the harness trainers, had grown up with an alcoholic father who, according to court documents, remarried approximately thirteen times, including once at the age of sixty to Dane's nineteen-year-old maternal half sister. Horses offered him a kind of solace, an escape from the chaos at home, and he had dropped out of school at sixteen to try to make it at the racetrack.[1] He was sentenced to thirty months in prison.[2] A horse owner associated with Navarro told the judge that it was a shame that Navarro "feels, as he puts it, 'he has to prove himself because he's brown.'" He wrote: "I would not try to defend him or make excuses, but I will say he is a product of being raised backside at the racetrack."[3] His mother-in-law told the judge that Navarro had "lost everything when they took his livelihood and his horses away from him. He has been through enough trying to prove his worth to all the upper classmen [sic]."[4]

Fishman and Servis elected to fight the charges. In the months following his arrest in the Miami airport in October 2019, the government said, Fishman continued his drug distribution business through Lisa Giannelli while himself keeping "a low profile."[5] In one unexpected development that seemed to hint that there could be some truth to the vet's boasting about his work for Dubai's Sheikh Mohammed, a lawyer claiming to represent a handful of Emirati organizations, including the "Presidential Camel Department" and the Dubai Equine hospital, filed a motion in a federal court in Florida arguing that they had purchased the drugs that the FBI had seized from Fishman, and that the US government had no right to hold them. The vials, they said, were for use during the camel and horse breeding season and were not intended for performance animals.

According to court documents, Fishman appears to have orchestrated this intervention behind the scenes. In December 2019, several months after his arrest and a few months before the court filing, he exchanged emails with a person named Adel, who was his distributor in Dubai.

"Please remember that products were also requested by certain vets working for private stables owned by HH," Fishman wrote to Adel, using a common reference to Sheikh Mohammed, or "His Highness." The issue would need to be raised with "the Palace," he said, "because there are likely implications that go far beyond any importer or hospital."

"My fears are that a few young and inexperienced US officials eager to make major headlines without understanding the politics will loose site [*sic*] of their objective quickly. In respect to the crown I think being overly proactive would be far more appreciated than reactive," Fishman said.[6]

The feds ultimately denied Dubai's request to have the products returned, and the entire episode appeared to fade away in US racing. Godolphin, Sheikh Mohammed's international racing and breeding operation, continued business as usual in the United States. In 2024, Godolphin had more than fifty horses in training in America.*[7]

Fishman's case went to trial in February 2022, but he missed the last two days of it when he was hospitalized for a week following an apparent suicide attempt. According to one source familiar with the matter, he swallowed a fistful of a common anti-anxiety medication in a move that law enforcement officials, rightly or wrongly, saw as calculated. During his sentencing, his lawyer asked for leniency because of his "substantial" psychiatric disabilities; his father told the court that Fishman never intended to do harm, but he "still exhibits poor judgment in making decisions. . . . Seth only sees black and white; he doesn't see gray. He is a complex person." A physician told the court that Fishman "has suffered from poorly managed symptoms of Bipolar II Disorder and Attention Deficit/Hyperactivity Disorder for the entirety of his adulthood that have been compounded by the abuse of various substances."

Judge Mary Kay Vyskocil was unmoved. She sentenced the vet to eleven years. Fishman's face was expressionless.[8]

"I have no desire to make another substance for a racehorse again," Fishman told the court.

---

* From 2009 to 2011, I was the beneficiary of a two-year management training program offered as a fully funded scholarship by Godolphin.

Vyskocil sentenced the last of the Thoroughbred defendants on a warm day in July 2023. Jason Servis sat in the stand, shrunken and turtled into himself like an old man. The shoulders of his sport coat were too big, inflated over thin shoulders. On a plain bench in the back of the grand courtroom in lower Manhattan, Shaun Richards, now retired, sat anonymously and listened.

Servis took the microphone to address the court. According to Rita Glavin, his well-heeled defense attorney, he had lost twenty pounds over the last three years.

"Um," he began. He gave a ragged sob, his shoulders shuddering, and Glavin pulled the mic away.

"Why don't we take a brief break," the judge suggested. But Servis wanted to proceed. He had memorized his statement but decided in the moment just to read it.

"There are no words to explain how remorseful and sorry I am for the decisions I made," he told the court, still sobbing. "The people I've let down and hurt, my wife especially."

Richards sat with his legs stretched out, crossed at the ankles.

"I am most truly sorry as I throw myself at the mercy of the court," Servis said.

That was all.

Richards had sat in, now, for three years' worth of trials, plea deals, and sentencings. It stunned him every time that the defendants, when given their chance to speak, would apologize to family, to staff, to owners—but never to the horse. They never apologized to the animal. Servis had been no different, and to Richards, he was no different.

Yet in a few key ways, Servis was different. His horses had not died of heart arrhythmias and broken legs. The two drugs he used, SGF-1000 and compounded clenbuterol, were marketed as a supplement, and perfectly legal in its FDA-approved form. Although he had taken steps to hide his drugs from regulators, he had exhibited none of the cavalier celebration of cheating that Navarro had. Although it's true that Servis potentially risked his horses' health by giving them compounded drugs that were not federally approved, it's not clear at all that he believed at the time or even later that those drugs posed any danger to his horses.

The picture that Glavin presented to the court to argue for leniency was an image of a naïf, an unsophisticated innocent misled by bad associations, someone whose conduct was so commonplace that even when it was brought to his attention that it was under legal scrutiny, he couldn't fathom stopping. When the state police approached him, she said, he lied about the extent of his use of SGF-1000 because he "completely freaked out." But, she said, he discussed getting a lawyer because he wanted an attorney to "clear things up," not lie on his behalf. When he split a bottle of clenbuterol between multiple horses without a prescription, he was merely following routine racetrack practice. There was a "fundamental decency" to Servis, Glavin insisted. He had made a mistake, he said, in trusting Kristian Rhein, who "lied to him" by representing that SGF-1000 was permissible and safe. The greatest regret of his life, she said, was being stabled next to Navarro. "That's how this happened," Glavin insisted. Navarro had led him astray.

The unstated current beneath Glavin's argument was that Servis had lived his life within the warped logic of the racetrack. He had done the best he could—perhaps better than others—and she suggested he could hardly be judged for being unable to see where the rules of his world collided with the rules the rest of the world lived by.

There is some moral relativism to this argument. But she was right that the courtroom on Pearl Street was as far from the backstretch of a racetrack as it was possible to be. It's almost hard to read the government's submissions with an old racetracker's eye. I can see where they are simply not speaking the same language. Even in open court, when the judge referred to Servis's years as a "valet," she mispronounced the word, using the technically correct "val-EY" rather than the correct racetrack pronunciation.

It might sound bonkers to the rest of the world, used to living by inviolable rules set by federal, state, and local government. But inside racing, there has always been a certain blurriness around the edges. Jason Servis had lived his entire professional life inside a regulatory scheme that was different in every state he operated in, where the rules changed constantly and so did the drugs, where there was never any real penalty for using even the really serious stuff—much less a drug that would have been legal but for a little paperwork—where in the old days, no one would have bothered you about a prescription for a goddamn *horse*. What mattered, culturally, was whether you were a good horseman and what mattered financially was whether you won races, and what mattered least was whether you followed every little rule to do it. Where everyone else was doing what you were, or worse, and if you wanted to pay the bills, you'd better keep doing it too. Where, within some unwritten reasonable limit, a little touch of larceny was all part of the fun. In the universe in which Jason Servis had lived his entire life, that "reasonable limit" had always been like the proverbial definition of obscenity. It was a matter of debate, to be had while leaning on the rail when the first set was just hitting the track.

"You cheated, you lied, and you broke the law," Vyskocil said. "You did endanger the horses in your care. Luckily, they didn't break down. You tried to gain an unfair advantage. I hope you accept that but I'm not sure you do."[9]

She was probably right.

In the online marketplace of equine drugs, you can today buy something called SGF-5000, from a company claiming to be based in Jacksonville, Florida, for two hundred dollars a bottle. The website promises that the little vial contains the "worlds [sic] most potent super growth factors" that will "take your horse . . . to a new level of competitiveness."[10]

There were things that nagged at Shaun Richards and Andrew Adams long after the case was done. Richards told me that New York regulators, for reasons that were unclear to him, would only grant him a license for harness tracks in the state, not Thoroughbreds—effectively preventing him from doing clandestine out-of-competition testing he wanted to do at Saratoga and Belmont in 2018.[11] Investigators had also never been able to develop any evidence that might allow them to figure out what Surick was talking about when he said he had helped make "six horses" disappear for Navarro. And they hadn't been able to get anywhere near Bob Baffert. The FBI hadn't specifically targeted Baffert, which isn't permitted under bureau rules, but they had certainly heard rumors and asked questions. Ultimately, none of the sources who brought so-called tips about Baffert to the bureau had anything that the FBI refers to as "actionable": information that is substantial enough to satisfy a probable cause warrant for a wiretap, for example. The bureau didn't learn anything concrete enough to be able to legitimately investigate. They were never able to develop sources who had current access to Baffert's operation. The allegations against Baffert remained what they had always been: supposition and rumor. After the indictments became public, the owners of Maximum Security sent the horse to Baffert to train.*

---

* Baffert told me that Maximum Security had been known as a difficult animal to handle when he was with Servis, but that in his barn, he was "just so quiet." Like everyone, Baffert had been following the indictments. He blamed the changes in the horse's demeanor on Servis's administration of "that high-powered Mexican clenbuterol"—not the SGF-1000, which he said he had heard didn't do much to a horse. Bob Baffert, January 2, 2023.

There had been some limitations on the FBI. To investigate Baffert, the bureau would have needed evidence that he had committed a crime that in some way touched the state of New York, where Richards and his team had what's known as "venue"—a court they knew would hear the case. Baffert was based in California. The scope of his activities, and the opportunities for catching him committing a hypothetical crime, were much narrower on the East Coast.

But within two years, 5 Stones would ink another important contract. Their client this time wasn't Stuart Janney and the Jockey Club but another one of racing's most powerful institutions. This time the intelligence firm's investigation had much bigger targets. Among them was Bob Baffert.

PART III

THE FINISH LINE

◆

It should come as no surprise that the sport's tragic flaw is the same volatile combination that did in the societal concept of "Americana" itself: Innocence, coupled with an unwillingness to change, eventually reveals itself in the long run as a sucker's bet.

—T. D. Thornton, *Not by a Long Shot*

CHAPTER 19

ALL HEART

The first thing Gail Rice noticed when she pulled into the driveway of her son Kevin's small Florida breeding farm was that one of her mares was lying down. This particular mare, a big bay horse named Mongolian Changa, was three weeks overdue to have her foal. Maiden mares are often late, but on this afternoon in early April 2018, Changa was very late. She had shown no signs of developing a bag full of milk. But when Rice reached her side in the paddock, it was clear to her that she had gone into labor. Rice checked under the mare's tail and found two things: The foal was positioned far too high. And the mare's vaginal opening hadn't relaxed.

She screamed for Kevin and Emily, her daughter-in-law.

When all goes well, horses enter the world front feet first. They dive out of their mothers in a Superman posture, with their noses cradled between two tiny hooves. When a mare goes into labor, the foaling manager will put a hand inside the mare to check that he can feel the two front feet and the round hump of the foal's soft muzzle. When the nose emerges, the foaling person will break the sack so the foal isn't deprived of oxygen. Once the shoulders clear the mare's pelvis, the hard work is done and the rest of the foal usually slides out in a single gush. There is something magical about the experience for even the most hardened horseman. The little wet foal shivers in a tangle of cartoonishly long limbs, stunned and dumb with the shock of new existence. The mare licks her baby dry, with a little help from the foaling person and a bath towel. Within an hour and a few lurching false starts, the foal will stand on splayed legs. The foaling person will plug him on to the teat if he gets lost. It is a beginning, full of innocence and possibility. There is a reason they call birth a miracle.

Gail Rice was worried that this birth was not going to proceed as Mother Nature intended. She coaxed the mare into standing and led her out of the herd of other broodmares and into another small, grassy paddock where she could deliver her foal alone. Emily had heard her call and come running out of the house to help. Her son, though, was heeding another call of nature and hadn't come. The two women hollered for him at the top of their lungs, to no avail. They called him, but his phone, on silent in the living room, went unanswered.

She could do this, Rice thought. While still married to her ex-husband, she had spent the last few years foaling out dozens of mares, and had handled some difficult births. She knew what to do.

"I'm gonna pull this kid out," she told Emily.

First she used her hands to stretch the mare's vaginal opening so it wouldn't tear. Then she had Emily take over stretching the mare while she reached inside to reposition the foal's feet so they were pointing down and out. Both women were still screaming at the house. *Kevin, come on, we're having a baby!*

Rice knew she needed to help pull the foal from the mare, lest he suffocate during a lengthy birth. She wrapped her hands around the foal's ankles and pulled with the mare's contractions, letting her dictate the pace. It's hellishly hard work, pulling a foal from a mare. Rice is laced with muscles from working with horses, but she's petite, just five-foot-five. She had Emily hold the mare's vagina open while she put a boot up against either side of the mare's rump and pulled for all she was worth. But she couldn't pull Changa's foal out herself.

Kevin, having exercised his male prerogative in such situations to take his sweet time, eventually came into the living room and noticed the missed calls on his cell phone. He stuck his head out of the door.

"Do you guys need me?" he called out.

Get out here now. We can't pull this baby out! The women were screaming. It took all three of them to get him out. The colt that would become perhaps the most argued-over Kentucky Derby winner in history slipped into the world in one final rush. He was dark brown, so dark that by adulthood he would appear black. He had just the faintest flicker of white between his eyes and a single white sock on his right hind foot. Even at birth there was something about him that caught your eye. He was mature-looking, strong, balanced. He had a kind and intelligent eye.

When horses are born, their hooves are soft. The soles are lined with rubbery, featherlike protrusions that are part of a capsule thought to protect the mother while the baby is in utero. Horsemen call them by a variety of names. One of those names is angel slippers. Rice felt certain that God had engineered the safe birth of this foal. He had been the tiny voice in her ear, telling her to drive home in time to find Changa lying down in the paddock. He had given her the tools and the experience to know how to deliver the colt safely. He had lined it all up.

The year Changa's foal was born, Rice was living in a Sunset Trail RV, parked under the bright blue overhang of one of the barns on Kevin and Emily's ten-acre farm. She was a long way from the grand breeding operations of central Kentucky. She had a handful of cheap mares, including Changa, and when she'd left her husband—a second marriage—she'd taken them with her, determined to make a go of it in the horse business.

Rice, who was originally from Pennsylvania, hadn't grown up with horses. In fact, she was scared to death of them. But she went to high school with Wayne Rice, the son of a horse trader and trainer who became the patriarch of a sprawling dynasty of trainers, jockeys, and horse traders. (Wayne's sister, Linda Rice, is a successful trainer in New York; Wayne was a jockey and then a Thoroughbred trainer; various other family members work in the bloodstock business.) Gail and Wayne lost contact after graduation, but reconnected years later when they ran into each other at the local hangout near Penn National Race Course. The bar was inside a Holiday Inn and was called the Winner's Circle Saloon. It was the kind of place that had a mechanical bull and played nothing but country music on the jukebox. Rice was twenty-one and working a computer job on a military base. Wayne was trying to make it as a jockey. He took her to the track and taught her how to muck a stall.[1]

Rice fell in love with horses. Wayne began working in the two-year-old business, preparing unraced horses to breeze an eighth or a quarter mile at auction, and for Rice, watching young horses grow up took hold of her in a way that would shape the rest of her life. "Oh, my God, it just got me," she said, years later. "My heart was in it. I just love them, and I haven't been able to stop."[2] When the couple split up, in the 1990s, she continued in the business.

More than anything, Rice wanted to make it as a breeder. She harbored, deep down, the dream of selling a million-dollar horse that she had bred. She had always been surrounded by babies. When she was married to Wayne, everything on the place got bred—the dog, the ponies, the quarter horse. She'd had three children herself.

But by the time Changa's foal was born, Rice was broke. She couldn't afford to keep all her horses, and she didn't want to get "a real job"—a job away from the animals she loved so much. Her life revolved around them. Her horses ate before she did. And so she made a difficult decision: to sell Changa and her foal, and one other foal from a different mare. It's the tragic paradox for anyone who chooses to make a living with animals because they love animals: at some point, those animals must make money, which often means letting them go. It was hard to do: she had grown attached to Changa's foal. He had an attitude with the other babies in the paddock. No one pushed him around. Rice loved him.

"He is gonna be a racehorse," Rice told Emily.[3]

Rice grossed $75,000 on the three horses.[4] But Changa's colt, the colt whose birth God had engineered, made only $1,000.

It made sense. He was a nice-looking foal, but he had no pedigree to speak of. In the market for unproven racehorses, there were better bets out there. The colt was purchased by Christy Whitman, who made her living by buying weanlings and yearlings and selling them as two-year-olds. Known as "pinhooking," it's a business model not unlike flipping houses. Buying cheap is one way to make money, especially if you think the horse's physical appearance might improve with time. It's a difficult and risky business—predicting how a young horse will mature is a crystal-ball endeavor, and, as always with horses, your investment might suddenly decide to run through a fence—but it comes with the tantalizing possibility of a big windfall.

Whitman took the horse to a July sale in Florida for two-year-olds in training. Rice was working the sale for a friend, and she stopped by her little brown colt's stall several times. She watched from across the street as he was led to the auction ring. *Good luck!* she thought. *I hope you make lots of money!*

The lot of the Thoroughbred—especially the modern Thoroughbred—is to move from place to place with the changing of money. Where he lives, how often he travels, in whose barn he resides and for how long is defined by what he is worth—or what someone decides he is worth. (Penny Chenery, the breeder of Secretariat, once commented, "The price does not always represent what a horse is worth. It is only what some fool thinks he is worth.")[5] Perhaps the only place he commands his own destiny is on the racetrack, whether or not he knows it.

Changa's colt changed his destiny at the 2020 Ocala Breeders' Sales Company's July sale for horses in training.

It was hot at OBS. The sun beat down on man and beast. Horses dripped sweat in skeins off their bellies. Bloodstock agents in dusty paddock boots and tennis shoes shuffled, sapped, from one barn to the next studying the more than one thousand horses scheduled to go through the ring over the next two days. They were looking for a horse they thought could win, a horse they thought they could afford, and a buyer to pay for it.

Changa's colt was slight, but he had what horsemen call a racy body. He still sported the dark, almost black coat of his sire, Protonico. When he was sent to the track to breeze, he sizzled through three-eighths of a mile in :33 flat. Bloodstock agent Gary Young was among those watching. He scribbled a note on the horse's catalog page: *Natural router stride.*

Still, the horse wasn't on his list. He was shopping for Amr Zedan, a Saudi Arabian businessman born in Los Angeles who had given him a $1 million budget. The colt by Protonico would bring nowhere near that. If he were by one of the more fashionable sires—Tapit or Into Mischief—he would have been far more expensive, but Changa's colt had to prove his worth on speed and looks alone.

Besides, Young was done shopping. He had already spent his budget on a gorgeous filly that cost $1.35 million.

But then Zedan called him.

Zedan was new to the sport. In his midforties, handsome, and intensely competitive, Zedan was also, certifiably, horse crazy. He played polo and liked fast cars, but what he really wanted to do was win the Kentucky Derby. He had bumped into Baffert on a layover in the lounge at the Dubai airport in 2020 and together, the two sketched out a plan on a cocktail napkin. The plan included the $1.35 million filly. (I will turn her into a $3 million horse, Baffert texted him when Zedan was backing off the bidding at $1.2 million.)[6] It did not, necessarily, include a no-pedigree colt by Protonico. But Zedan had received a phone call from a friend who owned the stallion. The friend had suggested that Zedan take a look at Changa's foal. Zedan sent the agent to look at the horse and ran the idea by his trainer. Young and Baffert both agreed that the little brown horse had some potential. Zedan told Young to bid on him.

And so Changa's foal changed hands yet again, this time for $35,000—still a pittance. The leggy brown colt was loaded onto an airplane and took off into the sky. He was headed for California, to Bob Baffert.

Eventually, anyway. His first stop was Los Alamitos, where Mike Marlow ran Baffert's two-year-old barn. Marlow would get the horses about 75 percent ready to run before they were shipped to Santa Anita, where Baffert would take over their conditioning.

Marlow was a lifetime horseman who had worked thirteen years for D. Wayne Lukas. He had tried training horses himself, but couldn't make a go of it and eventually wound up working for Baffert in the early 2000s. Lean and weathered as an old bois d'arc fence post in a ten-gallon hat, Marlow was an excellent horseman. He was friendly and quick to tease, but he was also blunt. He told you what he thought.

"Bob, what is this thing?" he said to Baffert. Most of the two-year-olds that came off the plane from the sales were monsters. They were tall, heavily muscled, and came from well-bred matriarchs. Marlow didn't know the pedigrees or the sales price for any of the horses that came into his barn, and he didn't much care. But he knew that the little brown colt known then only by his mother's name and his birth year—"Mongolian Changa '19"—wasn't much to look at. He was spare and narrow through the chest.

"What do you mean?" Baffert asked.

"Well, there's just not much there," Marlow said.

"Just train him and get him ready," Baffert said. Marlow had a good program. The horse would either show himself or not.

Marlow shrugged and went to work.

Los Alamitos is a good place to train two-year-olds. The track doesn't keep its dirt surface very deep because of the quarter horse races there, typically run on a harder, faster track, so young Thoroughbreds are able to skim over the track like birds. It's a forgiving surface.

Marlow gave the horse a day of just jogging so he could get used to his new surroundings. Then he started galloping him. He never expected too much right away from the horses that had come from the two-year-old sales. Most of them either regressed physically or their brains were so scrambled from the pressure of the sales environment and travel that they needed a little break. Just because a horse had blistered through an eighth of a mile in under ten seconds at the sale didn't mean he was fit, mentally or physically.

It just meant he had some natural speed, Marlow said, and "they jacked his ass up, and had him ready to sell because he's fast." Most racetrackers assume that they have routinely been given clenbuterol or other drugs to get them to peak during their breeze show at the sale.

Marlow followed the Bob Baffert school of thought for training Thoroughbred racehorses: he trained off his eye. Some trainers follow a strict routine, putting each horse through a standard calendar of gradually progressing workouts. Marlow wouldn't intensify a horse's workload until he asked for it.

"When they're coming down to the wire and the rider's like this"—Marlow mimed a rider's upturned hand, holding a horse that is pulling—"and they're dragging him down to the wire, they're ready to move forward," he said. "We don't allow the riders to push and shove—that's not in our program. We want the horses to do it on their own and the rider just to have a little pressure on the reins and let the horse take you for the ride."[7]

The goal was to get the horse fitter than his competitors. Both Marlow and Baffert were aware that Baffert's critics complained that his horses "re-broke" in the stretch, something they saw as evidence of blood doping. But Marlow and Baffert both insist that their horses are capable of doing that because they are just plain fit.

"For Bob, if he can't go to the gate and work three quarters in [a minute and twelve seconds], he's not ready—because for Bob, and I think there's a lot of truth to it, tiredness creates injury." The horse might be able to run, Marlow said, "but your odds are in favor of him getting hurt because you're pushing past his limit. That is very important with two-year-olds."*

Mongolian Changa '19—a terrible name, Marlow thought—got his first real piece of work on August 21, a four-furlong breeze. He had looked fine galloping, but nothing special. By September, Mongolian Changa '19 got his own name, and he started to show Marlow something in his weekly breeze. At first Marlow thought maybe he had just had a good day here or there. But by the time the colt had ticked off a few four-furlong works, in

---

* The racing industry is often criticized for running two-year-olds at all. Horses have hit most of the major markers of physical maturity, like the closure of growth plates in the legs, by the age of two. But they will continue to develop until they are six years old, and critics of the sport complain that running unformed animals leads to breakdowns. The science doesn't bear this theory out, however. Although it's obviously possible to push a two-year-old too hard, in general, studies have shown that horses that run at two stay sound longer. This is because of a process called "bone remodeling": the stress of training causes micro-injuries to the bone, which then repairs itself to become stronger over time.

48 seconds, 49 seconds, 48 seconds, and then 47 seconds, Marlow thought that this Medina Spirit horse might be a good one. Nobody was more surprised than Mike Marlow.

Medina Spirit was an easy horse to be around, even as a baby. Marlow remembered him as workmanlike on the track, a professional. In the barn, he was laid-back. Some of the big colts were so tough to handle that it took two hot-walkers, one on each side, to safely walk the horse around the shed row. Not Medina. He had what horsemen praise as "a good mind."

Normally, Marlow liked to give the two-year-olds their first five-furlong breeze from "the pole"—meaning that the rider simply cues the horse to speed up at a particular furlong marker, rather than having him start from a standstill by breaking out of the starting gate. But Medina Spirit had impressed him enough that Marlow sent him straight from the gate. Five furlongs was what separated the good horses from the mediocre. If they could work five furlongs in a minute and change while dragging their rider out of the saddle, they were probably good horses. Medina Spirit did it in 1:01. By the end of the month, he was covering the ground in a minute flat. Marlow put him on the van to Santa Anita on October 26.

He called Baffert, telling him: "Now, don't judge this horse when he comes off the van. Judge him for what you see on the racetrack."[8]

What Baffert saw on the racetrack was a runner. He saw it when he started working the horse.

"The really good ones, they don't have a bottom," he said later. "They just don't get tired. They just keep going."

Medina Spirit didn't get tired.

Baffert ran him for the first time in a maiden special weight at Los Alamitos in December 2020. Medina Spirit won by three lengths. On January 1, 2021, he officially turned three. He made his next start that month in the Grade III Sham Stakes at Santa Anita and finished under a length shy of a horse Baffert considered one of his top three-year-olds, Life Is Good. And he was gaining all the way. Baffert thought to himself, *Is this little horse this good? Or is Life Is Good not as good as I thought he was?*

Medina Spirit answered that question in his next start, the Grade III Robert B. Lewis Stakes. He went off as the even-money betting favorite, set the pace from the start, and held on gamely to win by a neck.

Still, he continued to be overshadowed by Life Is Good. Life Is Good had run only three times, but he was brilliantly fast. And he was by one of the most fashionable sires of the time, Into Mischief. He was everything

Medina Spirit was not: mainly, expensive. In March he beat Medina Spirit again in the Grade II San Felipe, this time by eight lengths.

Then, later that month, Life Is Good emerged from a routine workout lame in his left hind leg.[9] He was sent to Kentucky to have a chip surgically removed from his ankle, and although he would return by the end of the year and win the Grade I Breeders' Cup Dirt Mile, Life Is Good was off the Derby trail. Medina Spirit had become "the big horse."

Baffert entered Medina Spirit in the Grade I Santa Anita Derby, where he finished second by four lengths to a horse named Rock Your World. It was a valiant effort, but Medina Spirit was never able to get on the lead, where he excelled. "They get on the lead, they get brave," Baffert said.

Entry to the Kentucky Derby is based on a points system. Horses are awarded a certain number of points for first, second, and third place in a set of official prep races. Some races, like the Santa Anita Derby, offer so many points that winning that race alone effectively guarantees entry. Medina Spirit gained entry to the Derby the hard way: racking up enough points by winning multiple smaller stakes—and running second in one big one. When he shipped to Churchill in April 2021, no one, including Bob Baffert, really thought he was going to win. The night before the Derby, at a Louisville steakhouse, Baffert ran into Cris Collinsworth, the NBC sportscaster and former pro NFL player. Collinsworth asked him if he had a shot.

"I don't know," Baffert said. "I think I can light the board."[10]

Baffert thought that if Medina Spirit could get on the lead, he could take home a check. He certainly didn't expect to win the race. The chatter going into the Derby was that other trainers were going to send their horse to the front early to prevent Medina from getting loose on the lead. They weren't going to give him the race he wanted.[11]

The 2021 Kentucky Derby was run under a clear blue sky. The world was beginning to recover from the Covid-19 pandemic. Baffert felt he had put all that nonsense with the lidocaine positives in Arkansas behind him. It was almost fun to fly under the radar at the Derby for once. There was less pressure. The NBC broadcasters barely mentioned Medina Spirit. "Don't know if he's the best in this class, in this field," one of them remarked, before turning his attention back to the favorite, a big gray horse named Essential Quality.

In the paddock, D. Wayne Lukas, as cool as ever in his trademark aviators, gave the "Riders up!" call, given before all races but of particular moment in the Derby. Johnny Velasquez was lofted into the saddle. Medina Spirit, slim and unobtrusive, walked calmly to the post. His big, soft ears almost flopped back and forth.

Twenty three-year-olds entered the starting stalls. The big drama at Churchill Downs that year was the new starting gate, debuted the year before, which had narrower stalls. Medina Spirit fit in just fine. The bell rang and he snapped out of the gate smartly in the frantic cavalry charge that marks the start of every Derby. He went right to the lead. It was as if it had all been lined up for him.

He was challenged right from the beginning. A 26-1 shot named Soup and Sandwich pressed his pace, settled just outside of his hip going into the first turn. But Medina Spirit galloped along comfortably out of the turn and into the backstretch, no fuss, no drama, his big ears flicking back and forth as Velasquez's elbows drew and relaxed in rhythm with his low stride. This was a comfortable horse.

The pack made its way around the far turn. The roar of the crowd built to a crescendo. Soup and Sandwich couldn't maintain the pace and, in the horseman's dialect, "ran backwards." The big gray favorite, Essential Quality, began to make his move on the outside. The blue-blooded Mandaloun had ranged up to pressure Medina Spirit, attaching himself to his hip like a burr, then drawing abreast of him, matching him stride for stride coming out of the turn. Velasquez went to his whip, pumping, pushing, riding. The field fanned out in the stretch. Three other horses were making a bid for it as the finish line loomed. Watching from the paddock, Baffert felt sure: *Now is when they're going to swallow him.*[12] Zedan, in a booth in the grandstand, was praying: *Allah maeak. Allah maeak. God be with you. God be with you.*[13]

But then, they didn't swallow him. Mandaloun stayed glued to Medina's hip, gamely fighting for the lead. The little horse from nowhere wouldn't give it to him. He simply would not let them pass.

"Here's the wire!" cried race caller Larry Collmus, as Medina Spirit dove for the finish line, a neck ahead of Mandaloun, a length ahead of Essential Quality and Hot Rod Charlie, daylight between them and the rest, having never given up the lead from the moment he seized it.

"Bob Baffert does it again. Medina Spirit has won the Kentucky Derby!"

Zedan wept. In the boxes, Gail Rice nearly toppled the folding chair she was standing on. She leaped off it and ran madly for the winner's circle. On the way, she grabbed people by the arms: "I pulled him out of his mother!" she cried. "I pulled him out of his mother!" She couldn't stop saying it. She didn't have the right pass, but she didn't care. She blew past the security guard and into the winner's circle. *I'm gonna hug my horse.* By the time she got through the throng and into the crowded winner's circle, they had already taken the photo and Medina Spirit had been unsaddled. A white rind of dried salt ringed his eye. Rice tapped Baffert on the shoulder. She knew he didn't know her, but she didn't care. *I have to touch my horse. I have to.*

"Can I hug my horse?" she asked.

"Well—" Baffert said.

Rice didn't wait for him to answer.[14]

Amid the chaos, she went to Medina Spirit's head. She stroked his neck once so he wouldn't be startled, then put a hand on his poll and a hand across his nose and pressed her mouth to the long plane of his face.

Baffert had walked to the winner's circle holding his wife, Jill's, hand. He had just won the Kentucky Derby a record-setting seven times. And he had done it with a horse that once cost just $1,000.

Medina Spirit trotted back to the winner's circle on a loose line, ears pricked, unfazed by the screaming crowds. He looked relaxed, even happy. Velasquez, one hand on the buckle of the reins, patted him. The little horse had done it on all guts, Baffert thought. He had *heart*. What heart he had.

"If you have him on the lead, he'll fight," Baffert told the television cameras. "I cannot believe he won this race. That little horse—that was him. It was all guts."

Baffert was the iconic picture of himself: smart yellow tie, a thick hank of white hair flopped over his tan brow, rimless blue sunglasses under a brilliant Louisville sun, flanked by a millionaire and waiting to put his hand on the trophy for the Kentucky Derby. He seemed untouchable. Once again, for no particular reason Baffert could discern, fate had smiled on him.

"I'm the luckiest guy in the world," he told the TV cameras.[15]

CHAPTER 20

THE POSITIVE

Model planes and propellers dotted the brick walls of the LA sports grill where Bob and Jill Baffert had stopped to get a bite to eat. They weren't far from the tiny metropolitan airport where the private plane they were taking to Kentucky was being serviced. It was a week after the Derby. Medina Spirit was still in Louisville, where he would stay while Baffert made a decision about running the horse in the Preakness. He and Jill were on their way back to the bluegrass to watch him train, but there had been a problem with the plane and now they had some time to kill while the mechanics worked.

As he slid into his seat, overlooked by American flags and black-and-white photos of old planes, Baffert was feeling pretty good. It wasn't just that he had won the Kentucky Derby an unprecedented seventh time, breaking the previous record of six, which had stood for nearly seventy years. And it wasn't even the way he had done it, with a Cinderella horse that no one else had recognized or wanted, although that was a big part of it. It was how easy it had all seemed. He hadn't really expected to win with Medina Spirit, and so he hadn't put any pressure on himself. The Derby, for once, had been a relaxing experience, even fun. And it had stayed light and fun. Baffert was sixty-eight years old, his hard-partying days behind him. A moment of ease seemed to have come into the rodeo of his life.

Something was nagging at him, lurking in the back of his mind. Someone—one of the many *this guys* and *someones* in Baffert's narrative style—had told him that the *New York Times*' Joe Drape was working on a story about him, something bad. It seemed to Baffert that no matter how much he accomplished, his enemies would always find a reason to come after him. But he had put it out of his mind. What could Drape possibly have to say now?

Bob ordered a Diet Coke while Jill went to the bathroom. His phone jingled the Indiana Jones theme song, his ringtone for his assistant trainers—a signal that he should pick up. Baffert was running a handful of other horses at Churchill that day and so he wasn't surprised to see it was Jimmy, good old soldierly Jimmy, who was still out in Kentucky with Medina and the other horses.

"Hey, Jimmy, what's happening?"

"Something really bad is happening," his assistant trainer said. "Something . . . something really bad happened."

The Kentucky Horse Racing Commission was searching the barn, Barnes said. They had told him that Baffert had gotten a positive test result, for Medina Spirit.

The color drained out of Baffert's face.

"For what?" he asked.

"Betamethasone."

"You've got to be shitting me."

Betamethasone was the corticosteroid that the filly Gamine had received a positive test for in the Kentucky Oaks the year before—the one that he had been surprised to learn from Kentucky Horse Racing Commission steward Barbara Borden was now a "zero-tolerance" drug, one with no threshold level to account for a lingering presence in a horse's system. Over the next year, Baffert would testify under oath multiple times that after Gamine tested positive, he had instructed his vet, Dr. Vince Baker, that he was no longer to use any joint injection products containing betamethasone. (There are, of course, other corticosteroids.)

Baffert called Baker as soon as he got off the phone with Barnes. According to testimony Baffert gave under oath, Baker told him that there was no way the horse had received betamethasone.

Baffert's next phone call was with the three Kentucky Horse Racing Commission stewards. For more than ten minutes, the stewards spoke no more than a few half sentences while Baffert launched into a tirade. He barely paused for breath.

"This is gonna just do me in. . . . Something is not right with that. I don't know what's going on. I don't know if they're pissed-off at me or what," Baffert began.[1] It wasn't clear who "they" was supposed to refer to, but over the next ten minutes, he would return many times to the idea of some mysterious "them" who were out to get him.

"I'm telling you, this is gonna be the worst thing ever for me," he went on as the three stewards listened, mostly in silence. Unbeknownst to Baffert at the time, they were quietly recording the call.[2] "That little horse doesn't deserve this. He didn't get treated with that, and I don't deserve it and it's just bullshit and I don't know what to say to you guys, but somebody made a mistake in the lab or whatever. . . .

"Nobody's gonna believe me, but we got all the records. . . . There's something drastically wrong, something went wrong in the testing. . . . I'm in shock. I cannot believe I have to go through this crap again. This is wrong. . . . There's gotta be an investigation. . . . We do not use beta— We're not that stupid. . . . There's something going on in Kentucky that's not right. . . . It's a set-up deal."

He went on in that vein for a few more minutes. Then, as if a new theory had occurred to him, he leveled a different accusation. "Somebody fucked me in the test barn or something. There's something going on," he said.

Over and over, he told the three stewards, "This is going to be horrible."

"Not happy about it ourselves," Borden, one of the stewards, acknowledged during a rare moment in which she was able to get a word in.

Jill, next to Bob, suggested a few questions for him to ask. Was Medina the only horse that tested positive for betamethasone that week? Fresh in her mind must have been what their lawyer had told them when Baffert was fighting the lidocaine positives in Arkansas: that a third horse had tested positive for a small amount of lidocaine that day. Borden said yes, he was.

Jill, ferociously protective of her husband, kept going. "The problem is, they don't fucking care," she said, venom in her voice. "They don't care. They're going to hang you out to dry and they don't care."

"You guys are gonna hang me out to dry, and you guys don't care," Baffert echoed to Borden. "You guys better do a super-duper investigation on this because this is really gonna be a ugly scene here."

"It is going to be ugly," Borden agreed.

Baffert demanded that the racing commission immediately take a sample of Medina Spirit's hair for testing, a method that can sometimes offer some clues about when a substance was given but which experts say isn't effective at detecting corticosteroids like betamethasone.[3] Borden didn't immediately commit, telling Baffert that the commission had never done that before and she would need to discuss it with their lawyers. She asked Baffert to contact Amr Zedan before the commission called him to notify him of the positive test. The commission would notify the owner of the second-place finisher, Juddmonte, and trainer Brad Cox, to let them know it was a disputed race. She also promised Baffert that the commission, at least, wouldn't go public with the positive. But she warned him: "I'm sure it'll get out there."

In 1968, when Dr. Alexander Harthill gave Dancer's Image a dose of the common anti-inflammatory Butazolidin six days before the Kentucky Derby, it was legal for training. Bute, which horsemen often compare to ibuprofen, had been legal almost everywhere since racing commissions first started testing for the drug in the 1950s, although different jurisdictions had policies of varying strictness metering its use in advance of a race. Dancer's Image had a history of sore ankles, and Dr. Harthill had been employed to treat the horse leading up to the race. His veterinary bill from that period includes a $7.50 charge for Butazolidin administered on April 28.[4]

A week later, Dancer's Image won the Derby by a length and a half for the Boston automobile dealer Peter Fuller.[5] The victory was short-lived: post-race testing returned a positive result for bute. Because Kentucky had a zero-tolerance policy for the drug, Dancer's Image became the first Kentucky Derby winner to be disqualified for a medication violation.

If what Harthill said about how he treated the horse was true, the positive result didn't make any sense. Bute typically clears a horse's system in seventy-two hours.[6] Although, as with all drugs, individual horses metabolize bute at their own pace, there should have been no trace of the medication left in Dancer's Image six days after it was administered—unless Harthill had treated the horse a second time, something the sly young vet denied. Fuller, a man of deep enthusiasms, went to battle over the disqualification.

The Boston car man was an outsider in the bluegrass. He had sought security for the horse when he arrived in Kentucky because he had been receiving threatening letters after the public revelation that he had donated the purse from a big race he had won in Maryland to the widow of the civil rights leader Dr. Martin Luther King Jr., who had been assassinated just a month before the Derby. Racing historian Milt Toby wrote that Fuller was "considered a damn Yankee by many Kentuckians who were still fighting the Civil War."[7]

He was determined to reclaim his horse's victory. Fuller spent five years challenging the accuracy of the state's testing and the competence of its chemist, a twenty-eight-year veteran of the trade, in an effort to redeem Dancer's Image. The record of his appeal is densely packed with arcane scientific arguments and painfully technical parsing of testing procedures. Court records from the time note that witness examinations were "generally long and detailed, with the cross-examination being prolonged, repetitious, and argumentative," and that "there are numerous contradictions and even contradictions of contradictions throughout this entire record."[8]

Even if Harthill had lied and Dancer's Image had been given bute a second time, it is supremely unlikely that bute alone would have allowed the horse to prevail in the Kentucky Derby if he would not have otherwise. It's a little disingenuous to say bute is just Advil for ponies—it's generally accepted to be stronger than that—but it's not a narcotic.

Still, just because a drug wasn't "dope," did that mean that its use didn't constitute cheating? Even a trace amount of bute, detectable long past when it would have any pharmacological effect on the horse, was still against Kentucky's rules.

Fuller's bid to reclaim the Derby roses for Dancer's Image ultimately failed. More than fifty years later, the saga surrounding Medina Spirit would play out in an eerie echo of Dancer's Image. Baffert, like Fuller, was an outsider in the bluegrass. Racing scribes would debate whether the use of a commonly used therapeutic that was neither a stimulant nor a depressant could be termed doping. The court record would become a twisted snarl of narrowly argued debates over obscure testing procedures. The honesty of the horse's human connections would be questioned. The outcome would hinge on the same question: Did the winner of the Kentucky Derby break the rules? But in both cases, the answer to that question would do little to help anyone understand what truly had happened—or why it mattered.

The news of Medina Spirit's positive went public in less than twenty-four hours, not just on the backstretch of Churchill Downs but on national television. The uproar was instantaneous. Baffert fired the starting gun himself. At 9 a.m., he gave a press conference at his barn at Churchill in which he announced the positive and insisted once again that the horse had not been treated with betamethasone.

Today, Baffert says that he was trying to get ahead of the story.[9] He was in a paranoid state of mind because of what had happened in Arkansas—the two lidocaine positives that he believed were the result of contamination in the test barn—and because of the fallout from Justify's scopolamine positive, which he felt had been supremely unfair. Meanwhile, Baffert says, the news of Medina Spirit's positive was already all over the backstretch—he believes it was leaked by the racing commission—and he was thinking about Joe Drape. *He's just going to gut me*, he thought.[10]

Wearing a black vest over black sleeves and appearing a little shaken, Baffert faced a thicket of cameras, cell phones, and recorders. His voice hoarse, he denied that Medina Spirit had received betamethasone and asked, almost plaintively, why it always seemed to be *him* that wound up with "these contamination levels." He talked and talked.

"I'm not a conspiracy [theorist]. I know everybody's not out to get me, but there's definitely something wrong," he said. "Why is it happening to me, you know? There's problems in racing, but it's not Bob Baffert."[11]

The whole appearance was a disaster.

After the press conference, Churchill Downs executives met in a conference room at the racetrack. They talked about the repeated medication violations and what they saw as Baffert's refusal to take responsibility for the horses in his care. His staunch denial that Medina Spirit hadn't received betamethasone was deeply implausible to them because, frankly, the man had done the exact same thing with Gamine in the Kentucky Oaks with the exact same drug the previous year. And he'd been told directly by the stewards that the drug was illegal down to the limit of detection—no threshold—and so the idea that he wasn't aware of the rules just didn't pass the smell test. His public statements, executives felt, "could not be trusted."[12]

The whole thing was a "danger to [Churchill Downs'] brand" and put "the integrity of the 2021 Derby . . . under a cloud," Churchill president Michael Anderson later testified in court proceedings. He had harmed the track and its business by "blighting" its "two most prestigious events, the Kentucky Derby and the Kentucky Oaks, in back-to-back years."[13] Then there was also the matter of Justify, who had gotten a positive test in his last major prep race that had allowed him to run in—and win—the Kentucky Derby. But rather than accepting responsibility, Baffert had "publicly denounced medication guidelines in a press conference on Churchill Downs grounds," Anderson said.

Within hours of Baffert's press conference, Churchill leadership had decided that it needed to take immediate action. The decision ultimately rested with Bill Carstanjen, the silver-haired CEO of Churchill's parent company. Churchill Downs Inc., or CDI, was bigger than just the racetrack. It was a publicly traded company that also ran online wagering and casino businesses, and it had generated more than $1 billion in revenue the year before. Carstanjen may have been a racetrack executive, but he was not a racetracker.

He did not deliver the news himself. Longtime Churchill executive Darren Rogers, a racetracker, volunteered to talk to Baffert. The afternoon of the press conference, he called Baffert and told the seven-time Kentucky Derby winner that he had to vacate the backstretch of Churchill Downs, effective immediately. By the end of the day, the track had issued a statement announcing that it had indefinitely suspended Baffert from entering any horses at the track.[14] It was an unusual move. As a private business, Churchill had the right to bar entry to its premises or its races. But suspensions are usually meted out by the state racing commission, and only after a series of established investigative steps. At that point, the split sample had not even been returned. Churchill said it would await the results of the Kentucky Racing Commission's investigation before taking any further steps, but the swift suspension left the distinct impression that Carstanjen was fed up with Bob Baffert and the drama that always seemed to follow him.

Baffert went on a media blitz. He appeared on Fox News and MSNBC to defend himself.* On May 10, the day after his press conference at the barn, he appeared on Dan Patrick's radio show and told the host that the track had a "knee-jerk, cancel-culture kind of reaction" and had violated his due process. He insisted again that the horse hadn't been treated with betamethasone. But this time he was more specific, telling Patrick that not only had the horse not been injected with betamethasone, he also hadn't been treated with or exposed to any ointments containing betamethasone. He had made a similar claim to the stewards—"we don't use any ointments"—but not in his public press conference.

"We checked to make sure nobody had any special creams," Baffert told Patrick. "I'm learning about it right now, but nobody [who] handled the horse had any creams or anything like that."[15]

He'd had a lot of success over the course of his career, Baffert said, and a lot of people didn't like him.

---

* One of his lawyers also appeared on CNN, where I work. I was not involved in arranging, conducting, or producing that interview in any way.

"Racing has a lot of problems, but Bob Baffert isn't one of them," he told Patrick, repeating what he'd said in the press conference. "With success comes a lot of jealousy and animosity."

Within twenty-four hours, Baffert's story changed.

Throughout, he had been talking to his vet, Vince Baker. According to Baffert, Baker had told him initially that it was impossible for Medina Spirit to have betamethasone in his system. But also according to Baffert, sometime on the day he gave the interview to Dan Patrick—the interview in which he specifically said that the horse had not been exposed to any creams containing betamethasone—Baker called him back. He told Baffert that an ointment he had prescribed for the horse for a rash on his hindquarters contained the drug. Baffert said he spoke to Baker after the interview.[16] But he also insists that up until Baker called him, they had all assumed they were talking about betamethasone in its injectable form, making his insistence to both Dan Patrick and the stewards that the horse had received no "creams" appear oddly prescient.[17] The Dan Patrick interview became famous at the time because of Baffert's "cancel-culture" remark. But it stands out in retrospect as a strange foreshadowing that the narrative was about to shift like the winds at sea.

Baffert was pissed, he says now. "Vince," he recalls saying, "what part of 'I don't want betamethasone in my barn' didn't you understand?" It was like being hit with the news of the positive all over again. Up until now, he had thought that there might have been a mistake. There might be a way out of this. But if the horse had received betamethasone, well, he had received betamethasone. Baffert hadn't been fucked in the test barn. He hadn't been screwed by the lab. The positive, however infinitesimal, was real.

Yet it seemed supremely unfair to Baffert that he should be penalized for a dermatitis ointment. He had followed all the relevant rules surrounding *injectable* betamethasone, he maintained then and now. Twenty-one pico-grams per milliliter of blood—the concentration detected in Medina Spirit's sample—was minute and almost certainly would not have impacted the horse's performance in the Derby, Baffert argued. That was an impossible proposition to prove definitively, which is why rule-setting for medication standards in racing doesn't take impact on performance into account, but it was also a reasonable assertion.

None of that changed the fact that once again, Bob Baffert had received a positive test result. Once again, Baffert's conduct had become the news story after a big race. And this time, it was on racing's most important stage. Behind closed doors, the authorities that run East Coast racing—from the executives at Churchill Downs to those with the New York Racing Association—were hardening against the white-haired cowboy from Nogales.

Ten days after the Derby, Baffert issued a statement, revealing what he had learned and acknowledging that a skin ointment called Otomax, containing betamethasone, could have been the cause of the positive. He insisted that the 21 picograms of betamethasone "would have had no effect on the outcome of the race." Medina Spirit, he said, "is a deserved champion and I will continue to fight for him."[18]

That argument seemed to convince nobody. Baffert's insistence that the horse had been treated with Otomax sounded like so many excuses he had leveled before: Barnes's sweaty back patch. A groom urinating in a stall. It was no secret that Baffert used betamethasone for his joint injections; he had acknowledged as much with Gamine, and California state records reflected it.

The racing world divided into two camps: One group believed Baffert was flying too close to the sun on his withdrawal times by giving joint injections too close to a race. It was known to happen. Kristian Rhein recalled to me listening to one trainer in New York openly chuckling with other trainers about cheating the withdrawal window for clenbuterol, which he remembered to be ten days at the time. The trainer, Rhein said, would crow, "Been nine!" The next week, Rhein said, he would hear him boast: "Got one through on eight!"

"All of a sudden it becomes who can spit the furthest," Rhein said.[19]

But of course, eventually someone gets caught. Whether or not it was true, that was what some people thought Baffert had done with a joint injection.

The other group believed, without doubt, that Baffert was cheating on his withdrawal times and also using EPO or some other kind of illegal performance-enhancing drug. The group that was willing to defend Baffert—the group that thought his visceral reaction to the positive was evidence he was telling the truth, or believed that there was no way Baffert was foolish enough to deliberately try to sneak betamethasone by Kentucky regulators after what happened with Gamine—seemed to fade into the bushes like Homer Simpson.

As a practical matter, multiple different racing jurisdictions had decisions to make. The split sample confirming the betamethasone finding still hadn't come back and likely wouldn't before May 15, when the second leg of the Triple Crown would be run in Baltimore. As the clamoring built, it became a pressing question: Would Medina Spirit be allowed to run?

CHAPTER 21

THE *SATURDAY NIGHT LIVE* EFFECT

Pimlico Race Course, where the Preakness is run, is falling down. A stripe of railroad red runs across the top and bottom of the glass-fronted grandstand; at one end, a white metal staircase snakes back and forth like a gangplank, giving the whole building the look of an aging steamboat limping into port. 1/ST, Belinda Stronach's conglomerate, has been trying to rid itself of this decrepit old vessel for years. But for one day a year, Pimlico is the beating heart of the city of Baltimore. It has been the home of the Preakness since 1873, and the city has done everything it can to keep it there. And so it is that one of the most debaucherous days in Thoroughbred racing—and one of its most prestigious—is held in a liquor-store-and-locksmith part of Baltimore at a stadium that feels proudly run-down and stubbornly out of time. (Preakness is also known for its rowdy infield, and in particular a sporting event known as the "toilet run," in which drunken gladiators sprint across the tops of a row of porta-potties while people throw beer cans at them. It was a magnificent tradition that Pimlico eventually cracked down on.)

Two different parties had to decide whether Medina Spirit should be allowed to run at Pimlico. One was the Maryland Racing Commission, and the other was 1/ST—the same company that owns Baffert's home track of Santa Anita. Since the split sample had yet to be returned and the Kentucky Horse Racing Commission had issued no sanction, Maryland could hardly do so. But 1/ST, as the operator of the track, had some discretion.

One of the first steps executives took was to pull the vet records on Medina Spirit, who had spent most of his career until the waning days before the Derby stabled in California. Under California rules, vets must file an electronic record of any medication they administer to a racehorse on the backside by ten o'clock the following morning. You can't backdate prescriptions after the fact, according to California regulators.[1] Medina Spirit's record showed that Dr. Vince Baker had prescribed the topical ointment Otomax for a skin lesion, and that he had recorded it in real time.

"So we did have the direct evidence that preexisted the Kentucky positive that he had been administered betamethasone topically," a source with firsthand knowledge of 1/ST's actions at the time told me. "Our own veterinarians examined [Medina Spirit] and he had a lesion that certainly would have merited an application [of a topical medication]." This distinction— the question of whether the horse had been administered betamethasone topically instead of in a joint injection—would later become the central argument both in bar stool debate about the race and, for years, in the courtroom.

Four days before the Preakness, Pimlico and 1/ST struck a deal with Baffert to allow Medina Spirit to run. The deal would put the horse through a battery of drug screenings leading up to the race, and Baffert committed to making the results public. Craig Fravel, a 1/ST executive, said in a statement at the time that the decision had been made out of a sense of fairness, because the split sample had yet to be returned. It was a controversial decision, albeit one that was basically in line with racing regulations in every state. The daughter of Dinny Phipps—Janney's cousin, the former Jockey Club chairman—issued a statement on Twitter announcing that she had spoken to their longtime trainer, Shug McGaughey, and that Phipps Stable would not "run in any race at [Pimlico] this weekend where we don't feel like we are running on a level playing field."[2]

In fact, there was never any real consideration inside 1/ST of not allowing Baffert to run, the source with direct knowledge of the situation told me—for precisely the reason that the company stated publicly. The decision was made in a flurry of phone calls between 1/ST executives. To bar Baffert from running would have been a violation of the basic due process right offered to every trainer who gets a positive: you can ask for the test to be run again at a lab of your choosing. And at that point, a different source close to 1/ST pointed out, the only information the track had about the positive had come from Baffert himself—not the Kentucky Horse Racing Commission.

Mercifully for 1/ST, it also avoided a potentially uncomfortable problem for the company, at least in the short term. If Pimlico banned Baffert, it would immediately raise the question of whether he should also be banned from running at Santa Anita. The track already struggled with a dwindling population of horses to fill races, and Baffert made up an enormous percentage of fields in its stakes races.

And so, Medina Spirit would be heading to Pimlico.

Amr Zedan, Medina Spirit's owner, stood by Baffert. He issued a statement backing up Baffert's defense that the horse had been treated with a topical ointment and expressing his "full trust and support for Bob Baffert."[3] Privately, he told me that he considered Baffert something of a "father figure." If anything, he was a little starstruck. Baffert was a "folk hero" to the horse-crazy Zedan. He called him "boss," because his own father had admonished him never to be so informal as to call him "Bob."

But he also felt he had gained a keen appreciation of who his larger-than-life trainer was as a human being. He felt he understood him.

"There's the person and there's the persona," Zedan said. "There's a big gap between both. The person is a very shy person. He's very reserved. Everything is calculated." People confuse that, he said, with "the persona": the white hair, the charisma, the energy that flows into the room when Baffert blows in.

Baffert, he also knew, suffered from a particular affliction of genius: he was emotional. When it came to training horses, Baffert was "like an artist. . . . It's art, it's not science. It's gut.

"People who are artistic are emotional," he said.[4]

Zedan felt certain that because he understood Baffert, he could trust that he was telling him the truth.

Other owners weren't so loyal, and it became clear for the first time that the positive in the Derby could imperil the career that the seemingly invincible Baffert had built in Thoroughbred racing since the 1990s. Spendthrift, a juggernaut breeding farm that both sends prospects to Baffert to race and has stood many graduates of his stable at stud, decided to pull some of its horses from his barn, including a promising three-year-old named Following Sea that would go to Baffert's main East Coast rival, Todd Pletcher.[5] Pletcher was also a juggernaut, especially with his two-year-olds. He seemed to train horses with the lethal precision of an NCAA basketball coach, imposing on his players an infallible and unvarying regimen. (This was the trainer that Adrienne Hall came to believe Seth Fishman wanted to court as a client.) Spendthrift's general manager was quick to emphasize that Baffert had never had a positive test with one of their horses. This was only a "pause," the GM said, and the farm wasn't "ruling anything out in the future."[6] But it was still a huge blow. Just the year before, Baffert had trained a horse named Authentic for Spendthrift that had won the Kentucky Derby and the Breeders' Cup Classic and been named the 2020 Horse of the Year.

Baffert had been under industry scrutiny before. He had never known the kind of heat that comes when you draw the attention of cable news producers. He was asked direct questions about the positive. "God, I was not prepared for that," he told me, more with wonder than anger in his voice. "Man, they just eat you alive." There is an innocence to racing people when they are suddenly forced to confront the expectations of outsiders. It's as if they can't believe the world could be so unforgiving.

Medina Spirit underwent three rounds of out-of-competition blood sample testing in the week running up to the Preakness, with the last one drawn four days before the race. All three were reported clear and Medina Spirit was declared eligible to run.[7] Baffert was ambivalent about it, he told me, given the uproar. He was the kind of horse that usually needed a little time between races to recover, anyway. But Medina Spirit was training well and Zedan convinced him: if the horse is ready, let's run. And so Medina Spirit would go to Maryland—Stuart Janney's home state.

Baffert didn't go. He said in a long statement issued the day of the race that he didn't want to be a "distraction."[8] It had been, he said, an "extremely hard and emotionally draining" time for him and his family.

"For those who want an explanation for what transpired with Medina Spirit, I have tried to be open and transparent from the beginning. Our investigation is continuing and I don't have definitive answers at this point," he said. "What I do know is that neither my barn, nor my veterinarians, directly treated Medina Spirit with the anti-inflammatory medication beta-methasone. Even though it is allowable, it is just not something we have ever used with this horse. The only possible explanation that we have uncovered to date—and I emphasize the word possible—is that betamethasone is an ingredient in a topical ointment that was being applied to Medina Spirit to treat a dermatitis skin condition he developed after the Santa Anita Derby.

"I have been deeply saddened to see this case portrayed as a 'doping' scandal or betamethasone labeled as a 'banned' substance," he continued. "Neither is remotely true. Betamethasone is an allowable and commonly used medication in horse racing."

In one of the small ironies sometimes bestowed by the racing gods, the Preakness that year was held on a glorious sunny day. The turf course was lush from rain and the painted white walls of the old grandstand popped against a blue sky. In the infield, 1/ST had built a gargantuan two-story white tent so that the elites of Baltimore could avoid the teeming masses of ordinary drunks and gamblers in the grandstand; Baltimore Ravens and Washington Commanders drifted onto the deck with their wives, holding flutes of champagne.

Medina Spirit went off as the favorite. The gangly brown colt broke sharply and took up his usual position at the front of the pack, running with a loop in the reins and his mulish ears flopping with his stride. He changed leads as he was meant to around the final turn, vying for the lead with a horse named Midnight Bourbon. But as the length of the stretch yawned around and ahead of him, as the loam of the track percussed under his feet, it was clear that Medina Spirit, the little horse who never got tired, had nothing more to give. Midnight Bourbon skipped ahead and a second horse swept past Medina Spirit from behind. He cantered, heavy-legged, under the wire in third place, the fading performance of a horse too tired to finish the job. As he galloped out after the wire, head down and heavy on the forehand like a cow pony, his long ears almost appeared to droop. It only increased the perception that the horse had only won because he had been given drugs.

That night, *Saturday Night Live* devoted its "Weekend Update" segment to Baffert, with comedian Beck Bennett caricaturing him. He wore the trademark blue ombre sunglasses and smirked at the camera like a gangster. In a satirized news interview, "Baffert" was asked about the horse testing positive for "steroids." It mirrored much of the actual news coverage of the event, which had also routinely referred to betamethasone as a "steroid," incorrectly suggesting that the horse had received a mass-building anabolic steroid rather than a corticosteroid—an anti-inflammatory. Bennett referred to the horse as having "throbbing muscles, bacne, a perfect square Zac Efron jaw, baseball bat shaft, pea-sized balls."

He mocked Baffert's endless explanations of positive tests and his "cancel-culture" remark. "Of course I deny it. Bob Baffert's not stupid! I don't cheat—do I look like a shady character to you?" Bennett said. "Honestly, yes, Bob," Michael Che, playing the news host, said. "Yes, you do."

At the end of the segment, Che asked Bennett how the horse had run in the Preakness.

"Well, he fell apart out there—he's nothing without his 'roids," Bennett joked.

◆

Two days after the Preakness, a committee of the New York Racing Association's board, including Stuart Janney, held a meeting to discuss the Baffert
positive. According to Janney, NYRA management recommended that they
suspend Baffert. This would temporarily prevent him from entering races or
occupying stall space at NYRA-operated tracks—Belmont, Saratoga, and
Aqueduct—with a final determination on the length of the suspension to
be determined by the outcome of the Kentucky regulators' investigation.[9]
The board voted unanimously to do it. In a statement, NYRA said it had
"taken into account the fact that other horses trained by Mr. Baffert have
failed drug tests in the recent past, resulting in the assessment of penalties
against him by thoroughbred racing regulators in Kentucky, California, and
Arkansas."[10] The decision was even more unusual than what Churchill had
done because none of Baffert's positives had occurred in the state of New
York or at NYRA-operated tracks, and it did not go unremarked in racing
that NYRA had waited to make that decision until it had become clear
that there would be no potential Triple Crown winner at the Belmont that
year—always a big money draw for NYRA.

Two weeks later, the split sample came back positive from the University
of California, Davis, the lab Baffert had chosen. Even before Kentucky state
regulators had announced their penalty, Bill Carstanjen announced that
Churchill Downs would suspend Baffert for two years, citing his "record of
testing failures" and his "increasingly extraordinary explanations."[11] Baffert,
Carstanjen said, had damaged the reputation of the Kentucky Derby.

Behind the scenes, Baffert was doing everything he could to clear his
name. He was wrangling with the Kentucky Horse Racing Commission—
the only government regulatory body with jurisdiction—about additional
testing of samples drawn from Medina Spirit on Derby day that he hoped
would help him defend himself. As a result of all the back-and-forth over
testing, the KHRC wouldn't meet about the positive until February of
the following year. In the meantime, Baffert would be allowed to run in
the Breeders' Cup that fall. When it finally met, in February 2022, the
KHRC officially disqualified Medina Spirit from the Kentucky Derby and
suspended Baffert for ninety days—a penalty he could expect the state of
California to reciprocate.

Ninety days was bad enough. Baffert had never served a penalty longer
than two weeks. But the Churchill ban was even worse. It meant that even

when he could run again everywhere else, he still couldn't take any of his horses to the Derby—the cornerstone of his entire business model. The Derby King was out of the race for the next two years. In the end, it would be longer than that.

What came next, in many ways, was Bob Baffert's last stand. His reputation—the final repudiation of all the rumors that he took an edge, the vindication he craved for *being the best at what he did*—was riding on Medina Spirit's back.

"In the horse racing space, you see a lot of people who come and go. They're just looking for the quick return. You don't see that with Bob," Zedan told me. "He's not motivated by money. He's motivated by success."

It was what made the charges that he had cheated to win the Derby so difficult to take.

Over the next two years, drug testing would once again fail to offer either absolution or condemnation. Once again, the personalities and egos of the people in racing were going to dictate right and wrong. And once again, the horse himself would become an afterthought as everyone involved moved to protect their little piece of the humming engine of the business.

CHAPTER 22

21 PICOGRAMS

Shug McGaughey took the call from one of Bob Baffert's lawyers, a well-known horse racing gadfly named Clark Brewster, with a little surprise. Brewster wanted McGaughey to arrange a conversation between Baffert and Janney.

"I know if Stuart and Bob just sat down, this could all be resolved," Brewster said.

McGaughey and Brewster were friends, and he agreed to call Janney. Janney was confused by the request, if a little amused. The New York Racing Association, of which Janney was a board member, was preparing to hold a hearing on Baffert's suspension. Did Baffert want to essentially make his case privately in front of a single board member in advance?

"Hey, I just took the call," McGaughey said to Janney, in a way that suggested he was holding his hands up in the air.

Privately, Janney believed that Baffert's sins went beyond a certain sloppiness on withdrawal times. He believed he was a doper, according to a source familiar with his thinking at the time. But that was just a private opinion. Publicly, Janney had the air of a man singularly unconcerned with Bob Baffert and his problems.

"I never had a vendetta against Bob Baffert," Janney told me. "I, like a lot of people in the industry, was frustrated that he put himself in a very prominent position in the industry and then behaved in a way that didn't reflect very well on the industry. But that was the extent of my concern about Bob Baffert."[1]

What made the request strange was that Janney didn't have any official authority over Baffert. At NYRA, he was a single board member. He was not involved with the Kentucky state commission or Churchill Downs. The Jockey Club was the breed registry, not a regulator. The most Janney might have been in a position to do, officially, was put in a good word for Baffert, which he was very unlikely to do given that he thought Baffert deserved what he got. (He had voted in favor of suspending the trainer back in the spring.) Janney told the NYRA lawyers about the request from Brewster. They told him that the official channels for Baffert to negotiate a settlement in advance of the hearing were already open, so Janney decided that there was no need to involve himself in the situation.

It was clear that Baffert had fixated on Stuart Janney as the source of all his problems. He told me that he believes even now that Janney specifically told 5 Stones Intelligence to "target" him—something multiple sources with both the Jockey Club and 5 Stones deny—and that this was why he suddenly began to accumulate a rash of little positives in 2020 leading up to Medina Spirit's test in 2021. (This theory doesn't make much sense, even if Janney did specifically tell 5 Stones to investigate Baffert. Neither 5 Stones nor the Jockey Club has any formal authority over the Arkansas, Kentucky, or California state racing commissions, and it's unlikely any would act at their behest.* It's also worth noting that Baffert's positives happened in states where, according to my sources, 5 Stones wasn't able to get much traction.† Baffert also told me that he is convinced 5 Stones tapped his phone, something that the group, as a private intelligence company, does not have the legal ability to do, and there is no evidence that they did.)

In spring of 2022, Brewster tried again to get McGaughey to broker a meeting between Janney and Baffert. Baffert was at the Fasig-Tipton sale for two-year-olds in training, in Timonium, Maryland, traditionally held in the days following the Preakness. Was Janney there, and could they meet? By the time McGaughey relayed the message, Janney was already driving away from the sales grounds. He declined to turn around.

The two men did not know each other well. They had chatted briefly with each other from time to time at industry functions. Baffert believes that Janney bears a grudge against him because he wouldn't sign on to an industry effort to push for a Lasix ban, and because he would bring horses

---

* Arkansas, in fact, has directly bucked Jockey Club prerogatives by fighting the implementation of a new federal regulatory authority heavily backed by the breed registry. It's also not clear how much the state commissions knew about what 5 Stones was doing. One former racing commission official I spoke to complained that 5 Stones did not reveal what they were finding to state commissions in real time.

† Five Stones investigators did make multiple trips to Arkansas but felt that the backstretch had always been tipped off to their presence.

to New York and beat McGaughey's horses—Phipps horses—on their own turf. Janney, of course, denies this. In fact, it's not clear how often the two men have actually faced off on the racetrack in recent years. Baffert runs very few horses on the East Coast, typically just in the stallion-making Grade I's. Janney has some nice horses in his barn, but he doesn't always have a runner for that kind of race. It's obvious that the two men are strangers, shadowboxing each other across the country.

In some ways, their relationship typifies the way that racing's historically muddled, state-to-state regulatory schema left its constituents distrustful of the integrity of any given decision, creating an environment of paranoia that has persisted even after federal regulation was introduced in late 2020. Before that, racing commissions exercised a tremendous amount of discretion, and the regulatory structure of most states offered trainers ample opportunities to delay and dilute penalties. In some states, racing commissioners are allowed to own horses, giving them a financial interest in the industry they are tasked with regulating.* And, as the actions of Churchill and NYRA showed, private entities also have the power to act as de facto regulators, leading to dramatic variation in penalties for similar infractions. (Baffert also tried to arrange a private conversation with Bill Carstanjen, the CEO of Churchill. According to Brewster, discussions about arranging a face-to-face meeting broke down amid a debate over whether Baffert should be permitted to bring Brewster to the meeting. The meeting never happened.) It's easy to see why racetrackers might believe that personal politics plays a role in who gets penalized where—why some might believe Baffert is treated with kid gloves in California but penalized in New York, or that New York protects Todd Pletcher; why advocates for Rick Dutrow might come to suspect that syringes of xylazine had been planted by commission staff in his Aqueduct barn. Chicanery, after all, wasn't just the purview of the poor and the downtrodden. Sometimes it was the work of the well-heeled and the corrupt politician, the fat cats and the boss man.

By 2021, Janney—or at least the organization that he commanded—had succeeded in remaking the regulation of Thoroughbred horse racing in its

---

* In Louisiana, even the executive director of the state's racing commission—a person in a position to decide what cases the commission takes up—owns horses. https://paulickreport.com/news/ray-s-paddock/-voss-do-conflicts-of-interest-plague-louisiana-racing-commission.

own image. Just as Baffert's world seemed to be collapsing in on him, Janney was realizing his ambition to clean house within the industry.

After years of effort, Janney and the Jockey Club had gotten what they wanted: Congress, in the final few days of 2020, had passed legislation mandating a national regulatory authority to oversee anti-doping enforcement, medication, and safety at the racetrack. In the wake of the national uproar over the 2019 deaths at Santa Anita and the upsetting scandal of Jorge Navarro and Jason Servis, the Jockey Club and its allies had capitalized on the moment.

The major chit they had in their pocket was that the Senate majority leader, Republican Mitch McConnell, was from Kentucky and took a personal interest in the bill. Over the years, he had declined to move on different iterations of the bill because Churchill Downs, a business powerhouse in the state, had opposed the measure. The track seemed to fear that federal legislation would draw more negative public attention to the issue of racehorse welfare in ways that could damage its profitmaking, according to current and former congressional sources familiar with the dynamic. But Churchill, apparently, had come to recognize that the sport was in existential crisis. It needed to professionalize, it needed to clean up the messiness around drug rules, it needed to crack down on the endless parade of positive tests and, hopefully, breakdowns. This time, Churchill came to the negotiating table. Once Churchill was on board, the opponents of the legislation—like the major trade association representing trainers, the Horsemen's Benevolent and Protective Association (HBPA)—didn't stand a chance.

The bill was an unusual piece of legislation for a Republican to champion because it supplanted state-level regulation with federal rules (and would later be accused of violating a doctrine that had long been sacrosanct for Republican judicial nominees*). But horse racing was important to McConnell's state. He could hardly afford to ignore some of its oldest and wealthiest institutions and individuals.

---

* The so-called nondelegation doctrine is a "principle that holds that Congress cannot delegate . . . lawmaking ability to other entities." Republicans have long used the concept to argue against the delegation of rulemaking functions to administrative agencies. The new law created a private authority overseen by the Federal Trade Commission to administer racing's rules; for McConnell to support legislation that "delegated" authority in that way was an unusual break with the orthodoxy of his party. Legal Information Institute, "Nondelegation Doctrine," accessed September 23, 2024, https://www.law.cornell.edu/wex/nondelegation_doctrine.

McConnell "put a lot of political capital into it," a former aide who worked for him at the time said. "He worked his members on the floor between votes, saying, 'This is why it's important to me. You may not have racing in your state, and you may have a view that . . . less regulation in private industry is generally better than more. But this is special because it's incredibly important to my small state. And the current patchwork system just clearly is not working.'"

The new law formed the Horseracing Integrity and Safety Authority, and by 2023, it would take over regulation of medication rules at almost all racetracks across the country. It was a profound triumph for Janney. Beyond its lobbying efforts to pass the bill, the Jockey Club also exerted an enormous influence and indirect power over the development of the authority itself. It, along with the Breeders' Cup, Keeneland, and Churchill Downs, selected the members of the nominating committee responsible for naming HISA leadership. In some cases, these were close associates of Janney and the executive staff of the Jockey Club. Janney personally selected retired general Joseph Dunford, a former chairman of the Joint Chiefs of Staff who now sat on the board of Bessemer Securities, a private investment company also founded by Henry Phipps, in 1911. In a phone call, Janney told Dunford that he needed him "to do this little favor," according to a source familiar with the conversation. And because Congress didn't fund HISA—it only created the authority—the Jockey Club, along with the Breeders' Cup and a handful of other racing entities, also fronted the operational costs needed to get it off the ground.

Unlike the state commissions, HISA is a private organization. There is comparatively less public right to information about HISA rule-setting, leadership, or sanctions. HISA is not subject to the Freedom of Information Act; most of the information it releases is entirely discretionary. In short, the Jockey Club provided an unknown but significant amount of funding for the authority, and some of its closest allies selected its leadership—and there was no guaranteed way for the racing people it regulated to find out how it all happened or how the rules were set.*

One of HISA's first agenda items was to do exactly what the Jockey Club had wanted for years: do away with Lasix. The legislation banned the use of

---

* As a voluntary matter, HISA has released significantly more data on welfare and safety issues, issuing, for example, quarterly reports detailing fatalities by track in every state under its jurisdiction. This has lifted the veil on some states, like Kentucky, that had released comparatively little data on fatalities under the old system.

furosemide in all stakes races and two-year-old races, and mandated a total ban in 2026 unless the HISA board votes unanimously to continue to allow it.

There was instant revolt. The HBPA believed with righteous conviction that HISA was a bid by the Jockey Club to amass regulatory power over the industry and push through its long-held desire to ban Lasix. Whether it should be categorized as a performance enhancer remained a matter of debate—reading the studies on Lasix is a bit like reading the Bible: you can find evidence to bolster any argument in there—but many trainers viewed the drug as an indispensable part of getting a horse to the races regardless. Some horsemen came to see HISA as a power grab by the blue bloods of the sport at the expense of working trainers, those who did not have a string of replacements waiting to fill the stalls if one of their horses turned out to be a bleeder. (Look at California, Eric Hamelback, the CEO of the HBPA, said to me. The state had drastically reduced Lasix in the wake of the 2019 breakdowns. Now, he argued, "It's tough to fill races. There's an economic aspect to administering Lasix that I think is important.")[2] Ban Lasix, do away with the little guy, shut down the small tracks, and return racing to what it was meant to be: the sport of kings.* The first lawsuit against HISA was filed in March 2021.†

HISA quickly became the battleground for the class distinctions in Thoroughbred horse racing. The big and old institutions, the wealthy and the sophisticates, supported HISA and its Coubertinian ideal of a "level playing field," a drug-free chivalric vision splendid of Thoroughbred racing, where gentlemen met on the track to see whose horse was faster. The allowance trainer and the midlevel racetrack vet, who knew that vision was a hypocritical falsehood because everybody, at every level of racing, was looking to make money on this, rallied against it. The big breeders supported doing away with Lasix, some horsemen maintained, not because they were purists but because foreign buyers from countries where Lasix isn't permitted on race day were beginning to see the American product as inferior. This fight

* Janney, and the Jockey Club, vehemently deny the characterization of the organization as an elitist old guard seeking to do away with cheap racing. "We have no interest in" taking over the regulation of the sport, Janney told me. "What we have an interest in is seeing the sport is around in a form that we're either proud of or which we find to be successful. It looked to us five or six years ago that that was not going to happen." He added: "We're not focused just on the upper end of the sport. . . . All parts of it have to prosper."

† Ironically, horsemen argued that the law was unconstitutional on the same doctrinal grounds that typically would have kept a Republican like Mitch McConnell from voting for the bill in the first place.

was about business, not the horse. And just who should get to shape that business to their own advantage?

At the time of Medina Spirit's positive in the Derby, HISA wasn't yet the law of the land. The regulatory agency Baffert had to contend with was the Kentucky Horse Racing Commission, which had yet to issue a ruling. The two major organizations that had taken the toughest stance against Baffert were private organizations: Churchill Downs and the New York Racing Association. But for Baffert, they were tied up together.

Over the decades, Baffert had ascended to a social and financial stratum that would have been unrecognizable to the boy selling chicken eggs in Nogales. He lived now in the kind of mansion that is invariably referred to as "palatial," in a tony suburb on the edge of Los Angeles called La Cañada. It was California's version of an old-money neighborhood: out-of-the-way and quiet, with a restrained affluence compared to some of the flashier parts of Los Angeles. Horse-riding trails wound around its steep, tree-lined hills. Baffert's neighbors were the rich and famous: Vince Vaughn, Kevin Costner's ex-wife, and a private school that Haley Joel Osment had attended. In his house, Baffert kept a gleaming room dedicated to his trophies just inside the door, off a soaring foyer that was decorated expensively and tastefully. A giant gate with a keypad slid seamlessly open for him to come in and out. When he went to the races, he was recognized, raved over, beseeched by fans demanding autographs. Yet he felt keenly that he would always be standing on the outside of the world that Stuart Janney occupied,[3] a world where no one had ever been forced to scrabble for success and where power was wielded silently, subterraneanly, in ways that Baffert didn't wholly understand but was convinced held sway. Old money did not exercise its power through lawyers like Clark Brewster. It whispered it softly but directly in the ear of the judge.

Baffert felt certain that Janney and his ilk were using this positive—one that any other trainer would be given a pass for—to try to take him down. He was determined to fight back against what he perceived as a persecution by the elites, the petty and the jealous, the irrelevant holdovers who were resentful that a cowboy hat from a rough little town in the West was beating them at their own game. He wanted, he insisted then and now, justice for Medina Spirit—and himself. If quiet, backdoor conversations wouldn't resolve the issue, then he would marshal the law.

◆

From the start, the science surrounding Medina Spirit's positive test was contentious enough that you could draw whatever conclusion you liked about Baffert's guilt or relative innocence. The whole abstruse debate became a referendum on his character—and an exhausting illustration of the absurdity of drug regulation in racing.

Even before the Kentucky Horse Racing Commission had held a hearing on Medina Spirit, Baffert was in court in two states. He challenged the New York Racing Association's right to suspend him indefinitely. (NYRA had said only "temporarily," and had given no indication of how long that might be.) And he filed a civil suit against the Kentucky Horse Racing Commission demanding to test the split urine sample—the split blood had come back positive, of course—which at the moment sat in the commission's freezer. The goal was to prove through testing that the betamethasone positive had come from the use of the skin ointment Otomax, not from a joint injection. It was then a matter of dispute why that mattered, since Kentucky's regulations did not differentiate between injectable and topical administrations of betamethasone. At the time, the rules just said that "betamethasone" couldn't be present at any level in a horse's system on race day—perhaps simply because no one had thought of it, but it was the rule. Still, Baffert and his legal team believed that the distinction should exonerate Baffert. It's not an irrational point: if the purpose of the regulation was to safeguard the horse's safety by preventing him from running too soon after a joint injection, then the application of a topical ointment shouldn't be a concern.

The process was a comedy of errors from the start. After the primary testing process, what remained of the original blood and urine samples was sent off to a New York lab for additional testing, at Baffert's request. The vial containing the blood apparently shattered en route and, since the vial was in the same evidence bag as the urine container, it could plausibly have contaminated the urine sample—meaning that both were now basically useless.

More questions about sample integrity arose after a Kentucky judge granted Baffert's request to have the same New York lab test the untouched urine from the split sample, which was sitting in the commission's freezer. The lab in question was run by Dr. George Maylin, the same director who sources told me had, perhaps jokingly, perhaps not, advised Kristian Rhein to burn his documentation related to SGF-1000. Maylin's Equine Drug Testing and Research Laboratory has long been a curious case. In 2010, he had pushed for the lab to be moved from Cornell University to Morrisville

State College, which he told the state of New York would shave $500,000 off the lab's operating budget. This had raised some questions about how he could maintain testing standards on such a tight budget. His lab has historically returned positive tests at a far lower rate than any other state.[4] Maylin himself and his methods are deeply controversial within the industry. He is seen in some corners as a visionary, a man obsessed with tracking down unknown substances. In other corners, he is suspected of choosing not to report positive tests for controlled substances. In Maylin's own telling, he is simply not interested in inconsequential positives for trace amounts of legal therapeutics.

"Our focus is finding performance-enhancing drugs that are new, and not looking at things that are ho-hum on whether they have an effect or not," he told me.

And so Kentucky regulators weren't surprised when drama ensued over the Medina Spirit sample. After some legal dispute over precisely how many milliliters of the remaining fluid from the various samples Baffert and the commission should each be entitled to, the Kentucky judge ordered that the split urine sample be flown to New York, accompanied by representatives for Baffert and Amr Zedan, and two KHRC representatives: then-director Marc Guilfoil and Dr. Bruce Howard, the commission's equine medical director at the time.[5] The four climbed onto a private plane in Kentucky and sat knee-to-knee across from one another with a locked briefcase of horse urine between them.

"This sample is not leaving our side," Guilfoil said, according to a source present on the trip. "If one person goes to the bathroom, we all go to the bathroom."

While they were at the New York lab, Guilfoil and Howard were supposed to bring home whatever remained of the samples that had been sent to Maylin and arrived damaged. But according to court filings by the commission, Maylin, when asked to provide the samples, refused.

"No, I think we'll hold on to that," he said. Only when Howard produced the court order did Maylin show the two men a urine tube with "one or two milliliters of bloody fluid." The tube had been stored at room temperature rather than frozen. Guilfoil and Howard took what they could back to Kentucky—but they wanted to know what testing, precisely, Maylin had done on the samples. (Maylin told the two men at the time that his "word is honest and without compromise by either side in this case.")[6]

Maylin would ultimately report that he had found betamethasone valerate in Medina Spirit's sample, an ingredient in Otomax but not in the joint
injection form of the drug, which contained betamethasone acetate. Baffert
and his lawyers argued that this proved that the horse had been administered a topical ointment rather than a joint injection of betamethasone. It
would become the cornerstone of Baffert's defense during a six-day hearing
in August 2022. It is still his defense.

Later, some researchers would criticize Maylin's methodology and his
quality control measures, arguing that he had not met the basic scientific
standard necessary to establish even that Otomax had been used at all.[7] His
work would never be peer-reviewed.

There was also debate over whether the concentration of betamethasone found in Medina Spirit's sample was more consistent with a topical
application or a joint injection. Less than two weeks before the Derby,
Medina Spirit had tested negative for betamethasone during pre-race out-
of-competition testing, despite reportedly having been on the ointment
daily for nine days. But a little more than a week after that, in the Derby,
the drug was detected in his system. According to one racing regulator, "the
concentration that was detected is consistent with the concentration that you
would detect following an intraarticular injection of nine milligrams"—the
standard dose for a betamethasone joint injection—"like 48 to 72 hours
after an injection." But as a theoretical matter, said Sams, it's also plausible
that Otomax, dispensed daily for a month, could produce a 21-picogram
positive. The problem is there is no way to know because the appropriate
studies simply have not been done.

To inject a horse's joints with a controlled substance days before the
biggest race in the country would be an irrationally bold move—especially
given that Derby contenders are under 24/7 surveillance in the week
leading up to the race.[8] There is skirting the edge, and then there is doing
something that almost guarantees you will be caught doing it. One theory
has it that the Otomax was meant to be an elaborate cover-up all along—
that Baffert had Baker record the prescription of the ointment to cover
for the administration of a joint injection—but that theory is difficult
to square with the chaotic and at times almost amateurish way Baffert's
organization runs.

"This does not strike me as the barn that is capable of a caper—planning
ahead and saying we're going to record this horse had Otomax dispensed
twice and then we're going to inject his hocks three days before the Derby

and nobody will be the wiser? I can't give them credit for that kind of finesse," said the racing regulator.

Perhaps the best evidence to show that Medina Spirit was likely administered betamethasone in the form of an ointment for dermatitis is California vet records showing the prescription—and the numerous witnesses who confirmed to me and in court proceedings that the horse did have an obvious skin disease that it would be reasonable to treat with some form of anti-inflammatory.*

There is the fact that the day that the Kentucky Horse Racing Commission searched Baffert's barn at Churchill, they did not find any Otomax. Baffert has maintained under oath that the tube was tucked innocently in Medina Spirit's brush bucket. The KHRC, he said, simply didn't look there.[9] But if the groom was in fact slathering Otomax on the horse every day, as Baffert's team testified that he was, then he should have long run out of the size tube that California records say Baker prescribed. Baffert was arguing that his barn had somehow stretched two 30-gram tubes of Otomax for more than a month, giving it every day in quantities sufficient to produce a 21-picogram positive. "That has a credibility problem for me," the regulator told me.

There is one possible answer, one that only makes sense in the overhang of a shed row at the track. Record-keeping on the backside is notoriously poor; Baffert's vet, Baker, in 2023 would be one of several racetracks vets placed on probation with the California Veterinary Medical Board, in part over his paperwork—including a finding that he had failed to provide and document the required drug consultations when he prescribed Otomax to Medina Spirit.[10] There are any number of ways that more tubes of Otomax, a drug the Baffert barn clearly believed was an inconsequential topical, might have wound up in the barn, and not in the state record—and then, slathered liberally on a horse with a very real skin rash.

But that, of course, is speculation. As with every other minute overage of allowable therapeutics fought by trainers in jurisdictions across the country, there may never be irrefutable proof of how the drug wound up in the horse's system—whether it was an intentional effort to skate the rules or simply an honest mistake. Testing had offered no definitive answers. The

---

* Of course, this too is up for debate. I spoke to several trainers who were flummoxed at the choice of Otomax—"That's for a dog's ears, for Chrissake," said one prominent trainer. "I've never heard of a vet prescribing Otomax to a horse for a skin rash"—and others who said it was a perfectly reasonable and common drug choice for horses.

bigger question is whether the way the sport approaches the regulation of drugs—pick a long list of accepted "therapeutics," set "thresholds," offer poorly substantiated withdrawal times, and then test for them down to the picogram—makes any sense whatsoever.

It's important to remember that in the worst-case scenario—Baffert intentionally injecting one of the horse's joints too soon before the Derby for the drug to clear the animal's system—he was still using a drug that until recently was permitted by most jurisdictions up to two weeks before a race. (In some jurisdictions, it was less than that.) If betamethasone was such a serious medication, one worthy of disqualifying the winner of the Kentucky Derby over 21 picograms, why did the rules also say it could be administered just fourteen days out from the race? Were all of these different drugs, so tightly intertwined with the practice of getting horses to the race-track, necessary and ethical interventions for the horse? If they were, why the uproar? And if they weren't, shouldn't the rules be a lot more conservative than a fourteen-day stand-down? That question has been left unasked and unexamined in the excruciating back-and-forth over Medina Spirit.

Racing regulators say that most drug positives are mistakes, a reflection of a normalized lack of professionalism across the sport. It's easy to under-stand how it could happen: The vet truck comes around at the end of the morning, after training hours are finished. Sometimes the trainer is there, but sometimes he isn't. And anyway, the trainer has a barn full of sixty horses to care for. He can't remember everything. Perhaps he keeps good records, perhaps he doesn't. Perhaps the groom, who may speak little English in a barn run by a foreman who speaks little Spanish, pulls the wrong horse out of the stall. Mistakes happen. It's hard to forget the finding in the after-action review of the 2019 breakdowns at Santa Anita of the horse treated by two veterinarians who had no idea that they were treating the same animal. The two vets injected the same joint within five days of each other.

As the Kentucky proceedings dragged on through 2021 and 2022, a strange side act to Baffert's legal machinations occurred. Clark Brewster was an Oklahoma trial lawyer. He had a toothy grin and the kind of lank hair that made it hard to tell if it was gray or a pale, creamy blond. Like Baffert, he tended to overwhelm you with words. He represented a number of con-troversial horse people; Steve Asmussen, the trainer whose operation had been caught up in an undercover PETA investigation in 2014, was a friend and a client. Brewster also represented Stormy Daniels, the event rider and porn star who had become famous for receiving an alleged hush-money payment from Donald Trump.

In September 2022, Baffert was back at Keeneland for the sale. At the time, he was still in court in Franklin County, fighting the Kentucky Horse Racing Commission over Medina Spirit's disqualification. Clark Brewster was also at the sales grounds that week. Brewster had some reservations about the hearing officer in the case, a man named Clay Patrick, whom he found "conscientious" but believed had "obvious connections to the KHRC."[11]

Brewster also liked to own a few horses, and he bought five at Keeneland that year. One of them was a rich bay colt offered by Taylor Made Sales, a large commercial consignor of yearlings owned by a big roster of different clients. Brewster spent $190,000 on the colt.

Only later, he said, did he realize that the colt had been owned by Clay Patrick. The purchase created the obvious appearance of a conflict of interest, in which one of the parties to the litigation had paid the hearing officer tens of thousands of dollars. Patrick recused himself from the case.

Brewster rightly pointed out that the horse's catalog page made no reference to the breeder or owner, although the information was available in digital catalogs used by some buyers. "It was an honest and innocent decision to purchase [the horse] and if I knew Mr. Patrick had any connection or ownership interest I would have passed on bidding out of an abundance of caution to avoid any appearance of impropriety," he told me.[12] The animal, he said, had been short-listed for him by Steve Asmussen, who he said was also unfamiliar with the colt's provenance. Only after he had purchased the colt and started studying his siblings did he realize Patrick's connection.

"Believe me, when I buy horses, and you can talk to anyone at Keeneland or [Fasig-Tipton]—nobody is checking who the owner is," Brewster told *BloodHorse* at the time. "That's not a relevant fact on making a decision on a yearling."[13] He reiterated this point to me. (In my experience working for a major yearling consignor, this isn't always true. Some buyers absolutely seek out this information from consignors.)

Patrick is not a large breeder. Keeneland auctioned more than four thousand yearlings during the September sale that year. It was a remarkable coincidence.

◆

The eviction of Bob Baffert from horse racing was not uniform. 1/ST didn't follow Churchill and NYRA's ban. The Breeders' Cup allowed him to run without interruption. The Breeders' Cup rotates from track to track each year, and in 2021 it was scheduled to be run at Del Mar. There was nothing, technically, to prohibit Baffert from entering his horses. Still, the Breeders' Cup is a private company, and it had a decision to make. As 1/ST had done for the Preakness, it placed conditions on his participation, but allowed him to run.[14]

Another set of private entities was also still willing to allow Baffert to participate in the fall of 2021. Baffert attended the Keeneland yearling sale in September. He could be seen by the back ring, watching these colts walk up and down one last time, making a final judgment call on his gut alone. In the first days of the sale, Donato Lanni, a Kentucky bloodstock agent who often does Baffert's buying, purchased colts for George Soros's racing partnership, all between $325,000 and $850,000 each. Baffert—and his ability to make colts into valuable stallions—is an intimate part of the syndicate's business model.[15]

Even as some of them privately derided him as a doper, Kentucky's breeders were more than happy to take Baffert's money.

Baffert thought that he was being persecuted for not belonging. There may have been some of that. But as the hearings, court filings, and public testimony surrounding the positive continued to unfurl in 2022, Churchill and NYRA were forced to articulate their rationale for the extraordinary penalties they had levied on Baffert. It would become clear that Baffert wasn't being punished because of a medication violation. He was being punished because, for the giants of racing, he was a risk to the bottom line.

CHAPTER 23

THE BOTTOM LINE

Baffert won a temporary victory in New York. A federal judge froze the NYRA ban, ruling that it had deprived him of his right to due process by denying him the opportunity to defend himself in a hearing. And so, in September 2021, NYRA delivered a statement of charges to Baffert articulating its rationale for the suspension.

It accused him of conduct "detrimental" to the best interests of racing, the health and safety of horses and jockeys and, critically, NYRA's business operations. NYRA established a novel set of hearing rules and procedures for Baffert to respond to those charges and in January 2022 held a five-day administrative hearing. Baffert appeared over webcam, "tapping his feet in a fidgety way while sipping from a white coffee mug."[1]

The attorney for NYRA, Hank Greenberg, opened by accusing Baffert of a "rampage of doping violations." Baffert, Greenberg said, "took a wrecking ball over a one-year period to the integrity of a sport that was so good to him for so many years. He sullied and soiled, in one year . . . three of the great races in America: the Arkansas Derby, the Kentucky Oaks, and the Kentucky Derby. Throughout that period, not once did he take responsibility for his actions, did he express contrition. Time and again, again and again, six times, he would blame others to try to avoid responsibility for his own actions." Even after the Derby, Greenberg said, Baffert failed to "accept responsibility." Instead, he "trashes everyone he can think of. He trashes regulators. He trashes the media. He attacks everyone and everything, and he says he can't figure out how this could happen."[2]

The NYRA hearing, like the myriad hearings in other venues that would follow, devolved into an esoteric argument over whether 21 picograms of betamethasone in a blood sample would have triggered a positive in other racing jurisdictions or under different model regulatory schemas, whether it might have impacted the horse's performance or masked pain on the day of the Derby, whether there was sufficient science to support the conclusion that the positive test had arisen from the application of Otomax rather than a joint injection. Lawyers readjudicated the 2019 and 2020 positives, ticking through academic research on how quickly horses metabolize dextromethorphan, lidocaine, and bute and what impact the levels found in Baffert's horses might have on a horse's performance in a race. It was a master class in the overwhelming complexity, if not outright futility, of trying to regulate huge numbers of "therapeutic" drugs used in horses—living animals with diverse metabolisms operating under dramatically different conditions across the country—with a relatively low budget for research into the science underpinning those regulations. You can make any case you like, which both sides did. Brewster parsed bylaws in such minutiae that at one point the judge accused him of badgering the witness with the same question half a dozen times.[3]

But through the static, an answer to Baffert's plaintive question on the morning of his ill-fated press conference—why me?—was becoming clear.

Greenberg called a pair of witnesses that, in some ways, were surprising in a case about a drug violation. First he called Matthew Feig, the general manager for NYRA's wagering platform, which, in addition to New York, also took bets on races in California, Arkansas, and elsewhere—a total of thirty-one states. Feig testified that he had received "questions" from both underwriters and regulators "in passing" about Baffert. The day the news of Medina Spirit's positive became public, he said, customer service representatives at NYRA Bets had a "very large spike in volume . . . we weren't really prepared for."

"A lot of questions regarding 'Are you going to refund my wager,' 'I bet the second place horse, Mandaloun, are you going to pay me what I was owed,'" he recounted.

This was never going to happen. Amateur gamblers are often surprised to learn that racetracks do not reallocate payouts when the final order of finish is disputed after the race due to a medication violation. (It would almost certainly be impossible to do logistically; and, "under Kentucky law governing pari-mutuel wagering, the first official order of finish is final. . . . After the order is marked official, neither the stewards nor the courts can turn a losing wager into a winning one."[4] Occasionally, including in the case of Medina Spirit, bettors will try to sue for damages; it doesn't work.[5])

But for NYRA, the very real concern was that disillusioned gamblers might not return, or that new customers might be scared off by the perception that the game was rigged. Bettors are a subculture of their own within horse racing—they are not considered to be horsemen and often have no direct contact with the participants of the sport—but from the racetrack's perspective, their sentiments about the sport are of paramount interest.

Second, Greenberg called NYRA's vice president for marketing, Donald Scott. Scott testified that the day the news broke, "we were getting customer calls. . . . These customers were identifying themselves. Specifically saying, 'This is who I am and this is how much I wager with NYRA. And I'm very upset about this and I want to know what your position is.'" Baffert, he said, was the only trainer about whom his department had received specific calls or complaints. The calls "threatened all the brand equity that I had been communicating in financial investment [disclosures] to say we are the leader: You can trust us. Wager with us on the Kentucky Derby."

After the Derby, Greenberg mused to the hearing officer, "You would think" that Baffert "would have the good sense to sort of let things lie, allow his lawyers to see what they could do to help him out of this tight spot he was in, but no." Instead, Greenberg said, Baffert went on a blitz of media interviews, including the infamous "cancel-culture" interview. NYRA, he went on, "had an obligation to act . . . to protect the sport of thoroughbred racing."

"Institutions like NYRA, Churchill Downs, and other operators of racetracks have a social license . . . between them and the public, which holds those people who use horses for wagering opportunities, and what happens if those institutions do not use their very best effort, everything in their power to protect the safety of animals," he said.

"What happens is what happened to greyhound racing, which you no longer see. What happens is what happened to circuses where there were lion tamers. They don't exist anymore.

"So NYRA and institutions like that must do everything in their power to protect the safety of horses."

There it was, in black and white: Baffert was a risk to the long-term business of racetrack operators. In that brutally honest forum where lawyers defend the fundamental self-interest of their organization, what mattered was not the health and safety of horses for its own sake. What mattered was maintaining the customer base. Baffert, as the most recognizable face in horse racing, now made even more recognizable, posed a danger to that customer base.

Churchill Downs would make a similar argument. Both Churchill and NYRA would cite the *Saturday Night Live* skit, with Greenberg pointing out that it would be viewed by "customers and potential customers of New York Racing Association."

Another of Baffert's lawyers, Craig Robertson, would point out that his client had never received a single violation in the state of New York in thirty years of racing horses there. Just three years previous, Robertson noted, NYRA had inducted Baffert into their Saratoga Walk of Fame, calling him one of "the greats of the game." He pointed out that all the positives that Greenberg had ticked through had been adjudicated with no suspension for Baffert—and that NYRA had expressed no outrage at the time. NYRA was only acting now, Robertson alleged, because "a handful of NYRA board members" had "some personal vendetta against Mr. Baffert."[6]

"Do they not like him, are they jealous of him, or perhaps because they own horses that race in New York, they're tired of Mr. Baffert coming to New York and beating them in New York races. And they want to eliminate a competitor," Robertson said. The Kentucky Horse Racing Commission—the only regulatory body with jurisdiction—had not yet issued its ruling on Medina Spirit, he pointed out. But the NYRA board members "don't care about the evidence. They don't care about due process. They're on a mission. They know what they want to do, and they want to kick this man out."

Elsewhere during the hearing, Greenberg had heavily suggested that Baffert had gotten a soft deal from the Breeders' Cup because twelve of its fourteen board members had owned at least a leg of a horse he trained,[7] and from the California Horse Racing Board with Justify's scopolamine positive in 2018 because the chairman owned a piece of a horse in Baffert's barn. Yet despite the clear parallel, he dismissed Robertson's arguments that NYRA board members—also competitors in the sport now acting in a quasi-regulatory capacity—might also have had a personal incentive to act as they did. Greenberg called such suggestions "offensive" and "ridiculous," insisting that there was "not a scintilla of evidence" to support them.[8]

It was a distraction. The hearing officer assigned to the case ruled that NYRA had proved that Baffert's "implausible excuse[s]" for each of his violations unleashed a "torrent of negative media coverage on the sport," and that NYRA had "reasonably concluded that it will not condone Baffert's reckless practices, outrageous behavior and substance violations, each of which compromises the integrity of the sport."[9] It was Baffert's insistence on drawing attention to racing's biggest vulnerability, medication, and thus the danger he posed to the ledgers of its stakeholders, that mattered. The little black colt, born in a field in Florida, faded into an afterthought.

That was it. Baffert's team made a few failed efforts to appeal the decision, but ultimately, he was out of New York for one year.

A month later, in February 2022, the Kentucky Horse Racing Commission finally held its hearing. Brewster presented the Otomax defense. Days later, the racing commission suspended Baffert for three months, fined him $7,500, and officially stripped Medina Spirit of his win in the Kentucky Derby.

When Kentucky knocked Baffert out of the game for ninety days, California followed precedent and barred him from racing horses for the same length of time. Baffert's horses were transferred to other trainers, including to Tim Yakteen, his old assistant, who now trained under his own name but remained a staunch defender of his former boss. The jumbled cacophony of colorful signs tacked on the end of Baffert's barns at Santa Anita, painted placards celebrating trainer titles and Triple Crown victories, signs emblazoned with horse names and race wins, was pulled down. Baffert went home.

For the first time since his career at Rillito took off, he had no horses to train and nothing to do. Jill tried to keep him busy, getting him on the exercise bike. Baffert is a restless man. She called it "Bobby-sitting."[10] It was the longest he had been idle in his entire career, maybe the first real vacation since he took his first wife, Sherry, to Hawaii after getting a positive for Robinul in 1991. "I don't take vacations," he said. "Our vacations are when we go to these races."

He would ultimately fight the Kentucky Horse Racing Commission's disqualification decision for two years. The outcome was the same: Mandaloun remained the official winner of the 2021 Kentucky Derby.

Baffert "didn't rob a bank," said one source familiar with the commission. But he wouldn't let it go. "It's a therapeutic overage. Fall on the sword, tell everybody you're sorry. It's a forgiving world." Instead, the source said, he "dragged us all through the mud."

Baffert also sued to get the Churchill Downs suspension overturned so that he could compete in the 2022 and 2023 Derby. This effort also failed.

All of that lay ahead of Baffert on December 6, 2021. He had yet to be suspended by Kentucky. The signs were still up at the end of the Baffert barn, the first barn on the left as you entered the Santa Anita backstretch. His status in New York and Kentucky remained uncertain, a matter of intense litigation, but on that morning, he was feeling, for the first time in a long time, a glimmer of hope. George Maylin had just issued his findings that the substance found in Medina Spirit's sample was betamethasone valerate, not acetate—definitive proof, Baffert and his attorneys felt, that the horse had not been injected to relieve joint inflammation. It had been the ointment all along.

That morning, Baffert ascended the steps of the Santa Anita grandstand and took a seat in his usual spot, a box right in front of the wire. He had little talismans that marked him a horse trainer: his binoculars, his two-way radio, his stopwatch. This was his whole identity. If he couldn't train horses, be around horses, inhale the warm scent of their flesh and their breath, as indescribably sweet as the top of a baby's head, then who was he? What would he do?

Medina Spirit, with Juan Ochoa in the irons, stepped onto the loam of the track. The rider would have checked his girth and set his bridge in the wide rubber reins, pebbled in his hands. He would have picked up a trot and then an easy gallop to warm the horse up. He would have clocked, perhaps without even thinking about it, each flick of Medina Spirit's long brown ears and made imperceptible adjustments based on what he felt through his hands, his seat, his legs; seeking balance, stillness, steadiness. Seeking, perhaps, a touch of greatness.

"That horse never got tired," Baffert told me. "He never was blowing hard, he never corded up, he never—he wouldn't get tired. He could go a mile and a quarter, go a mile and a half, easily."

Medina Spirit died at the seven-eighths pole, a furlong past the finish line. Baffert, sitting in his box looking down at the track, did not need his binoculars. The horse died in front of him.

CHAPTER 24

HATE THE GAME, NOT THE PLAYER

At some point after the Justice Department announced charges against Navarro, Servis, and the others, the role that 5 Stones Intelligence had played became known in the industry. Later, some horsemen would turn against Janney and his efforts to clean up the sport, accusing him of using 5 Stones to target innocent trainers. But in the aftermath of the indictments, with the industry reeling, the publicity appeared to help the group ink a new contract with a new client. The target, once again, was top trainers suspected of cheating. This time 5 Stones was going to investigate Bob Baffert for real.

The client was Churchill Downs, according to multiple sources with direct knowledge of the work.*

It's not clear whether the racetrack and wagering behemoth put Baffert's name on the contract. But he was indisputably one of the top targets, if not the top target, of a short-lived probe, according to these sources. On at least one occasion in spring of 2022—a year after the Medina Spirit positive and not long after Baffert had sued Churchill to overturn the track's two-year suspension—Dave Tinsley sent a handful of investigators to California to run down actionable intelligence. Five Stones personnel surveilled the outside of Baffert's gated home in La Cañada and tailed his grooms. They dug through Tim Yakteen's trash in the middle of the night. Yakteen, who had just taken over training his old boss's horses while Baffert served his ninety-day suspension from the Kentucky Horse Racing Commission, said he was awoken at 1:30 a.m. at his home in Monrovia. When he checked the footage from his security camera, he saw at least two men in a dark pickup

---

* One 5 Stones executive with direct knowledge of the contract told me that the racetrack worked through a law firm.

truck taking photos of his house and, most curiously, stealing his trash from the curb. It frightened him: he thought someone was casing the house in preparation for a home invasion. Yakteen and his wife have children. He filed a police report.

This activity went on for months. Then Churchill—inexplicably, to the 5 Stones crew—shut the whole thing down.

"Churchill didn't have the appetite to go after the dopers," one of the sources insisted.

Churchill did not respond to my numerous requests for comment on this episode. But it's difficult to credit the suggestion that the track was willing to hire 5 Stones to find evidence that Baffert cheated, only to back away when they found what they were looking for. In the years after the 2020 indictments became public, 5 Stones would face some pushback for its handling of Saffie Joseph—and none of the group's leads on any other trainers appear to have panned out. Much of what 5 Stones was turning up in California seems thin, while some of their tactics seem invasive. And once again, their understanding of common racetrack practice is open to question. Five Stones investigators were deeply suspicious that Baffert's long-time groom Eduardo Luna owned his own home and drove a new vehicle, on what they assumed was a paltry groom's salary. Luna is renowned across the country for his skill with horses; at one point in reporting this book, I asked a few racetrackers who the most talented groom working today is. I got only one answer: Eduardo Luna. Five Stones investigators seemed to believe that it was possible Baffert was rewarding Luna for helping him dope horses; the Occam's razor explanation is simply that he pays an extremely valuable employee well enough to retain him. It appears that, once again, those seeking proof that Baffert dopes his horses had come up empty-handed.

There is no evidence that Baffert intentionally uses banned substances on his horses.* He is one of the most closely monitored trainers not just in California but anywhere in the United States. There are 1,100 cameras covering sixty barns at Santa Anita, including a view of the exterior of every stall on the property. In a control room in the grandstand, a security official sits in front of a bank of television screens pumping in the live feed. It looks

---

* Other than, of course, the morphine positive that he received in the 1970s when he was in his twenties. Some critics will also point to the morphine positive in 2001 and the scopolamine positive in 2018. These were banned substances rather than regulated therapeutics. In both instances, there is compelling evidence that the positives could have arisen from accidental exposure originating outside of the Baffert barn rather than intentional administration.

like the US military's mission control center in Baghdad, used for live drone strikes. It works: California officials had been tipped off by the state vet that horses in the barn of a trainer named William E. Morey had some unusual blood work results that might be suggestive of doping. A security official began to watch Morey more closely. Over time, he saw that Morey entered the stall of every horse right before it raced with a plastic grocery bag and a tube of paste in his back pocket—the same procedure, every race. Morey was ultimately suspended for giving an illegal supplement called "Blood Buffer" and kicked off Santa Anita.

Not once, track officials told me, have they caught Baffert or his staff doing anything—and "I have a list of people in my brain that I like to keep a closer eye on than others," the security official told me. California regulators that I spoke to, both current and retired, were dismissive of the suggestion that Baffert has been able to hide a routine use of banned drugs. In New York, Baffert says, his horses are monitored by track security from the moment they arrive on NYRA property.

Nor, it seems, were the FBI and 5 Stones able to develop any actionable intelligence on Baffert's operation to pursue. In more than two years of reporting, the only people I could find who were willing to state definitively that Bob Baffert dopes—or even that he cheats on the withdrawal times for legal drugs—are people who have no firsthand knowledge of his operation.

It is impossible to prove a negative, of course. Critics argue that the proof is the bevy of positive tests and dead horses. Just as there is no evidence—at least that I found or that is reported officially—to support the conclusion that Baffert uses banned substances, there is also no denying that between 2019 and 2021, he received a high number of positive tests for legal therapeutics. What's less clear is whether Baffert's record is unusual. The truth about Bob Baffert appears painfully more pedestrian: that when it comes to drugs, he is no better and no worse than most other trainers in America.

Todd Pletcher may be one of the single most boring interview subjects for turf writers. Famously monotone, Pletcher always comes off as neatly pressed and tightly controlled in public. He has won the Eclipse Award for top trainer eight times since 2004 and, from his home base in New York, is one of the dominant trainers on the East Coast. He often runs upwards of a thousand horses a year and consistently wins 20 percent or more of the races he enters, making him among the most important and successful trainers in the sport. Outside of racing, he is virtually unknown.

In 2012, one of Pletcher's trainees, a four-year-old gelding named Coronado Heights, broke down one furlong into a claiming race at Aqueduct, one in the succession of fatal injuries at the track that winter. Subsequent investigation by the state revealed that the horse had received seventeen perfectly legal injections in the week leading up to his final race. He was given intraarticular joint injections of hyaluronic acid and the powerful corticosteroid Depo-Medrol five days before the race (neither was reported as required under state regulation). He was treated with two anti-inflammatories and Legend, another hyaluronic acid. He was given Adequan, another joint treatment. The conclusion of the state task force that examined the breakdown was unequivocal: Pletcher's "aggressive pre-race medication protocol . . . may have masked clinical signs of lameness and confounded" the examination given to the horse prior to the race to determine his fitness to compete safely. "This medication practice may have represented a missed opportunity to prevent this injury," the task force wrote.[1]

According to the state report, "the trainer reported that the pre-race medication program for this horse was standard practice for all of the horses in his stable." This series of injections, it appears, was given to all horses in Pletcher's barn. This was "pre-racing": legal and common across the track, with variations between barns. There was no suggestion that any of the drugs that Pletcher had given Coronado Heights constituted "doping." His career continued.

In less than a year between 2022 and 2023, Pletcher racked up six positive tests, most for common therapeutics—bute, and the anti-inflammatories dexamethasone and ketoprofen—and one in a Grade I race for meloxicam, an anti-inflammatory that is not approved for use in racehorses in racing or training that Pletcher says his barn did not administer. Six positives—including several in New York—and yet there was no whisper of NYRA moving to penalize Pletcher beyond whatever penalty the state meted out.

"It can't escape notice that while Baffert's violations did not take place in New York, NYRA still felt compelled to act against him. Two of Pletcher's cases originated there, but he is also one of the largest barns on the NYRA circuit, if not the very largest and one of the most successful," noted the Paulick Report's Natalie Voss.[2] "Baffert ships horses for high-profile graded stakes races in Kentucky and New York, but his presence at those facilities isn't a deciding factor in whether races fill. It would be a tough business decision for NYRA to exclude Pletcher, who has already run roughly a quarter of his 445 starts this year at their facilities."

In that moment, it was difficult to distinguish Baffert's sins from his major East Coast competitor's. Yet while Pletcher quietly carried on with the business of winning races, Baffert was barred from two of the largest racing jurisdictions in the United States.

Not unlike Baffert, Pletcher believes he received a rash of positives in multiple states for reasons outside of his control. At the time, HISA was in the process of selecting the labs it would use to test racing samples. Pletcher told me that he believed "the labs were trying to show how low can we test for, trying to win those contracts."[3] Also like Baffert, he chose to fight the findings: He hired Karen Murphy to challenge the meloxicam positive—a test result that, much like Justify's positive in the Santa Anita Derby, only became public when the *New York Times'* Joe Drape reported on it—and benefited from testimony from Dr. George Maylin that the amount of medication found in the horse's sample was so low as to suggest it had been given long before the race.[4] It was a page out of a well-worn playbook from a trainer whose operation is both militantly professionalized and, the evidence suggests, run-of-the-mill in its use of medication. The difference between Pletcher and Baffert was that Pletcher, silent to the press and anonymous outside of racing, posed no worrying risk of scaring off potential customers. There was no need to publicly penalize Todd Pletcher, because nobody outside of racing was paying attention to Todd Pletcher. He had given no press conference, no round of disastrous cable news interviews. He was not racing's most famous face and infamous ambassador. Baffert had endangered racing not because his use of medication was unique but because, a superstar worried about his reputation and incapable of staying silent, he had endangered the moneymaking.

Since 2000, Baffert has received around 16 medication violations,* with only a few exceptions, like Nautical Look's morphine and Justify's scopolamine, for anything other than legal therapeutics. Pletcher has received approximately 12 violations during the same time, including one for betamethasone. Steve Asmussen has received at least 28.† There is a big caveat to this data, which is

---

* I am including Justify's scopolamine positive and Charlatan and Gamine's lidocaine positives.

† All of these numbers are drawn from data collected by the Association of Racing Commissioners International and provided to me on request. Because ARCI collects that data from state commissions, rather than generating it independently, those records may be incomplete. They do not represent findings since HISA assumed regulation of medication violations in 2023.

that Pletcher started more than twice as many horses as Baffert in that time, Asmussen more than four times as many. And most importantly, this is not to say some trainers don't get it right—Graham Motion, for example, appears to have been cited only twice over the course of his career.

Baffert has also faced public criticism for his fatality rates. In the maelstrom after Medina Spirit's positive test, the *Washington Post* wrote a damning piece that found Baffert to have the highest death rate per start of trainers in California. It is extremely difficult to draw meaningful nationwide comparisons on horse deaths between trainers because only two states, New York and California, publicly name trainers in their fatality statistics. Baffert's team took issue with some of the data analysis done by the *Post*. But based on California state data alone, it's correct to say that he has one of the highest fatality rates among California trainers, when training and racing deaths are included. Still, as an absolute number*—and based entirely on the limited data that's available publicly—his fatalities aren't out of line with other major trainers in and out of the state. At the time of this writing, Baffert has had 41 deaths in California since 2007; by comparison, Todd Pletcher has had 36 die in New York since 2009.[5] (Pletcher, unlike Baffert, also runs a significant number of horses in other states that do not report fatalities by trainer, and so it's possible that his rate is higher than the New York numbers alone suggest.) Some lower-level claiming trainers—invisible outside of racing—have far worse records. Since he began training in New York in 2010, while running far fewer horses than Pletcher, trainer Rudy Rodriguez has had 50 horses die.[6]

Because he runs comparatively fewer horses than Pletcher, measured against number of starts, Baffert's fatality rate is higher. But the simplest explanation for this discrepancy may be the rigor of Baffert's training program, not drugs. The same high-intensity program that means his horses are fitter, and more successful, on race day could also be translating to a high rate of attrition. Research suggests that a certain amount of high-speed work is critical to maintaining soundness, because it promotes bone remodeling. The hard part is striking the right balance between rest and work. Although

---

* I have chosen to use absolute numbers rather than the per-1,000-start rate commonly used as the benchmark in racing, because that statistic fails to account for the number of timed workouts a trainer conducts or the time frame in question; and because it can be misleading to compare trainers who start relatively fewer horses with trainers like Pletcher or Asmussen, who often run more than one thousand horses in a single year. It also doesn't account for the impact of fatality "clusters" like the one that took place in Santa Anita in 2019, which can dramatically skew a trainer's fatality rates.

this continues to be an active area of study, horse training still has a touch of the unknown about it.

Baffert and his team insist that they listen to the horse and ensure an animal is fit before they increase its workload. Baffert also told me that he is aggressive about telling owners: *Your horse isn't going to make it at this level. Don't try to force it to.* He is known for sending horses with training injuries to the farm for rest and recovery—something he has the luxury of doing because there is always another expensive horse to fill the stall. ("I'm always telling people, if you have a horse that's off [lame] for three days, and you can't find [the source], stop immediately because something bad's getting ready to happen," he said. "You just stop.")[7] From what I observed in his barn, this appears to be true. I saw no evidence that Baffert's team is insensitive to the health of horses; Baffert himself has an obvious affection for the animal. "You know what really got me?" he said to me, putting his hand on a horse's halter and pressing his face to the animal's muzzle. "Smelling around the nostril—that smell? I just love that smell. The soft part."[8]

But Baffert, like all trainers, is running a business that is based on getting horses fit enough to win races. In a grim way, he may simply be "better" than the competition.

"Not to pick on Bob, because everybody picks on Bob, but you have these quarter horse trainers like Lukas and Baffert come over who just train the holy bejesus out of these horses," Rick Arthur said.[9] That model can have a cost. (Lukas has, in the past, also faced allegations of having too high a rate of attrition.)[10]

It doesn't follow that *how* Baffert uses medication—what drugs he is giving his horses and how much of it he is giving—is out of the ordinary. The drugs he has given and the concentrations at which they have been found suggest that Baffert's use of therapeutics is basically in line with that of other major trainers—even if he has failed to ensure that these medications are not present in a horse's system on race day. Some of his advocates say that he is conservative about which therapeutics he uses, although without access to proprietary veterinary data, this is impossible to adjudicate. Baffert told me that he believes there are "too many" allowable therapeutics, and that trainers should be able to get by on bute, Lasix, and a handful of others. Arthur in his 2013 report on the 2011 deaths called Baffert's use of medication "moderate."[11]

"Just in my own experience working with Bob, he did not use an awful lot of therapeutic medication," said Eoin Harty, a former assistant trainer who now trains under his own name. "His pre-race medication was bute the night before and five cc's of Lasix on race day."[12]

The question of exactly what happened in the Baffert barn—in 2011 when seven horses died of heart attacks in less than two years, in 2019 and 2020 when he racked up half a dozen positives in a little under two years, and in 2021 when Medina Spirit tested positive in the Kentucky Derby and then died less than a year later—has no single answer.

At least one of those positives—the lidocaine—may have been outside of Baffert's control. Many of the others seemed to be simple, sloppy errors, what regulators call "poor medication control." Failing to better train grooms not to urinate in the stall. Injecting both of a filly's hocks when the threshold and withdrawal time were based on a single injection of 9 milligrams into a single joint. A vet who came to the barn too late in the day. A vet prescribing an ointment that contained a regulated drug. It's true that many of those mistakes do appear to be errors by the veterinarian—but Baffert employs the vet, and the ultimate responsibility rests with him.

Those who know Baffert best—the regulators who have overseen his operation in and out of California for decades, some of his family, former employees—see him as a flawed genius who can't get out of his own way. One former employee who knows him well called him an idiot savant when it comes to training horses. Baffert likes to talk, and he likes to be liked, and he likes to train horses. He cares about his reputation and he is driven by success. He's not interested in the details—he has hired people for that—and some of the details slipped. When he talks, he obfuscates on little things, rearranges facts in his own memory, adjusts the narrative to suit his vision of himself. It's hard to credit him, as the racing regulator said, with carrying out a sophisticated plot.

"I think he's an excellent horse trainer," Rick Sams told me. He paused. "I think he's very naïve when it comes to drugs. He has far too many positives—but I think that's more of a management problem than anything else."

Steve Lewandowski, the former state steward in New York, suggested that those who suspect Baffert and many other top trainers of doping are wildly overestimating their ability to pull it off. In this Lewandowski sounded very much like a source connected to the Jockey Club who in a conversation with me called trainers "farmers."

"Would you rob a bank with any of these trainers? No," Lewandowski said. "I don't see the sophistication where they continuously dope horses."[13]

Baffert's defenders say that his astronomical success is hardly the result of drugs, because, they say, he doesn't need them. Not only is he a preternaturally good horse trainer—something even his critics don't dispute—but he purchases the best young stock available and has an exceptional eye for talent. Most of the horses in his barn aren't diamonds in the rough like Medina Spirit or Real Quiet—not anymore. They are the top prospects with the best pedigrees and the best physicals.

"If you look at Bob's horses going to the track and then look at anybody else's, it's looking at the 49ers and then the junior varsity team," said the former employee. "His bad horses move better than most people's best horses. They look bigger. They look stronger. He's drafting the top picks every year."

Baffert, quietly, pointed out to me that his team spent $6 million on two-year-olds at a sale in 2024. "That's why my stable is so strong."[14] *Money*.

Critics argue that 1/ST and the California Horse Racing Board are protecting Baffert. There are very real conflicts of interest in the horse racing business model—just as Pletcher fills races for NYRA, Baffert fills races for the Stronach Group, so they have an incentive to keep him around. The state of California, meanwhile, permits regulators to participate in a sport they regulate.* But both conflicts are a pervasive problem in racing across jurisdictions. Stuart Janney owns racehorses. Members of the Breeders' Cup board own racehorses. Members of the Kentucky Horse Racing Commission own racehorses. Other NYRA board members own racehorses.

When you put Baffert's case in that context, he begins to look less like the singular villain of horse racing that he has been painted as and more like just another horse trainer in a bad system. The penalties he has received begin to look like a marketing effort—*Look, we've gotten rid of our most notorious doper. Come bet on our product*—one that conveniently ignores that Baffert's sins are the industry's. His ceaseless complaint—why me?—appears reasonable against the backdrop of the sport's handling of Pletcher, among others. His mistakes—and they are many—begin to seem logical in a culture that has through most of its history managed to defy any real efforts at professionalization and reform.

In 2014, after an undercover investigation by People for the Ethical Treatment of Animals (PETA) into Steve Asmussen's barn revealed his routine

* Here again, the financial model is partially to blame: a seat on the racing commission is a political appointment in California rather than a salaried position. Barring board members from participating in the sport would likely make it harder to attract qualified candidates willing to do the job for free, one racing executive posited to me.

use of legal medication and showed his assistant trainer using derogatory
expletives to refer to horses, Dinny Phipps, then the chairman of the Jockey
Club, said publicly that Asmussen should "stay away" from the Kentucky
Derby that year "for the good of the game." Otherwise, Asmussen's "pres-
ence and participation would indicate that it's just 'business as usual' in the
Thoroughbred industry," Phipps wrote.[15]

Of course, it *was* business as usual.

"It is wrong to characterize Asmussen as a bad apple. It is unfair to
single him out for stigmatization," Andrew Beyer wrote in the *Washington
Post*. And it was "thoroughly disingenuous" for Phipps to suggest that if
Asmussen, alone and singly, were not present, it would show that racing
had rejected "'business as usual."

The same could be said of Bob Baffert.

When I first talked to Baffert about the positive in early 2023, standing in
his box overlooking the wire at Santa Anita, the spot where Medina Spirit
had dropped, he was defiant. He was a horse trainer in command of his
craft. His suspension was behind him and he had a number of promising
three-year-olds in his barn. A sharp bay colt burly with muscle named
American Lion breezed past us. In the barn, Baffert had switched to shavings
in his stalls because he didn't want the risk of another scopolamine positive
that he feared might come hidden in straw bedding. He was defensive:
some of the positives he had received were "sloppiness," but they weren't
his sloppiness. They were little mistakes by his staff and others that other
trainers got a pass for.[16] His commentary pattered like rain on a tin roof.
Into the radio: "11 and two, that's beautiful. Shut her down, boy!" Another
colt started his work. "12 and three, that's a little slow . . . now he's movin'."
After a moment, to no one in particular: "I should have worked him in
company." Another pause. Then, like the winds shifting, he was talking
about Medina Spirit and the grave injustice that he perceived had been
dealt to him and the horse.

"The bias against me, it's just horrible," he said. "The only thing that gets
me through this is I know we didn't do anything wrong. We were treating
the horse for a skin rash. It's not what they said it was."

But by the spring of 2024, something indefatigable in Baffert seemed
to have given way a little.

The necropsy for the horse had come back. There is something uniquely horrible about equine necropsies. To see an animal as majestic and beloved as the Thoroughbred split open and splayed out on the table feels like a terrible violation. Even the language is humiliating and vulgar, a heartless account of the indignities of Medina Spirit's last moments on the earth. His body had "blue stained tape bandages at the level of both fetlock joints," which were "soiled with dirt." "There are scant, soft feces oozing from the anus. There are multifocal, 1 to 3 cm scratches on the upper left eyelid and the adjacent skin of the forehead. The skin of the left side of the head and neck is abraded and with dry blood." There are photos of Medina Spirit's organs attached to the report.

The results of the necropsy offered none of the solace that might have come with answers. It was like the seven 2011 deaths all over again. Investigators could not officially establish a cause of death, although it had probably been a heart arrhythmia. He was scanned for a battery of drugs, including betamethasone, EPO, and clenbuterol. All that was found was a common anti-ulcer medication and Lasix, both perfectly permissible.

In January 2024, Baffert had finally dropped the appeal of the Kentucky Horse Racing Commission's decision to disqualify Medina Spirit.[17] It was three and a half months before the 150th running of the Kentucky Derby. Under the original two-year ban, Baffert should have been allowed to participate. But Bill Carstanjen had already extended the ban for another year, citing Baffert's continued defense of Medina Spirit. Baffert, the track said, had continued "to peddle a false narrative concerning the failed drug test of Medina Spirit. . . . A trainer who is unwilling to accept responsibility for multiple drug test failures in our highest-profile races cannot be trusted to avoid future misconduct."[18] Baffert's decision to drop the suit did not change Carstanjen's mind.* Zedan alone would later sue for the right to enter one of his horses in the Derby, but Baffert would not participate in the suit. It failed anyway.

Baffert called the test result "just a stupid, foolish positive" and a "mix-up"—acknowledging for the first time, at least to me, that the positive test had been legitimate.

"I never apologized publicly for, you know, for having that positive. I should have been more . . ." he said. In classic Baffert fashion, he left the

---

* According to Clark Brewster, Carstanjen had told Baffert during a meeting in late 2023 that if he dropped his various challenges of the outcome of Medina Spirit's Kentucky Derby, he would be allowed to participate.

end of the sentence unfinished, the kind of murky hole in his thinking that has always allowed his listeners to fill in whatever conclusion they wished.

Baffert still believed the horse shouldn't have been disqualified.[19] "It was such a gallant effort by him. He had so much heart," he said. Medina Spirit, given the chance to show his mettle, had fought for the win. "It just shows you how competitive these horses are."[20]

But Baffert was tired. He and his family were scarred by the events of the last two years.

"It's gonna go on and on. And just, it's just not—it's just dragging and dragging. I'm tired of answering questions about it. You got to put it behind you. I want to just live a nice, quiet—I'm done with all the fighting and all that, you know?"

He was still angry. He still believed that the families that ruled the Jockey Club had engineered his downfall. He relayed endless rumors he had heard about Janney, about Dinny Phipps's son, Odgen Phipps II. Janney had won the Derby in 2013 with a horse named Orb, and Baffert had heard that the horse had had a positive test that the KHRC had covered up. (There is no evidence to support this story that I could uncover, but it is true that the horse received a legal corticosteroid around the time of the Triple Crown that was not properly recorded with state authorities—a violation that was quietly reported only under the vet's name, rather than the horse's, allowing owner and trainer to avoid public scrutiny.)* Phipps II, Baffert said, had told one of his owners that Baffert was using EPO. "This dumb fuck," Baffert called him, in some of the most abrasive language I'd ever heard him use. Racetrack talk is always punctuated by blue language, but Baffert is pretty tame by local standards, and his ad hominem attacks are usually relatively gentle. He tends toward the suspicious more than the outright vitriolic. Yet here his voice rose: "He doesn't even know who I am! And they're part of the Jockey Club! They're part of NYRA. And they're telling *my owner*!

---

* According to Lewandowski, who was a steward in New York at the time, and George Maylin, the New York lab director, Janney's vet gave Orb a legal corticosteroid between the Preakness and the Belmont. The drug was given appropriately and outside the withdrawal period, both said. But under New York regulation, the vet was supposed to record with the state that the drug had been administered. He failed to do so and received a citation from the state of New York. The citation does not name the horse, and the matter appears not to have been publicized. Janney, in an on-the-record interview, confirmed this account. "My understanding is that [the vet], who does not practice in New York, maybe did not do the paperwork on that," he told me. Shug McGaughey, when I asked him for comment on this, accused me of making up rumors. Omertà.

If he's telling him, they're telling everybody! And it's all rumor mill. They can't believe how this guy keeps winning. I've been doing this a long time. I work hard at it."

By spring of 2024, Janney was facing his own reckoning in the sport. The CBS News program *60 Minutes* had aired a piece in late 2023 that heavily linked breakdowns to a pervasive culture of doping. The show interviewed Janney and quoted him as saying that the regulation of racing had failed to clean up the sport. In describing hiring 5 Stones, he explained to host Cecilia Vega that he told the group "to go after the important people that I think are corrupting the sport."[21] People within the industry—including Baffert—interpreted Janney to be admitting that he had sicced a private investigator on certain trainers he disliked. Janney indicated later that he was trying to say that he had told 5 Stones to go after big players in general, not specific big players,[22] but that explanation didn't satisfy his critics. Few in the industry opposed the prosecution of Navarro or Servis, and so left unsaid is whom Janney is meant to have unfairly targeted.* But the narrative took hold, and all of the quiet distrust of the Jockey Club and its blue-blooded, closed-door clubbiness was suddenly a matter of public debate.

A well-liked Fasig-Tipton executive publicly called on Janney to "change the structure of the Jockey Club so that industry stakeholders have the opportunity to elect the members and board."[23] Mike Repole, the billionaire maker of the sports drinks Vitaminwater and BodyArmor, declared himself a "national commissioner" for racing and now frequently takes to social media to lambaste Janney as out of touch, calling him "Stuart Little Janney" and proclaiming that he "hasn't done anything for racing."[24] Midcareer horsemen who I spoke to complained that Janney has fixated on the drugs issue, which some see as overblown, instead of trying to proactively grow the sport, by spearheading client relations initiatives to make racing a more attractive experience for high-dollar owners and gamblers, for example.

---

* "What 5 Stones did was to create a body of work to take to the federal government that said here is what we found and suggested that a lot is going on in this industry that shouldn't be happening and that is big enough and important enough that you should be interested. After that, the federal government was in charge. To suggest that I targeted anybody is really to misunderstand how the process worked," Janney said in an interview with the *Thoroughbred Daily News* shortly after the *60 Minutes* piece aired. https://www.thoroughbreddailynews.com/addressing-the-60-minutes -piece-a-q-a-with-stuart-janney-iii/.

Chad Brown, the New York trainer whom 5 Stones had investigated, believes Janney begrudged him his success because he is self-made and wins races. "There's class warfare" in racing, he said. The old private stables have dwindled into memory, and brash new money has come to dominate the sport. "I think that's an uncomfortable adjustment for someone like Stuart Janney," Brown said. "He can't get his head around how this is where the sport has gone, and how people are successful, and not doing it the way his family did for generations."[25] Brown may be projecting, but the sense of grievance he feels is shared by many horsemen I spoke to.

Janney's efforts on behalf of the sport have been largely positive. The FBI would not have taken note of horse racing without 5 Stones; HISA may have its flaws, but it was at least an effort to replace a broken system. Still, whether out of hubris or naïveté, he appears to have overestimated the sport's tolerance for fundamentally antidemocratic action. Five Stones got the FBI to take notice—but it also appears to have investigated Chad Brown and Bob Baffert in ways that at best were unsuccessful and at worst were overly aggressive. HISA may be a good-faith effort to solve "the drug problem" in racing, but its structural lack of transparency has left it open to suspicion.

He is also only human. Janney exists in the same whorl of paranoia that grips most of the sport, possessed of the utter conviction that *somebody is cheating*—he just can't prove it. That, in a person of authority who is at least perceived to operate as though he still lives in a time where the landed gentry are responsible for managing the working class, has stymied his efforts at leadership and damaged his reputation with some members of the industry.

In many ways, Baffert's career is a parable of the big forces buffeting racing. He stands at the crossroads of the undeniable classist tension between the affluent old stables and the money-grubbing new guard. Racing, one longtime executive said, "throws together virtually every walk of life, from the very, very tops of the socioeconomic strata on down to the very bottom." That comes with "the social resentments that are going to be natural in an environment like the one that our sport exists in." The shadow war between Bob Baffert and Stuart Janney, two men profoundly distrustful of one another, who came to the top of the sport by very different pathways, speaks to the simmering antipathy for the Jockey Club, the Phipps family, even the old Kentucky breeders like the Hancock family, on one side;

and on the other side, the powerful suspicion of a privileged few that the sport's brash, ambitious working class could not possibly be doing so well on their own.

But most graphically, Baffert is a symbol of racing's failure to reckon with the foundational business model it has built around the horse, a model that may have finally outlived its time.

CHAPTER 25

"WE'RE ALL JUST WHORES"?

In 2018, Eric Hamelback sat down in a chair facing members of the powerful House Energy and Commerce Committee. Hamelback had been a high school football star in Louisiana when a back injury ended his plans to play ball in college, but he still went, studying animal science. He moved to Kentucky shortly after college to work on a Thoroughbred farm, eventually advancing to general manager in Frank Stronach's breeding empire. Hamelback was a big man, a hardworking former linebacker who describes himself as a loyal husband and a proud father, and one can imagine him coaxing skittish yearlings into behaving on sheer mass alone.

A few years before, Hamelback had left the barn to become the CEO of the Horsemen's Benevolent and Protective Association, the loose confederation representing Thoroughbred trainers across the country. The HBPA had staked out its uncompromising opposition to the passage of what became the Horseracing Integrity and Safety Act, legislation that the Jockey Club and its allies were then still lobbying Congress to pass, and now Hamelback sat before the committee, spitting mad. Stuart Janney sat at the same table and appeared, as always in the hallways of power, at ease and arguably a little smug.

Unbeknownst to Hamelback or anyone else in the room except Janney, the original 5 Stones probe was underway. Janney knew about Seth Fishman. He felt, at that point, completely and entirely confident that he had firm evidence of doping in Thoroughbred racing that was going undetected by state regulators.

Hamelback, in his opening statement, told lawmakers unequivocally that data compiled by the state regulators had showed "conclusively that doping of racehorses in the US is rare."

"The horse racing industry spends millions of dollars on comprehensive testing each year. In 2017, there were over 354,000 biological samples taken by regulators in the US. Only 169 of those tests were positive for drugs that had no business being in the horse," Hamelback said. "So to put it plainly, 99.9 percent of all tests were negative of any doping substance. That's a record that should be the envy of every sport that tests for illegal drugs."[1]

It was an embarrassingly credulous claim to make for anyone who insisted, as Hamelback did during the hearing, that he was opposed to the doping of racehorses. The existence of untestable "designer drugs"—drugs that had a single molecule toggled to make it equally effective but invisible to drug screening—was not a secret, even if Seth Fishman's operation had not yet been made public. It was not unlike defenders of Lance Armstrong claiming that because he had never tested positive on a drug screening, he was therefore innocent of doping.* It was also well-known that different labs screened for different drugs at varying levels of sensitivity—and that labs can adjust the sensitivity of their testing for particular substances. (Truesdail, for example, had long been known as the budget option for testing, "doing the bare minimum, charging the bare minimum, and not reporting [any positives], and then there are the laboratories that have access to" better technology, "and they're reporting new stuff and at lower concentrations," Rick Sams said.) Ed Martin, the head of the Association of State Racing Commissioners International, also testifying at the hearing, put the problem a little more honestly: when it came to catching dopers, "racing does as good a job or as bad a job as the Olympics or any other sport," Martin said.

But it would become a refrain from the HBPA and other opponents of HISA: racing doesn't *have* a doping problem, because no one had caught any dopers. Those arguments persisted even after the 2020 indictments, miraculously. Karen Murphy, the lawyer who was working with MediVet and SGF-1000, is outraged, even today, about the entire federal case, which she thinks should have left Thoroughbred trainers out entirely. "It's all fucking harness. The whole thing is harness. Navarro is training for harness, they tapped his phone based on his training for harness," she said to me. The indictment that prosecutors would ultimately file, she said, "had nothing to do with Thoroughbred racing. Nothing."[2]

---

* Elsewhere during the hearing, Hamelback did acknowledge the need for more research into designer drugs, an appeal that is difficult to square with his insistence that there was no evidence racing had a bigger problem than the 99.9 percent clearance rate on drug screening might suggest.

The notion that the case didn't have anything to do with Thoroughbred racing is patently counterfactual. Jorge Navarro, of course, was a prominent Thoroughbred trainer who was actively doping his Thoroughbred horses. And the unspoken suggestion that Navarro is the only Thoroughbred trainer to ever use illegal substances is laughable. The day after the 2018 congressional hearing, federal authorities arrested three Thoroughbred trainers (and a track clocker) in Pennsylvania for rigging races,[3] one of whom was charged with drugging horses.[4*] It's impossible to quantify how prevalent doping is in racing—we don't know what we don't know—but we know how long Seth Fishman's designer products went undetected. Now racing regulators are concerned not just about untestable drugs built by tweaking individual molecules; they are worried about developing tests for a burgeoning class of substances called "selective androgen receptor modulators," or SARMs, which mimic the effects of anabolic steroids. "The challenge is knowing which ones to look for," said one racing chemist.

Still, that was how the HBPA and its allies seemed to view the problem of "doping" in Thoroughbred racing: invisible and, therefore, nonexistent.

"Plain and simple," Hamelback said. "There's no proof [that] what we are doing currently needs further oversight."[5]

Hamelback and the other opponent of the bill testifying before the committee, industry lawyer Alan Foreman, also firmly stated that the horse racing industry didn't have a problem with therapeutic drugs. Much of the hearing, intended to consider a comprehensive piece of legislation covering medication and safety regulation broadly in racing, zeroed in on a single drug: Lasix.

Baffled lawmakers read prewritten questions they didn't understand, clearly fed to them by different stakeholders, that illuminated nothing. One side held that Lasix was safe and effective (largely true), and that it was inhumane not to give it to racehorses (a matter of debate). The other side argued that it could mask both injury and PED use (probably not true) and potentially weaken the breed (maybe true). The entire debate was reduced to an incoherent back-and-forth about the impact of Lasix on animal welfare.

---

* For another example: HISA had been in charge of medication regulation for roughly a year at the time Murphy and I had that conversation; during that time frame, horses under the care of three (low-level) trainers tested positive for cobalt. Cobalt has long been banned across jurisdictions, and there is a clear test for it. https://www.thoroughbreddailynews.com/monte-gelrod-latest-parx-trainer-to-have-cobalt-positive/.

What was more notable about the hearing was what it didn't discuss: the culture and economy of the racetrack that underpinned the widespread use of Lasix, or any other medication, legal or illegal. Only Foreman came close.

"If there is a move to eliminate Lasix in this country, it's going to force owners out of the business," Foreman said. He contemplated a system in which sales companies would force sellers to disclose bleeders. "Can you envision buying . . . a product where you're told at the time of sale that this product may have a problem [but] you're not going to be able to fix it in a way that you can use it? Are you going to buy that product?"

Doing away with Lasix, he said, would "chill sales."[6]

It was strikingly honest language to use in public. Most of the time, racing folks called racehorses "athletes" or "animals" when they were communicating with the public. But here was Alan Foreman calling racehorses— animals conceived solely for this purpose—a "product." He understood, and was brave enough to articulate, the truth about what racehorses are to the industry and how they are treated. It is their status as a "product" that dictates the care they receive.

Foreman went on. If horses who bleed can't get Lasix and therefore can't run, he said, their owners will leave the sport. "Where are those horses going to go?" he asked. And what would happen to the tens of thousands of people employed to care for them across the country?

"That's the welfare crisis that I'm talking about, and I'm sure many of you have heard about from constituents who are in the industry, and what effect what you think is a simple change will have on the economics of the horse racing industry," Foreman almost thundered.

He had just hit on the very heart of racing's welfare problem, and it was far bigger than Lasix or even drugs in general. He was asking, in effect, what happens if the cost of treating horses as anything more than a "product" is too high for most industry participants to bear. Would those horses, now worthless, be sold in kill pens and go to slaughter in Mexico? Some might be adopted by hobbyists and go on to second "careers," but not all. Was the economic impact generated by racing—the livelihood of the groom living on the backstretch, the farrier shoeing horses at training farms in Pennsylvania, the trainer with just ten or fifteen claimers in his barn in West Virginia— worth some compromises to the purest ideal of care for every horse?

Representative Bob Latta, the chairman of the subcommittee holding the hearing, said only, disinterestedly, "Thank you," and moved on to a prewritten question about milkshaking.

◆

In 2014, researchers at the University of Texas at Austin wrote a paper about interactions between humans and domesticated animals that was published in the *International Journal of the History of Sport*.[7] The paper examined the case of Dancer's Image, the horse that won the Derby in 1968 and was disqualified for bute. Decades later, the researchers wrote that the horse was simultaneously anthropomorphized and commodified. Dancer's Image was ascribed "a human-like moral code centered on the noble pursuit of athletic victory. When stripped of his victory, Dancer's Image is shown in these representations as suffering a tremendous emotional blow." Peter Fuller described the horse as having been "libeled" and insisted that as his owner he had to "clear the horse's name."[8]

And yet, the UT authors wrote, "alongside such instances of anthropomorphism . . . one can find numerous cases in which the horse's disqualification is discussed in purely monetary terms." Fuller, before the Kentucky Horse Racing Commission, also talked about the money that he stood to lose because the horse's value as a stallion prospect would be less if the disqualification stood.

Racetrackers insist on calling the horse "an athlete," but it is not. Athletes have agency. The horse is a financial asset. That reality governs its fate. This is not inconsistent with affection for the animal and indeed, many Thoroughbred horses are beloved. They also receive a highly attentive and sophisticated standard of care. But that care is centered not on the horse's well-being for its own sake but on enabling the animal to run and breed. Although the racing industry has increasingly created structures and institutions for aftercare, while the horse is still in use as racing or breeding stock, with a few exceptions, husbandry is performed not for its own sake but as a fiduciary duty to the animal's owners. I am not accusing (most) horsemen of being callous or unfeeling about the animals they work with; quite the opposite. Most horsemen I know show a tender loyalty for the horse. Welfare is a factor, of course, and most decisions are made within an Overton window of acceptable care. But their choices are necessarily governed by the accounting ledger. Small, seemingly inconsequential choices on a day-to-day basis are made with a necessary attention to the balance between cost and revenue. It is not one single evil, but the accumulation of small harms in a diffuse, historically underregulated capitalist system. This same problem faces many large, complex systems, like the health care industry.

The common misconception is that if you just did away with drugs, that would fix the breakdown problem. It's not true, although certainly medication, like joint injections, plays a role. Drugs and breakdowns are both a symptom of the same ailing system.

This problem goes beyond the racetrack, to the real moneymakers in the sport: the breeding farms. In 2021, a breeding stallion at one of the major commercial studs in central Kentucky, WinStar Farm, died after he was administered a fatal shot of multiple expired off-label vitamins and iron "in excessive amounts." The stallion was given the shot because he had been refusing to breed mares for two days and seemed lethargic. "There was hope," the Paulick Report wrote, "the vitamins would give him renewed energy to breed." The stallion, Laoban, had struggled with soundness issues that apparently made it painful for him to breed. "Despite these problems," the Paulick Report said, "Laoban's report of mares bred maintained in WinStar's records indicates he bred two mares a day for much of the breeding season, covering 126 mares, some of them multiple times in the season."[9] His stud fee was $25,000.

Stories like this put the lie to the racing industry's insistence on calling these horses "athletes." They are working animals, an asset that is not precisely analogous to livestock bred for consumption—but certainly not pets. A pet would have been given a rest from the job he was being asked to do, even if it cost his owner money. An asset must be rehabilitated to perform. The standard of care may be incredibly high in terms of the attention and intervention the horse receives. But the *purpose* of the care is the animal's performance.

As a culture, we have accepted this revenue-driven standard of care, with a few limits, for animals that we use to provide the essential function of feeding us. But the horse doesn't feed us and it doesn't carry us to war or plow our fields anymore. Although the Thoroughbred creates jobs, its basic function is the entertainment of owners and gamblers. It raises the question of whether the standard of care should be brought in line with the standard for pets: divorced from the financial incentive.

Many horsemen I know will be incredibly frustrated by what I have written here. They will, rightly, point out the individual horses they have rehomed that weren't suited to racing; the horses they have loved and connected with over the years; the times they have forgone profit or forked over income to give a horse what it needed; the obsessive care they have given to every horse in the barn. This reality is not incompatible with what I've written. I am not writing about the individual horsemen who are doing the best they can by the horses in their care. I am writing about the regulatory, social, and economic system they exist in—and the ways it can be abused. It's a system that not only allowed Jorge Navarro to successfully drug his horses for years but may also have pushed him to think he had no other choice. A system that offers that many opportunities for abuse is also a system that can lead even the best horsemen to make decisions for individual animals that may not live up to the highest ideal of care.

Good horsemen—and there are many—will put the overall good of the horse before the bottom line, particularly in extreme and obvious cases. But it's not the extreme and obvious case that concerns me. It's the accumulation of small compromises made every day. These are not compromises made with the big greed that we associate with Washington Irving's Tom Walker, selling his soul to the devil in exchange for Captain Kidd's worldly treasure. They are little compromises, made to make ends meet, or with a child's college education in mind, for some; but for others, with a vague dream of a bigger house or an annual vacation in the Virgin Islands hovering as the unspoken motivator—the American dream. They are compromises made from a drive to keep up with the Joneses, an ambition to move up in society, or a fierce desire simply to *belong*. Sometimes they are compromises made because, as racing has grown less popular and the pool of money available to run it has shrunk, it is increasingly difficult to make a living at it. They are compromises made by individuals and by racing's biggest corporate structures, compromises made at the racetrack and in the sales and breeding sector. Compromises like: the decision to put screws in a yearling's knee so he is more salable at auction. The decision to put every yearling in the barn on Thyro-L. The decision to inject a horse's ankles with Depo-Medrol to get him to the races. The decision to give a two-year-old in training clenbuterol between races or before a sale. The decision to try just one more shot of vitamins to see if you can get an obviously tired and sore stallion to breed.

Perhaps the most appalling display of brute commercial self-interest at the expense of the breed—and make no mistake, the soundness of the *breed* is a welfare problem—was the wholesale rejection by some of the big Kentucky breeding farms of what is known as the Mare Cap. In 2020, the Jockey Club moved to restrict the number of mares that registered Thoroughbred stallions were allowed to breed, to 140 a year. This would have been in line with the way that the breeding business used to work, before advances in veterinary science allowed stallions to breed upward of 200 mares a year in some cases. Because stallions could only breed so many mares per year—40 used to be considered a "full book"—if a stallion's offspring turned out to be unsound or otherwise unsuited to racing, its impact on the overall gene pool was limited. But now, when big commercial nurseries allow first- and second-season sires to breed more than 200 mares a year to make good on large purchase prices, "we've concentrated all our eggs," Seth Hancock told me.[10] Suddenly there may be hundreds of unsound young horses from a single unproven stallion headed to the racetrack—with no plan B for those animals if they can't stand up to the rigors of racing. Because there are so many of them, those same horses may themselves wind up being bred. In this system, one unsound horse has the potential to create many more.

Several farms are known for breeding particularly large books of mares, including Coolmore, the empire than Robert Sangster built. It, along with Spendthrift and Three Chimneys, immediately moved to kill any effort to limit their right to breed as many mares as they damn well pleased. The three farms sued the Jockey Club in federal court, alleging an "anti-competitive restraint" that threatened the free market of the bloodstock business.[11] The Jockey Club was later forced to rescind the rule after the Speaker of Kentucky's House of Representatives cosponsored a bill that would have prohibited it from "restricting the number of mares that can be bred to a stallion" in the state of Kentucky.[12] There were also quiet threats that Kentucky might move to establish its own stud book, an effort that would have utterly fractured the industry but was nevertheless an effective deterrent. The profit imperative had won the day.

The racetracks are among the worst bad actors in this flawed system. Racing secretaries at some tracks will write a condition book with more races than the track has horses to fill, then see which races attract the most entries. Those races, which will earn the track the most money, will be the ones that "go." Races that don't fill don't run. This makes it impossible for trainers to plan a campaign for a horse. Either the animal must be kept at peak fitness constantly or hustled into the starting gate without the proper conditioning. It's a profit maximization tool for the racetracks, but it's a recipe for injury for the horse. And there continue to be troubling allegations that suggest some racetracks are still pushing horses to run that shouldn't to maximize field size. In Illinois, a state-licensed veterinarian has accused track officials (as well as state regulatory officers) of overruling her in multiple instances when she tried to scratch unsound horses prior to a race, something she said was part of an effort to increase betting revenue. (The track denies the allegations.)[13] Other tracks, meanwhile, have been accused by horsemen of failing to spend the resources to maintain a safe racing surface.[14]

You can also lay fault at the feet of owners, who continue to buy faster and faster two-year-olds, or send horses to trainers with known records of drug positives—or worse. In a conversation recorded by the FBI between one of the operators of a racing stable in California and Navarro, the owner asked Navarro if a horse called Nanoosh was getting "all the shit."

"He gets everything," Navarro assured him.[15]

Racing has been telling itself a comfortable lie. Only now has public scrutiny forced the sport to grapple with its great paradox. John Williams, a former sales consignor and onetime general manager of Spendthrift, recalled something that a breeder once said to him.

"John," he remembered the breeder saying, "we're all just whores."[16]

Racing has made lurching efforts to improve itself in recent years—and it has made profound progress that suggests there is great reason for hope. As HISA has tightened and standardized many of the rules governing veterinary oversight, testing, medication guidelines, and best practices on the backstretch, fatalities in the states it governs have dropped dramatically. In the first quarter of 2024, racing-related fatalities dropped by 38 percent[17]—a testament not to a single cure but to a broad effort to professionalize the sport. Individual tracks saw even more pronounced improvements: in 2023, nine horses died during racing at Saratoga;[18] in 2024, one died.[19] This progress must be sustained, but it's a significant step in the right direction that hasn't received enough attention outside the sport.

Racetracks have increasingly turned to sophisticated screening technology to try to diagnose underlying injuries before the worst happens. Both Churchill Downs and Santa Anita now have PET (positron emission tomography) units, high-tech imaging machines that are particularly useful in spotting damage to a horse's fragile ankle. Some racetracks have experimented with biometric sensor technology to detect minute changes to a horse's gait that might help identify early warning signs. The industry is developing increasingly sophisticated data analytics tools to spot at-risk horses who might benefit from further diagnostic scrutiny or veterinary oversight. The hope is that early detection may help trainers manage horses better and prevent breakdowns.

Perhaps for the first time, the regulatory model governing racing may be acting as a deterrent. HISA has instituted tougher, mandatory penalties for banned substance violations and has pledged to expand out-of-competition testing. It has made it far more difficult for trainers to drag out the adjudication of positive tests. And it has issued rules requiring horses that are scratched by a state vet before a race to pass a blood test and a vet evaluation of a workout to be eligible to race again. It's early, but multiple horsemen I spoke to reported that trainers are being forced to take a more conservative approach to both medication and soundness management—even if some of them complain about it.[20] Equally importantly, it has jurisdiction over the racetracks, and can effectively prohibit tracks from exporting the feed of their races out of state or taking online bets—huge penalties to revenue—if the track isn't satisfying safety regulations.*

Meanwhile, HISA has sought to standardize the labs, a key part of creating a level regulatory playing field across the country. George Maylin's lab was not selected as a HISA lab; the University of Kentucky in spring of 2024 had its accreditation removed while its lab director was placed under investigation. In September, the drug enforcement arm created by the new law released a report that found the director, Scott Stanley, had charged for some tests he hadn't performed, including a confirmatory analysis on a sample that initial screening suggested contained EPO. The machinery he would have used to test for EPO, in fact, was "inoperable."[21] According to the Paulick Report, a separate review by the university also found that the director had the ability to change test results without anyone knowing. Stanley denied any wrongdoing and blamed the challenges on "real, systemic issues involved in shifting regulatory frameworks" between the old state system and HISA that he said went ignored by the new regulators.[22] It appeared

---

* To take that step, HISA would have to revoke the "accreditation" of a covered racetrack, something it declined to do in September 2024, when horsemen complained after a fatal breakdown that the turf course at Parx had been poorly maintained and the track, which also runs a casino, was unwilling to spend the money to fix it. (Parx, in a statement denying the charges, noted that it was at the "forefront" of the fight against "the rampant and pervasive use of illegal substances by unscrupulous trainers on their horses.") HISA evaluated the track, met with Parx officials about their mediation plans, and "will continue to closely monitor" the safety of the surface. Natalie Voss, "Despite HISA Oversight, Parx Turf Course's Seasonal Bow Had a Bobble," Paulick Report, September 23, 2024, https://paulickreport.com/news/thoroughbred-racing/despite-hisa-oversight -parx-turf-courses-seasonal-bow-had-a-bobble.

to be a stunning validation of every racetrack "conspiracy theory" about lab testing; every time Baffert had said to me: "These labs can really screw you, if they want you."[23] (Of course, it also raised questions about whether Baffert and others had inadvertently been the beneficiary of lax testing procedures in California, where Stanley had run the state lab until late 2018; many of Baffert's high-profile positives have been for horses running in other states.)[24] The whole mess—including the basic fact that the labs from the two biggest racing jurisdictions in the country were not considered up to scratch—was a broad indictment of the professionalization of the industry. HISA's effort promises to close a loophole: in theory, trainers will not be able to use more medication in one state than another simply because the testing is less sensitive there. For the first time, the sport could have a consistent picture of the scope of the use of both therapeutics and known PEDs.

Horse racing is essentially a fractious confederation of thousands of small businesses. Not all trainers, racetracks, or races are created equal: A McKinsey study commissioned by the Jockey Club found that from 2018 to 2022, just 50 trainers (out of roughly 4,500 with at least one start)[25] accounted for 13 percent of all North American fatalities. (The study did not name those trainers.) Those 50 trainers demonstrated more than twice the average fatality rate. The same study found that tracks that perform an additional vet screen for horses after they are entered in a race have a 30–40 percent lower fatality rate. Claiming races had a 25 percent higher fatality risk to horses.* Those are numbers that suggest not just problems, but clear opportunities for improvement.[26] They also suggest that some racing entities are doing things right already: critics of US racing often point out that fatality rates in the United States are much higher than those in many other racing nations, but that's a national average. At some tracks the fatalities are in line with international standards, Del Mar, Gulfstream, and Santa Anita among them.

There are some states that are challenging the constitutionality of HISA in federal court, including Texas, Arkansas, and Louisiana, among others.

---

* Why claiming races are more dangerous is a hotly debated topic. In general, claimers are lower-quality horses that run more frequently and can change barns often. In some states, the purse in a given race can be much larger than the "tag"—the set price a horse can be claimed for, and thus its market value. This can create an incentive to take a chance on running an unsound but cheap—and thus expendable—horse to try to cash in on a big purse. There is evidence that when the purse/tag ratio gets out of whack, fatalities increase. https://paulickreport.com/horse-care-category/racing-safety-whatever-happened-to-that-purse-to-claim-price-ratio.

These states, not under HISA's authority as a result, are currently demon-strating much higher fatality rates. It's an argument in favor of HISA's approach, but also a reminder that the sport remains at war with itself; that HISA is a technocratic solution to a cultural problem. HISA doesn't pretend to fix all the industry's problems, and although it has forced some real improvements in fatality rates, its successes are not enough for the sport to claim victory.*

The industry must address the cultural failing that is racing's original sin: its view of the horse.

The racing business—the entire industry—must make a readjustment toward thinking of the horse as a "pet"—not an investment, not an asset, not even an "athlete."† Only then can it tackle the myriad small adjustments that will necessarily cut down on the income of participants but will safeguard the horse. Tightening the number of permissible therapeutic medications is only one of a thousand small adjustments that might be made. There are regulatory changes that could force better husbandry of the breed. One example that comes to mind: German breed authorities must approve all stallions that go to stud. Prospective stallions must not only meet certain physical standards that indicate soundness, but they must meet a high standard of performance on the track and have never run on bute, Lasix,

---

* Horsemen from HISA-run states often express frustration that despite the dramatic improve-ments to fatality rates in 2024, negative stories continue to be written about horse racing. Even though there is a jurisdictional divide between HISA states and non-HISA states, in a very real way they still belong to the same industry. There is evidence that horses that don't meet HISA's standards for safety and soundness are simply shipped to non-HISA states, where the rules are looser. That isn't just a regulatory failure in Arkansas or Texas. It's a broader industry failing to protect these animals, bred and sold by its participants for this purpose. Different industry groups operating within the HISA system are aware of the problem, and there has been some discussion about what to do about it, but because of this basic commonality—the Thorough-bred horse—I have declined to separate "HISA states" from "non-HISA states" or to parse the differences between the two.

† I want to be clear that I am not advocating for changing the legal classification of horses to "pet" and away from "livestock." My recommendation to think of racehorses as "pets" is a cultural one. As a legal matter, most US states and, since 2018, the federal government recognize horses as livestock. https://www.usda.gov/farmbill. Changing that would have a host of downstream effects that probably would make it logistically and financially prohibitive for many people to own and use horses. It would also impose regulation that would make it difficult to practice good-faith herd management care practices, and would have important consequences for the regulation of slaughter (a controversial topic beyond the scope of this book, but suffice it to say that there is a welfare argument in favor of legalizing and regulating it in the United States, primarily to prevent animals from being bought by kill buyers and shipped across the border to be slaughtered in a setting where the US has no regulatory power to protect these animals in their final moments).

or any other medication. Germany, perhaps not by accident, is known for breeding tough, sound horses that are able to maintain lengthy careers.[27] Janney told me that the Jockey Club in 2023 began to look at how best to reform the claiming game to better protect horses from a predatory system and develop a functioning market for lower-level animals.

As with any systemic change, the ripple effect must be managed and unintended consequences anticipated. Adequate investment in horse after-care will be important, because animals that can't compete on the racetrack cannot be left to the mercies of the open marketplace. The basic economic framework of racing must be fixed so that horsemen *can* make a living while maintaining the appropriate standard of care. Janney, in advocating for reforms to the claiming game, points out that the volatile financial nature of running claimers is part of the reason why yearling sales for horses that aren't obvious stakes horses worth hundreds of thousands of dollars are "such a disaster." There's "no market—and there used to be. Not every horse can be a $300,000 yearling."[28] Right now, while horses at the top of the market can bring eye-popping money at the sales, horses at the lower end are often overlooked and unprofitable for their sellers. In theory, if the purse structure was reformed to create a reliable calendar of competitive races for horses of varying levels of ability, there might be a more robust market for cheaper horses that would benefit horsemen.* There will also probably need to be a long-term resolution to a 1978 federal law that has left racetracks earning a smaller percentage of the money wagered on their races at off-track facilities than that spent at the racetrack where the races are being run. In the modern era, so-called simulcast wagering makes up the bulk of most tracks' business; the result is smaller purses, so the problem trickles down to how horsemen make their living too.[29] Finally, and perhaps most importantly, the sport will have to do as horsemen say: address how to better attract and maintain both fans and gamblers.

"The whole business of racing, the economics of racing, the loss of support in various jurisdictions—that's the next challenge, and that isn't HISA," Janney said. "HISA does not do that."[30]

Right now, the Jockey Club seems to be providing some of the only meaningful intellectual leadership on the big-picture problems facing racing.

---

* This is a massive oversimplification of a complex issue, the particulars of which are also beyond the scope of this book. The Paulick Report, among other industry publications, has done some good work on the nuances of the problem that I encourage readers to seek out.

But it has faced revolt at every turn: HISA has been an uphill battle and continues to face stiff resistance from horsemen.* Big stud farms sank the Mare Cap. A past effort to get racetracks to better coordinate post times to avoid cannibalizing each other's gambling dollars also met with failure. Janney himself is now portrayed as an elitist villain, accused of loosing private investigators on trainers he didn't like. Racing is a sport that values its traditions. The wholesale resistance to change of any kind may augur the end of those traditions.

So the basic prescription that I am offering isn't technocratic or regulatory. It's a modesty of ambition. It must be enough to raise and race these beautiful animals, without attention to the return on investment. If you want only to maximize the value of a potential stallion or bolster the price of your yearling at auction, or eke "just one more race" out of a tired claimer, then you shouldn't do it.

There is a cost to this prescription, not just for the big farms and racetracks whose private owners and corporate boards I acknowledge are supremely unlikely to compromise their earnings without regulation. It's an especially harsh prescription to offer racetrackers: if you cannot afford to manage your stable to the standard of a beloved household pet, then you shouldn't be participating. There will be horsemen, good horsemen, who can't meet that standard. It risks consolidating the industry in the hands of wealthier participants—a grudging return, perhaps, to "the sport of kings." But if the industry doesn't embrace that litmus test, in time those people won't have jobs at the racetrack anyway. Recasting the racehorse as a "pet" isn't just a moral calculation. It's also a financial one.

Racing in some states is at very real risk of being ushered out of existence. The risk isn't just legislators responding to constituent outrage about the breakdowns. (Although racing should take heed of then-Senator Dianne Feinstein's outraged reaction to the 2019 breakdowns at Santa Anita, for example, and the stark warning in the *Washington Post* after the 2020 indictments that racing should be ended entirely.) The equally

---

* One egregious example: Louisiana, one of the states that has gone to the courts to avoid submitting to HISA, in 2024 briefly adopted rules that significantly loosened restrictions around the use of clenbuterol and a concentrated corticosteroid whose misuse has been linked to catastrophic breakdowns. The state quickly rolled back those changes amid an industry backlash. Natalie Voss, "At Emergency Meeting, Louisiana Commissioners Vote to Walk Back Changes to Regs on Clenbuterol, Depo-Medrol," Paulick Report, June 4, 2024, https://paulickreport.com/news/the-biz/at-emergency-meeting-louisiana-commissioners-vote-to-walk-back-changes-to-regs-on-clenbuterol-depo-medrol.

urgent threat is waning public interest, and with it the loss of gambling dollars that underpin the sport's existence. It's not in any immediate danger in a state like Kentucky, where the economic impact the industry has on the state is so huge. But Kentucky isn't just a racing state, it's an export state. If California horsemen, for example, no longer spend millions on yearlings produced by Kentucky breeders, even the citadel of American breeding will shrink.

In the 1970s, horse racing was among the top spectator sports in America. One of the challenges the sport now faces is that, for most of America, horses are not seen as "livestock" or "assets." They are seen as what they are: fiercely intelligent, sensitive, sentient beings. This is particularly acute as the number of people who have any day-to-day interaction with animals beyond cats and dogs shrinks.

"The relationship with horses and people from the beginning of time has been so different than any other animal and nobody can explain why. They've been one of the most important things for humanity," said one leading horse trainer in Kentucky. But, he said, "you got to realize that horses have gone from being cattle and sheep, to being dogs and cats in people's eyes." It is not enough for racetrackers to say that outsiders simply "don't understand" the care these animals receive. They understand. They just don't approve.

Racing is aware that its social license to operate is dwindling. The term itself is now a buzzword in the sport. But the industry has approached the problem as if the only solution needed is "marketing." Grassroots organizations have sprung up to promote positive messages about welfare in the racing industry. Their impact is difficult to measure, but it's fair to say it's been limited at best—probably due to the basic disconnect between how racing talks about its horses to the outside world and how it handles them internally. *We message them like pets, but we treat them like livestock*, one racing professional said to me. No marketing campaign can cover up that discrepancy.

"There is a need to balance the economics of the industry with society's expectations of the acceptable or ideal use of animals in both sport and production," a group of New Zealand researchers wrote in a 2023 study.[31] It's an approach already common in other regulated industries that use animals. Cattle farmers must respond to cultural expectations for the standard of care for their livestock, even though some of those standards may be in opposition to the maximization of profit, the writers noted.

To improve the welfare of the horse, they wrote, the industry needs to focus on "optimising the system as a whole." Their implication is clear: the sport is out of balance. It has given too much attention to profit and not enough to husbandry of the living animal. It's a familiar tale.

Horsemen like to say that the Thoroughbred loves to run, that the good ones know when they win or lose. Anyone who has spent any time around them knows that this is true. They call it the look of eagles: ears flicked forward in anticipation, the wide space between the animal's eyes marking a rare intelligence, and all the while his keen and generous eye on the horizon, searching for worlds to conquer. After Seabiscuit had trounced the great War Admiral in the 1938 match race widely considered to be one of the greatest horse races of all time, his jockey George Woolf looked back: "I saw something in the Admiral's eyes that was pitiful. He looked all broken up. I don't think he will be good for another race. Horses, mister, can have crushed hearts just like humans."[32]

But at its worst, the justification that Thoroughbreds "love to run" can become an excuse for any number of abuses. Horses also run when they're panicked and hurting. Anyone who has watched a Thoroughbred with a shattered ankle desperately trying to escape its handler and keep running on nubby bone knows that is true, also.

Like most racetrackers, Bob Baffert has his head down in the atavistic internal politics of Thoroughbred racing, obsessed with picograms and thresholds. He feels betrayed by the sport—and perhaps disappointed. After all these years spent winning the biggest races, he is still the farm boy from Nogales, the quarter horse guy, a man whose personality felt too big, at odds with unspoken rules he didn't understand.

Baffert, like so many racetrackers, seems obsessed with the notion of belonging to this sweet, seductive world, where men stand shoulder to shoulder with greatness. He had always felt lucky, he told me. Yet at the end of his career, Baffert sits alone in his box in the Santa Anita grandstand. In the bluegrass they are playing "My Old Kentucky Home" while twenty three-year-old horses parade to the post. In Nogales, Arizona, chickens still scratch and peck the ground. Baffert is somewhere in between.

"If you weren't born in the right stall in Kentucky, you're gonna be an outsider," Baffert said. "They're never gonna let you in. I will never be accepted. I'm not—I'm from Arizona. I'm a quarter horse guy. *Lukas* was never accepted."[33]

Medina Spirit, and his trainer, had been a symbol for racing's great paradox. Baffert had insisted that it was the horse that had been violated, dishonored, degraded by the disqualification. Yet in the end he had jumbled up his personal disappointment with the animal's. Medina Spirit didn't know he had been disqualified, or that his trainer had been ridiculed on national television and drummed off the most famous racetrack in America. The horse was buried at a farm for those few famous retired racehorses that do not become breeding stock. For more than three years, Baffert had been made out to be the cartoon villain of Thoroughbred horse racing, on national television, in the pages of newspapers, and within the sport he loved more than anything. It had been a degrading, painful, and traumatizing time. His sins were real, but they were not exceptional. He had been singled out, by a sport desperate to save itself and by a wider world that was leaving the old ways behind. He is still fumbling for how it could have all happened to him. There is something very innocent about it.

"I always thought what I loved about horse racing is such a pure—" he started. "Everything is settled on the track."

He trailed off.

EPILOGUE

In 2023, Baffert won the Preakness for a record-setting eighth time with a horse named National Treasure. Earlier in the day, he ran a horse named Havnameltdown in the Grade III Chick Lang Stakes. Midway through the race, Havnameltdown's left front ankle gave way beneath him. His jockey, Luis Saez, was catapulted over his head and into the dirt. Havnameltdown kept running with the pack, his nose bobbing down to the dirt like a pendulum with every stride, his hind legs staggering, out of alignment with his front end. These were the final moments of his life.

As usual, it couldn't have happened at a worse moment. Seven horses had just died in the week leading up to the Kentucky Derby. Not all of them were catastrophic breakdowns. One horse flipped over in the paddock—a freak accident—while two trained by Saffie Joseph died of sudden death. (Churchill Downs moved to suspend Joseph, who is based in Florida, "indefinitely until details are analyzed and understood"; he was ultimately reinstated when nothing was found.)[1] Havnameltdown's death would be major national news.

When the Paulick Report made the medical records for Havnameltdown public, it revealed that Baffert had injected the horse with betamethasone.[2] It had been recorded appropriately in state vet records and it had cleared the horse's system before race day. There was no allegation that Baffert had broken racing's rules. In fact, since May 2021, he had received no medication violations of any kind. Clark Brewster, in a statement to the Paulick Report, said Baffert had gone back to using betamethasone when HISA rules were about to come into effect in May of that year.*

But it was an unsettling reminder that Baffert, like so many trainers who had run afoul of racing's petty regulations before, had simply gone back to business as usual. After all his proclamations about getting betamethasone out of his barn, he had ultimately determined that it was the most effective tool to prepare horses to win races. After all, it was legal. On April 16, about a month before the Preakness, Dr. Vince Baker injected Havnameltdown's stifles (a hind-end joint) with hyaluronic acid and betamethasone and his hocks with hyaluronic acid and another corticosteroid called Kenalog. He had also at different points received Banamine, Torbugesic, and Dormosedan, a combination of common pain relievers and sedatives, according to the Paulick Report. Trainers everywhere use them. Baffert was breaking no rules.

Just hours after Havnameltdown was euthanized, Baffert accepted the trophy for winning the Preakness. In the gloaming, he walked back to the barn. It was crowded, as drunk horse people moved in currents around him. Out of the crowd, an intense man with close-clipped hair gray at the temples snagged him. It was Shaun Richards. He stuck out a hand.

"I'm Shaun Richards. I'm the new director of intelligence for HIWU," he told Baffert, referring to the Horseracing Integrity and Welfare Unit, the antidoping and medication control authority created by HISA.

What happened next is a matter of dispute. Baffert told me that Richards issued an aggressive warning: *I'm going to be coming out there and I'm gonna be watching you guys, and you better not mess up because I know how to find you.* Baffert said that he told him, "I'm easy to find if you want to talk to me." Richards, he said, replied: *Well, I'm not easy to find. But I'll be watching.* According to Richards, he merely introduced himself: "It was fabricated, other than I said hello."[3]

Shaun Richards now faces the same problem that racing commissions had: If he didn't know what to test for, how could he catch the dopers in the act? He had done it before, with Navarro and Servis, but it took Title III wiretaps. He no longer had that authority. He leaned heavily on his training in the FBI to develop sources and build "enterprise" investigations.

---

* "HISA enactment has clearly made great strides in providing more reliable information and scientific guidelines to all treating racetrack veterinarians. Based upon the [HISA] rules and studies Bob has placed his confidence of proper medications use on those experienced experts," Brewster said. https://paulickreport.com/news/the-biz/dead-horses-medical-records-cast-light-on-bafferts-evolving-relationship-with-betamethasone.

He'd had some wins—like an Ohio veterinarian suspended for two years for administering a non-FDA-approved blood builder[4]—but he had busted no more prominent trainers. The testimony of other racetrackers—rumor and innuendo, that indestructible haunt of the racetrack—still held sway.

If nothing has *really* changed with drugs at the racetrack, it's because nothing has changed. HISA has, so far, offered no fundamental rethinking of the economic model that underpins medication use at the racetrack, the model that is crumbling beneath the sport just as surely as Havnameltdown's legs crumbled beneath him in a Grade III on the undercard of one of the biggest races in America. It's still trying to set an expanding list of acceptable drugs and regulate them down to the picogram, rather than asking questions about *why* there are so many drugs in use on the backstretch. It's doing nothing to address the complaint that the sheer number of permissible drugs is likely doing harm to the animal; variously, by replacing good horsemanship, enabling horses to run that need rest or retirement instead, or perhaps, in some unknown combination, causing sudden death. (It's not really working for horsemen either.) When I asked Todd Pletcher if his approach to the use of medication had changed over the years, he said he had gotten more conservative—as the rules had changed. "A lot of it is determined by withdrawal times and what standards they set," he said.[5] This tired approach still assumes that all is fair on the open marketplace, as long as it technically abides by the rules. This was glaringly on display in a filing by Coolmore, intended to persuade the Jockey Club of Saudi Arabia to permit Maximum Security—owned in part by the breeding farm—to retain a win in a $20 million race there.[6] As part of its bid, Coolmore submitted sections of a report by Scott Stanley, the University of Kentucky lab director who was removed after an investigation by HISA, insisting that SGF-1000 "contains no prohibited substance." This was a year after Jason Servis had gone to prison for his use of the drug.[7]

Despite its limitations, HISA is probably the best hope that the industry has to force some of the millions of small changes necessary to protect the animal. Regulation, at its best, is designed to insulate the innocent from the brute force of the marketplace.

But whether HISA will be the beginning of true change in the Thoroughbred industry will depend entirely on whether the industry will consent to be regulated. The HBPA continues to fight tooth and nail against HISA, with states like Louisiana trying to loosen rather than tighten drug rules. The law's survival is not guaranteed: At the time of this writing, the legal challenge to the new regime appears poised to be heard before the US Supreme Court as early as 2025. And even if HISA is both successful and accepted, it is not the magic bullet. It has no authority to regulate the sales and breeding industry, for example.* Different entities in racing have sought to provide the kind of inspirational leadership necessary to transform the sport as a system, with mixed results. The Jockey Club's efforts have been rejected as elitist, authoritarian, out of touch, and, to some, corrupt. ("Management of the Jockey Club reminds me of that knowing father who tells his children, when pressed on a topic, 'Now, now, this is nothing you need to know,'" Ray Paulick wrote.)[8] Janney—whose efforts have been mainly aimed at reining in the sport's excesses—is now seen as a villain within some corners of racing as surely as Bob Baffert is seen as a villain outside of it. In November 2024, he stepped down as chairman. He recommended his own replacement,[9] an Oklahoma native named Everett Dobson. Dobson did not come from a legacy racing family, entering the business in the 1990s, but he has quietly assumed senior positions in all of the traditional organs of prestige in racing—including the Keeneland Association, the Breeders' Cup, and the Jockey Club. Whether he will be able to restore some of the Jockey Club's popular legitimacy remains to be seen. The Jockey Club may be trying to lead, but it's not clear it can anymore.

"What bothers me is I think it's a diversion from getting on with the decisions that have got to be made about racing," Janney said of the criticism he has faced. "And I'm not sure we have the luxury of diverting ourselves rather than focusing on getting things fixed. I think we're running out of chances."[10]

The same could be said of Baffert, whose public pillorying for the past three years has felt more like a scapegoat for racing's bigger problems than a solution—a deliberate confusing of the symptom with the disease.

The survival of the sport will depend on its ability to reckon with the animal at its heart—and whether it is able to accept any true limits in service of that animal. I hark back to the words of another famous Kentuckian, the environmental and cultural writer Wendell Berry, who has lived most

---

* HISA has engaged in some voluntary discussions with sales companies in Kentucky and elsewhere about creating some kind of standardized approach, but HISA CEO Lisa Lazarus said in early 2024, "We can only do what the statute allows us to do and right now the statute specifically provides that a horse becomes a covered horse upon its first workout." Bill Finley, "HISA Not Positioned to Police Sales," *Thoroughbred Daily News*, February 28, 2024, https://www.thoroughbreddailynews.com/hisa-not-positioned-to-police-sales/.

of his life in Port Royal, an hour and a half northwest of Lexington, and wrote of soil loss in 1991: "It is lost a little at a time over millions of acres by the careless acts of millions of people. It cannot be saved by heroic acts of gigantic technology, but only by millions of small acts and restraints, conditioned by small fidelities, skills, and desires. Soil loss is ultimately a cultural problem; it will be corrected only by cultural solutions."[11]

I am hopeful. Some horsemen have quietly told me that they have seen attitudes toward the animal begin to shift—perhaps because horsemen have been driven by HISA to be more conservative to avoid regulatory scratches, perhaps because they are facing the prospect of the demise of their way of life, perhaps because the unrelenting national criticism of horses dying on the track has forced a reckoning. Particularly among horsemen of my generation—the horsemen I grew up alongside—there is a recognition that the way we were taught might not have been right. A gentler, more thoughtful approach to in the horse business may be on the rise. Whether that change will happen fast enough to catch up to the outside world's expectations remains to be seen. And horsemen, of course, were never the only ones to blame.

In July 2024, Churchill finally dropped its ban against Baffert. It had gotten through its marquee event, the 150th running of the Kentucky Derby, without incident, and Carstanjen and Baffert, it seems, came to an understanding. Baffert issued a public statement that he "accept[ed] responsibility for Medina Spirit's positive test" and for "any substance found in the horses I train." Baffert had finally figured out why Bill Carstanjen cared so much.

"It wasn't personal with Bill," he said. "It was just business."[12]

Baltimore had turned out the day Baffert won the Preakness with National Treasure. Football players and their wives were partying in Belinda Stronach's infield tent. The governor was in attendance. Among horse people, the amusement of the afternoon was watching the wife of one of the younger football players try shamelessly to get herself invited to the exclusive, and presumably more glamorous, second floor of the tent. She did this largely by buttering up horse people, none of whom themselves had received wristbands from 1/ST to get up there. She was an outsider. She didn't know how this world worked—and she was laughed at.

The last race of the night was run under a lowering sky, gray and pregnant with coming rain. In the infield, a crowd was building as people from the fancy party tents lined up at the crosswalk to leave. A few heavy drops began to fall, splattering darkly on bright hats and silk pocket squares. The crowd pressed denser and denser against the railing, as if their impatient mass might induce the track workers to run the walkway across the dirt track to the parking lot right away. But horses were still running and they had to wait. The six-horse field passed under the wire, and then in front of the crowd waiting to cross. A gray horse with an awkward flagged tail chased the pack, his legs churning helplessly. From somewhere inside the crowd, a drunk man yelled, "*No one cares!*"

A few minutes later, the gray horse would be the last to walk back to the barns, led alone by his groom. Track security had let most of the thronging crowd across, but a few stragglers were still on the walkway.

"*I need you to STOP*," one of the security guards said, his voice pitched with frustration. "I have *horses* here."

"We're stopping, we're stopping," a man said, offended.

The groom led the gray horse past, bracing his forearm against its shoulder to keep it from getting loose. The horse's ears swiveled madly as it was led between the chaotic gauntlet of people, none of whom knew his name—or cared. The groom kept his gaze forward, to the barns, where, long after the crowds had dispersed, long after the body of Havnameltdown had been removed from the track, after Baffert and the syndicate that owned National Treasure had celebrated the $1.5 million purse from the Preakness, this gray horse would still need to be fed, bathed, and walked until he was cool.

ACKNOWLEDGMENTS

This book would not exist without the hundreds of horses that have been my teachers since I first put foot in iron, but most especially Buckie, who was technically only half-Thoroughbred but who taught me what it was to have the look of eagles (and what it was like to ride a horse that knew how to kick a hole in the sky). Rest in peace, old man. But there were so many more: Redmond '07—later, Spectacular Sight, but who lives in my memory as "the Redmond filly." Pitcrew. Harley—officially, Donji Is Lucky. Cigar, who I was lucky enough to get to fool with in his older years at the Kentucky Horse Park. (How else to spend your one day off a week from rubbing yearlings but by rubbing the greatest racehorse of my lifetime?) Ridley. Surprise Package. (Also not a Thoroughbred; also taught me to ride a horse that bucked.) Mr. Hooker. The three or four of Doug Fout's that routinely dumped me in the summer of 2007. There is no animal more noble than the Thoroughbred horse. Let us try to do better by them—and be grateful when we have.

This book would also not exist without the scores of very fine horsemen who taught me most of what I know about the Thoroughbred, and a lot of what I know about life. Some of them are no longer with us, and I miss them. There are too many to name here, but I will try. In no particular order: Brian, who taught me attention to detail and how to stand a horse up. Jesse, who taught me that if you are good to the animal, he will be good to you. Sherri, who tried and failed to teach me how to put poultice on a horse without getting it all over myself. Nestor, who taught me how to make my way around the big colts without getting my shit rocked. Woodberry, who, even when I blew by with a handful of too much horse, kept legging me up. Ferris, who first handed me a leather shank with a Thoroughbred

319

at the end of it. Noel, who was incomparable in all ways. Bill, who taught me to look for balance above all things. Dennis, whose wit, good cheer, and enthusiastic support are missed by many. Debbie, whose patient guidance, enthusiastic encouragement, and legendary kindness saved me from disaster with horse and human over the years. The groom in Dubai whose language I didn't speak and thus whose name I never learned, but who spent countless hours kneeling next to a horse with me ensuring that I learned to wrap a leg properly: even, secure, and safe. Multiple generations of Bance women, whose fearlessness in the saddle and unrestrained passion for the Thoroughbred has inspired (and occasionally terrified) me since I was a child. Pam, who told me to have some "style" when I rode. Richard and Colleen, who have kept the Thoroughbred in my life in recent years, and always encouraged me to kick on. And to many other friends and former colleagues in the horse business, whose work I admire, respect, and support. I hope, when this is all done, that there will still be a place for me if I want to give up journalism and take up horses again.

Most especially, I am grateful to the horsewoman who began it all for me, my mother, Robin. Mom, you got me my first job walking hots at Colonial Downs when I was sixteen, made sure I followed hounds with Noel Twyman, sent me to the finest yearling man alive, Brian Graves. You insisted the Colonial stewards interview all my dates, helped me move in and out of a million barn apartments, answered phone calls in the middle of the night from Australia, and in countless other ways made it possible for me to chase every dream I ever had with horses. And then, when I said I wanted to write instead, you supported that too. But most importantly, you showed me what it looks like to wrap your toes under the belly of a rogue and stick like a cocklebur. I have watched you in the back of the field stuck to an orangutan at creek crossings, and stared at photos of you on Timely Boy at Clay Camp's with nothing on your head but a stocking cap, or riding a home-bred mare over timber in a full snowstorm. I have seen you hop on a strange horse and put it over a three-six vertical in *shorts* (not even the one we wound up buying, as I recall). I've seen you laugh fit to bust when Buckie or Saylor or any one of the long line of bucking horses you've bred turned himself inside out with you in the irons. If I am brave at all, it's because of you. "I used to ride racehorses. What are these guys gonna do, break my arm?"

A profound thank-you to my racing insider, who will go unnamed here but is an incomparable horseman who, from the first day I called about this project, encouraged me, acted as an invaluable sounding board for the ideas in these pages, and helped me translate incomprehensible racetrack speak. ("Why must horse people just leave out words all the time?" "You forget that you are a 'horse person.'") You were the first person to say to me: *I want this sport to continue to exist. Write it as it is.*

Thank you to my CNN colleagues, who have tolerated periodic interruptions to the business of covering national security to listen to me speechify about horse racing (or, in Kasie's case, consent to literally *go* to the racetrack). Callahan, Natasha, Alex, Zack, Haley, Kylie, Sean, and Adam: thank you all. Thank you to Fuzz, for reading this thing and making it better. And a special thank-you to Matthew Philips, whose peerless editing of my work for CNN has made me a better writer and a better reporter in ways that have unquestionably improved this book.

I am grateful to my first editor, Sean Clancy, who, when I was twenty-one years old, told me, "I know you want to sell horses, but you were born to write." It took me a minute to come to that conclusion, but point taken, boss.

I have been lucky, also, to have great friends who have shared my passion for this sport over the years. Natalie (Mr. Insider), Allaire, Jodie, Jenny, Vicky, Kyle, Evan, Jak, Scott, Catherine (Peril and Sin). The rest of an entire herd of Clancys across generations. You have all, in different ways, helped me refine ideas and pushed me to treat the sport with compassion and nuance. And you've been there for every bad bet and questionable decision for more than a decade (including my quest to run around the turf course at every major North American racetrack, and some in the Southern Hemisphere). It's been a hell of a ride.

A shout-out to the very fine reporters at the Paulick Report, whose rigorous, independent, and clear-eyed coverage was an irreplaceable resource for this project and provides an incredible service to the sport. A special thank-you to Natalie Voss, whose sage advice and endless enthusiasm for late-night text conversations about, like, peptides kept me from getting too lost in the woods. I'll meet you at Colonial this summer.

Thank you to my readers, all of whom brought different perspectives to the manuscript and made it better: Samantha Koon, whose friendship and fearless honesty when it comes to the written word it has been my privilege to enjoy since we were babies on the desk at the *Cavalier Daily*. *STAYING OUT ALL NIGHT LONG . . .* while reading Faulkner; Dr. Adam Cawley of Racing Analytical Services Ltd., who graciously agreed to read hundreds of pages for a complete stranger out of nothing more than an honorable commitment to making sure the information the public receives about racetrack testing is accurate; and one more racing insider who shall go unnamed but whose experience and fundamental sense of fairness were invaluable. I will be forever grateful to you all.

And to Michelle, my kidney friend, whose brilliant and restless mind—and decades spent gamely attending horse races from Kentucky to New York with me—worked overtime in service of helping me figure out how to translate "horse things" for regular people. Thank you to Janet Byrne, my indefatigable fact checker, whose eagle eye for error was awe-inspiring and whose enthusiasm for this project made me excited even on days I wasn't.

A deep and abiding gratitude to my agents at WME, Sabrina Taitz and Eve Attermann, who saw the potential in this project when it was nothing more than two pages of *horse stuff* and helped me bring it into the world; to Dana Canedy, LaSharah Bunting, and the rest of the Simon & Schuster team, who first took a chance on a national security reporter who wanted to write about horse racing. I am profoundly grateful to my editor, Stephanie Frerich, who embodies what good editing should be: patient, true to the project, and challenging in all the right ways (including reminding me that not everyone in the world knows what a maiden special weight is). I never even had to send her for the key to the quarter pole.

Most of all, I am grateful to my husband, without whose endless support—including many hours of solo parenting so I could report and write—this project would not have been possible. Mike, you are the love of my life. You had my heart even before you took me to Charles Town to drink Bud Light and put two-dollar paddock bets on a bunch of platers. It is a privilege and the greatest source of joy I have ever known to share this life with you.

Finally, I want to say thank you for everyone, named and unnamed, who agreed to speak with me and helped me tell the stories in these pages. A special thank-you to Bob Baffert, who took a risk in choosing to talk to me. He was generous with his time and his candor throughout this process, which I know was nerve-racking for him and his family, and he should be commended for what I believe took some courage. Bob has been made out to be a cartoon villain in Thoroughbred racing. I have not shied away from pointing out his flaws. He is a human being, and like all of us, he has many of them. But it is my personal belief that this characterization is deeply unfair. I hope I have done better.

AUTHOR'S NOTE

This book is exhaustively sourced. I conducted dozens of interviews over more than two years of reporting, reviewed thousands of pages of documents drawn from the public record and provided to me by sources, and read (and reread) more books about racing than I can count. Some of my interviews were on the record, but many of my sources, for various reasons, would speak to me only anonymously. On some occasions I have provided some identifying information about sources in the text, such as organizational affiliation; elsewhere, to protect the identity of those who trusted me with their story, reporting that is drawn from interviews is not endnoted or sourced in the text.

This is a work of reported nonfiction, and none of the assertions it contains are made up in any way. When I characterize people's thoughts or emotions, I have relied on their direct testimony to me and to others or on descriptions of their mindset by multiple sources who knew them at the time of the episode in question.

Descriptions of the investigative process that led to the 2020 indictments—the work of 5 Stones Intelligence and the Justice Department—have been recounted based on sources with firsthand knowledge and on publicly available records. The group of people who knew about any one stage of the investigation wasn't always large, but it was large enough that I was able to confirm each piece of reporting either through documents or interviews with multiple sources. There are no citations in the endnotes to much of this reporting, and it is not sourced in the text; it has been drawn from anonymous sources. In an extremely small number of instances, I relied on the testimony of a single source with firsthand knowledge of the event in question. I did this only when I judged that the source's testimony was credible and consistent with a broader body of reporting, and when their depiction of the event was not denied by any other sources with knowledge of it.

Confidential informants who cooperated with the federal investigation are not named because in all instances, my sources declined to name them to protect their identity. Although they are described by occupation or contribution to the investigation, I did not, as the reporter, know their identity. In each instance, I confirmed their role with multiple sources.

All of the major subjects in this reporting had an opportunity to respond prior to publication to the assertions and characterizations that relate to them. There was an awful lot of guessing about who had told me what; I was often amused by how frequently the guesses were wrong. I offer that as a caution to industry readers who may make assumptions about the provenance of some of the reporting in these pages.

Bob Baffert was incredibly generous with his time and his candor. I have drawn extensively from on-the-record interviews with him beginning in January 2023 and continuing into the spring of 2024. I also leaned heavily on a 1999 autobiography he wrote with industry reporter Steve Haskin. In some instances I tested Bob's recollections against those in his book; they were remarkably consistent. When I was able, I worked with a fact checker to corroborate Bob's own telling of his early history with publicly available documents, including contemporaneous news coverage. I also checked Bob's recollections of some of the key episodes reported here against his brother Bill's memory; again, I found them to be consistent. As a result, much of the reporting about Bob's youth and early years as a quarter horse trainer are drawn exclusively from Bob's own telling, to me and to Steve Haskin.

Baffert disagrees with some of the characterizations of his actions and motivations in this text, although not all. He has also challenged the relevance of some of the reporting. Where possible, I have tried to let Baffert's own words—to me and to others—speak for themselves. Once again, I wish to reiterate his professionalism and courtesy in our interactions throughout the entire process of the reporting, writing, and publication of this book.

I engaged directly with many of the defendants in the Southern District of New York federal case. Nearly all in some fashion or other agreed to tell me their side of the story, sometimes on their own and sometimes through an attorney. Some did not. Because many of these people are still either in federal prison or under supervised release, they are necessarily in a position of vulnerability. In cases where I was able to clearly establish an agreement that we were speaking on the record—or in which I was instructed to "write whatever you want"—I have quoted them directly. In other instances, I have treated any engagements as background information that contributed to my characterization of the person in question.

Many of the assertions and characterizations herein are drawn from my own experience working in the Thoroughbred racing industry. While I had met some of the major subjects before I began reporting—including Bob Baffert, whom I interviewed for a racing paper in 2011—I had no sustained or meaningful relationship with any of them. But I was in a unique position from the outset, in that I had both deep cultural exposure to the world of racing and a degree of subject matter expertise. While writing, I often stress-tested my own recollection of the culture and character of the sport against the thoughts and impressions of professionals still working in it today. I have tried to signal to readers when a particular observation is drawn from personal experience. I also engaged several readers with decades of experience in different parts of the industry to review the manuscript prior to publication and flag any factual inaccuracies, faulty logic, or bad-faith judgments. They have asked to remain unnamed, but I am grateful for their help in ensuring that I presented an authentic picture of a complicated and often misunderstood sport.

I engaged a technical reader with deep experience in lab testing and toxicology in the racing industry to review, for scientific accuracy, the assertions made in these pages about drugs—doping and therapeutics. I deliberately chose a reader from another major racing country—Dr. Adam Cawley of Australia's Racing Analytical Services—to ensure that this person was independent of the internal politics of the sport in the United States. Any errors, of course, are mine, not his.

A word on language: As addressed in a footnote early in the text, I have in nearly all cases defaulted to the masculine in my descriptions of horse people. I refer to the "track man" and the "men of the Jockey Club" and "horsemen." I have done this for two reasons. The first is that, as with the term *horseman* or *track man*, this is how racing talks about itself. It was very important to me in writing this story to remain true to the texture and character of this unique subculture; nowhere is any culture more evident than in its choice of words. The second reason is that while there are a great many women who work in horse racing and breeding, there are still relatively few in positions of leadership or authority. There is still a stunningly small number of female trainers, despite an enormous number of women in skilled positions at the racetrack. When I left the industry in 2013, I was shocked (and relieved) to find that the misogyny so normalized that it went unremarked inside racing was seen as unacceptable outside of it. I'm pleased to see that this is changing, particularly as my generation enters leadership positions. I am proud of my friend Jodie Vella-Gregory, who has been one of the driving forces behind an annual summit dedicated to promoting and supporting women in the sport. The fact that the current CEO of Keeneland is a woman speaks volumes about the progress the industry has made.

NOTES

PROLOGUE

1 Bob Baffert, January 4, 2023.
2 "Tales from the Crib: Medina Spirit," Kentucky Derby, accessed September 9, 2024, https://www.kentuckyderby.com/horses/news/tales-from-the-crib-medina-spirit/.
3 "Tales from the Crib: Medina Spirit."
4 Joe Pantorno, "Bob Baffert: Controversial Kentucky Derby Winner Medina Spirit Victim of 'Cancel Culture Kind of Thing,'" amNewYork, May 10, 2021, https://www.amny.com/sports/bob-baffert-controversial-kentucky-derby-winner-medina-spirit-victim-of-cancel-culture-kind-of-thing/.
5 Editorial Board, "Opinion: Horse Racing Has Outlived Its Time," *Washington Post*, March 13, 2020, https://www.washingtonpost.com/opinions/horse-racing-has-outlived-its-time/2020/03/12/5dd48e46-6476-11ea-acca-80c22bbee96f_story.html.
6 Paul Mellon, *Reflections in a Silver Spoon: A Memoir* (New York: William Morrow, 1992), 254, http://archive.org/details/reflectionsinsil0000mell.

CHAPTER 1 THE BEST AT WHAT YOU DO

1 Bob Baffert and Steve Haskin, *Baffert: Dirt Road to the Derby* (Lexington, KY: Blood-Horse, 1999), 52.
2 Betty Barr, "Memorial Race to Honor Bill and Ellie Baffert," Nogales International, April 3, 2013, https://www.nogalesinternational.com/the_bulletin/news/memorial-race-to-honor-bill-and-ellie-baffert/article_6dacbd6e-9c75-11e2-b6de-001a4bcf887a.html.
3 Joe O'Connor, "Canada's Greatest Racing Horse Still an Influence in the Sport of Kings," *National Post*, accessed September 20, 2024, https://nationalpost.com/news/canada/canadas-greatest-racing-horse-still-an-influence-in-the-sport-of-kings.
4 Muriel Lennox, *Northern Dancer: The Legend and His Legacy* (Toronto: Beach House Books, 1995), http://archive.org/details/northerndancerle0000lenn.
5 Andrew Beyer, "Northern Dancer: Call Him Sire," *Washington Post*, https://www.washingtonpost.com/archive/sports/1982/07/24/northern-dancer-call-him-sire/eb7cd597-a259-4173-a00b-9706931933e2/.
6 "Sparkman: Northern Dancer the Biggest Little Horse," *DRF*, accessed September 10, 2024, https://www.drf.com/news/sparkman-northern-dancer-biggest-little-horse.
7 Don Hedgpeth, *They Rode Good Horses: The First Fifty Years of the American Quarter Horse Association* (American Quarter Horse Association, 1990).
8 Baffert and Haskin, *Baffert*, 65.
9 Bill Baffert, June 12, 2023.

10 Baffert and Haskin, *Baffert*, 65.

11 Carlo Devito, *D. Wayne* (New York: Contemporary Books, 2002), 53.

12 Bill Baffert, June 12, 2023.

13 "About," Permanently Disabled Jockeys Fund, accessed September 20, 2024, https://pdjf.org/about/.

14 "Los Alamitos Race Course," accessed September 10, 2024, https://www.losalamitos.com/.

15 Bob Baffert, January 2, 2023.

16 Bob Baffert, January 4, 2023.

17 Bill Baffert, June 12, 2023.

18 Bill Baffert, June 12, 2023.

19 Bob Baffert, May 25, 2023.

20 Bob Baffert, May 25, 2023.

21 Bob Baffert, May 25, 2023.

22 Bob Baffert, January 2, 2023.

23 Baffert and Haskin, *Baffert*, 88.

24 Bob Baffert, May 25, 2023.

CHAPTER 2 **GO WEST, YOUNG MAN**

1 "Los Alamitos Race Course," accessed September 10, 2024, https://www.losalamitos.com/history.aspx.

2 "Los Alamitos," OffTrackBetting, accessed September 10, 2024, https://www.offtrackbetting.com/racetracks/LA/los_alamitos.html.

3 "Los Alamitos Race Course."

4 Quoted in Chamberlain, "April 15," *Quarter Horse Journal*, https://en.wikipedia.org/wiki/Go_Man_Go.

5 "Los Alamitos Race Course."

6 Bob Baffert, January 4, 2023.

7 Baffert and Haskin, *Baffert*, 84.

8 Paul Moran, "Moran: A Sign of the Times," ESPN, April 2, 2012, https://www.espn.com/horse-racing/story/_/id/7766140/a-sign-times.

9 Thomas Tobin, Joan Combie, and Ted Shults, "Pharmacology Review: Actions of Central Stimulant Drugs in the Horse II," Publication No. 48 from the Kentucky Equine Drug Research and Testing Programs, University of Kentucky, March 1979, http://www.thomastobin.com/archive/048%20-%20Actions%20of%20Central%20Stimulant%20Drugs%20in%20the%20Horse%20II.pdf.

10 Bob Baffert, January 4, 2023.

11 Bob Baffert, May 25, 2023.

12 Baffert and Haskin, *Baffert*, 84.

13 Bob Baffert, January 4, 2023.

14 Bob Baffert, May 25, 2023.

15 Bob Baffert, January 4, 2023.

16 Bob Baffert, January 4, 2023.

17 Baffert and Haskin, *Baffert*, 84–85.

18 Baffert, January 4, 2023.

19 Baffert and Haskin, *Baffert*, 86.

20 Baffert, January 4, 2023.

21 Baffert and Haskin, *Baffert*, 89.

22 Bill Baffert, June 12, 2023.

23 Baffert and Haskin, *Baffert*, 91.

24 https://www.tucsonaz.gov/files/preservation/rillito_racetrack-chute_final.pdf.

25 http://atba.net/pdf/atba-rillito.pdf.

26   Baffert and Haskin, *Baffert*, 95.

27   Baffert and Haskin, 95.

28   Joe Drape, "Hard Work, Failure and Passion: How a Horse Trainer Made It," *New York Times*, March 24, 2017, https://www.nytimes.com/2017/03/24/sports/bob-baffert-horse-trainer-career .html.

29   Bob Baffert, January 4, 2023.

30   Bob Baffert, January 4, 2023.

31   "Bob Baffert: Going for the Gold," *Speedhorse*, September 17, 2020, accessed September 10, 2024, https://www.speedhorse.com/m.blog/1898/bob-baffert-going-for-the-gold.

32   Bill Baffert, June 12, 2023.

33   Bill Baffert, June 12, 2023.

CHAPTER 3 **THE COWBOY HAT**

1   Baffert and Haskin, *Baffert*, 110.

2   Baffert and Haskin, 110.

3   "Triple Crown: Now That's Something to Celebrate—Mike Pegram's Horse Gets Ready for Race and Party," *Seattle Times*, accessed September 10, 2024, https://archive.seattletimes.com /archive/?date=19980606&slug=2754693.

4   Bob Baffert, May 25, 2023.

5   Baffert and Haskin, *Baffert*, 110.

6   DeVito, *D. Wayne*, 62.

7   Bob Baffert, May 25, 2023.

8   Bob Baffert, January 4, 2023.

9   Baffert and Haskin, *Baffert*, 114.

10   "Tired of 'Just Breaking Even': Trainer Ron Faucheux Wins Fair Grounds Title Before Launching Jockey Agent Career," Paulick Report, April 10, 2023, https://paulickreport.com/news/people/ tired-of-just-breaking-even-trainer-ron-faucheux-wins-fair-grounds-title-before-launching -jockey-agent-career.

11   New York Racing Association in the Matter of Robert A. Baffert, New York, January 24, 2022.

12   Joe Drape, "A Horseman's Lawsuit Puts Trading Practices in the Spotlight," *New York Times*, May 3, 2006, https://www.nytimes.com/2006/05/03/sports/othersports/03jackson.html.

13   Jay Privman, "For Lukas Family, the Highest Stakes; Trainer Sees His Son Through Grueling Recovery from Track Accident," *New York Times*, January 23, 1994, https://www.nytimes.com /1994/01/23/sports/for-lukas-family-the-highest-stakes-trainer-sees-his-son-through.html.

14   Bill Finley, "How 'Super Trainers' Have Come to Dominate the Sport," *Thoroughbred Daily News*, June 19, 2018, https://www.thoroughbreddailynews.com/how-super-trainers-have -come-to-dominate-the-sport/.

15   DeVito, *D. Wayne*, 172.

16   William Nack, "Another View from the Top," *Sports Illustrated*, May 9, 1988, accessed September 10, 2024, https://vault.si.com/vault/1988/05/09/another-view-from-the-top -just-four-years-ago-gene-klein-fled-the-nfl-and-lit-into-racing-with-a-daring-strategy-and-a -big-bankroll-now-hes-americas-most-successful-owner-of-thoroughbreds.

17   Nack, "Another View from the Top."

18   Joseph B. Hickey Jr., "The Grand Old Man of Windfields Dies at 29," Mid-Atlantic Thoroughbred Stallion Directory 1991, Maryland Horse Breeders Association, 1991, http://archive .org/details/nslm-midatlantic-thoroughbred-stallion-directory-1991.

19   "Robert Sangster," *Times* (London), April 9, 2004, https://www.thetimes.com/article/robert -sangster-gnvfrg8srdf.

20   "Lady's Secret Dies from Foaling Complications," *BloodHorse*, accessed September 10, 2024, https:// www.bloodhorse.com/horse-racing/articles/183376/ladys-secret-dies-from-foaling-complications.

21 Nack, "Another View from the Top."

22 DeVito, *D. Wayne*, 77.

23 Bob Baffert, January 2, 2023.

24 "Mythbusting Lawn Jockeys: Untangling History from Lore," YouTube, 2021, https://www
.youtube.com/watch?v=QNDFDozfjRM.

25 Charlotte Squire, "Opinion: The Lawn Jockey Cannot Stand as a Symbol of Racism at Skidmore," *Skidmore News*, August 3, 2020, http://skidmorenews.com/new-blog/2020/8/3/opinion
-the-lawn-jockey-cannot-stand-as-a-symbol-of-racism-at-skidmore.

26 Natalie Voss, "Something's Missing Here: Explaining Ridglings," Paulick Report, https://
paulickreport.com/news/ray-s-paddock/somethings-missing-here-explaining-ridglings.

27 Baffert and Haskin, *Baffert*, 116.

28 Baffert and Haskin, 116.

29 Baffert and Haskin, 116–21.

30 Bob Baffert, January 4, 2024.

31 "R. D. Hubbard: AFG Founder Flexes Takeover Muscles on Own Company," *Los Angeles
Times*, April 4, 1988, https://www.latimes.com/archives/la-xpm-1988-04-04-fi-330-story.html.

32 Baffert and Haskin, *Baffert*, 121.

33 Baffert and Haskin, 122.

34 Baffert and Haskin, 122.

35 Baffert and Haskin, 123.

36 Baffert and Haskin, 123.

37 DeVito, *D. Wayne*, 62.

38 Baffert and Haskin, *Baffert*, 139.

CHAPTER 4 **DERBY FEVER**

1 Chris Kenning, "'My Old Kentucky Home': Why the Kentucky Derby Anthem Remains
So Controversial," *Courier-Journal*, May 2, 2019, accessed September 10, 2024, https://www
.courier-journal.com/story/entertainment/events/kentucky-derby/2019/05/02/my-old
-kentucky-home-song-controversial-lyrics-derby-anthem/3643822002/.

2 Jay Privman, "Long Shot Mine That Bird Smells Roses at Derby," ESPN, May 2, 2009, https://
www.espn.com/sports/horse/triplecrown09/news/story?id=4128286.

3 Baffert and Haskin, *Baffert*, 17.

4 Baffert and Haskin, 18.

5 Baffert and Haskin, 12.

6 Bill Christine, "A Charmed Life: For Bob and Beverly Lewis, It's a Silver Colt That Helps
Them Celebrate a Golden Anniversary," *Los Angeles Times*, June 3, 1997, https://www.latimes
.com/archives/la-xpm-1997-06-03-sp-65241-story.html.

7 Baffert and Haskin, *Baffert*, 28.

8 Baffert and Haskin, 34.

9 Baffert and Haskin, 29.

10 Baffert and Haskin, 32.

11 Baffert and Haskin, 32.

12 Baffert and Haskin, 34.

13 Baffert and Haskin, 34.

14 Baffert and Haskin, 157.

15 Baffert and Haskin, 157.

16 Baffert and Haskin, 39.

17 Baffert and Haskin, 40.

18 Baffert and Haskin, 40.

19 Baffert and Haskin, 161.

20 Baffert and Haskin, 46.

21 Baffert and Haskin, 138.

22 Baffert and Haskin, 46.

23 Baffert and Haskin, 46.

24 Bob Baffert, May 25, 2023.

25 Baffert and Haskin. *Baffert,* 47.

26 Baffert and Haskin, 88–89.

27 William Nack, "The Almighty Bob Baffert," Stacks Reader, accessed September 20, 2024, http://www.thestacksreader.com/the-almighty-bob-baffert/.

28 Baffert and Haskin, *Baffert*, 165.

29 Bob Baffert, January 4, 2023.

30 Baffert and Haskin, *Baffert*, 162.

31 Baffert and Haskin, 145.

32 Baffert and Haskin, 21–22.

33 Baffert and Haskin, 22.

34 Chris Smith, "Smith: Cavonnier Now Holds Court in a Meadow," *Santa Rosa Press Democrat*, April 28, 2016, https://www.pressdemocrat.com/article/news/smith-20-years-later-cavonnier -holds-court-out-in-a-meadow/.

35 Natalie Voss, "'This Is About Taking Care Of Horses': Rescue Mare Has Claiborne Mulling Policy Changes," Paulick Report, September 13, 2024, https://paulickreport.com/horse-care -category/this-is-about-taking-care-of-horses-rescue-mare-has-claiborne-mulling-policy -changes.

36 Chris McGrath, "Vocation Beats Vacation for the Ultimate Horsemen's Vet," *Thoroughbred Daily News*, April 22, 2024, https://www.thoroughbreddailynews.com/vocation-beats-vacation -for-the-ultimate-horsemens-vet/.

37 Bob Baffert, January 2, 2023.

CHAPTER 5 **FREE FROM EVERY MORTAL SIN—INCLUDING BUTAZOLIDIN**

1 Baffert and Haskin, *Baffert*, 42.

2 Baffert and Haskin, 41.

3 Baffert and Haskin, 41.

4 Baffert and Haskin, 42.

5 Ryan Goldberg, "Secret to Success: A Derby Win and Racing's Doping Addiction," ProPublica, May 2, 2014, https://www.propublica.org/article/secret-to-success.

6 Milton C. Toby, *Unnatural Ability: The History of Performance-Enhancing Drugs in Thoroughbred Racing* (Lexington: University Press of Kentucky, 2023), 188.

7 Toby, 182.

8 Goldberg, "Secret to Success."

9 Toby, *Unnatural Ability*, 184.

10 Toby, 188.

11 Goldberg, "Secret to Success."

12 Goldberg.

13 Corrupt Horseracing Practices Act: Hearing Before the Subcommittee on Criminal Law of the Committee on the Judiciary, United States Senate, Ninety-seventh Congress, Second Session, on S. 1043 . . . May 26, 1982.

14 Toby, *Unnatural Ability*, 15.

15 Toby, 78.

16 https://www.thoroughbreddailynews.com/pdf/magazine/Magazine-Drugs%20in%20Racing -Part%20I.pdf; Toby, *Unnatural Ability*, chapter 8.

17 Goldberg, "Secret to Success."

18 "Lasix: A Timeline of the Drug in Racing," *DRF*, accessed September 10, 2024, https://www
    .drf.com/news/lasix-timeline-drug-racing.

19 Victor Ryan, "Lasix-Free Stakes Racing Comes to Fruition in 2021," Horse Racing Nation,
    December 31, 2020, https://www.horseracingnation.com/news/Lasix_free_stakes_racing_
    comes_to_fruition_in_2021_123.

20 Christopher Kremmer, "Racing Chemistry: A Century of Challenges and Progress," *Drug
    Testing and Analysis* 9, no. 9 (September 2017): 1284–90, https://doi.org/10.1002/dta.2147.

21 Toby, *Unnatural Ability*, 193.

22 Toby, 192.

23 Association of Racing Commissioners International, "Uniform Classification Guidelines for
    Foreign Substances and Recommended Penalties Model Rule V.17.0," December 2023, https://
    www.arci.com/docs/Uniform-Classification-Guidelines-Version-17.0.pdf.

24 Kenneth W. Hinchcliff, Paul S. Morley, and Alan J. Guthrie, "Efficacy of Furosemide for
    Prevention of Exercise-Induced Pulmonary Hemorrhage in Thoroughbred Racehorses," *Journal
    of the American Veterinary Medical Association* 235, no. 1 (July 1, 2009): 76–82, https://doi
    .org/10.2460/javma.235.1.76.

25 Toby, *Unnatural Ability*, 193; Byron Rogers, "The Lasix Debate: The Scientists Muddy the
    Waters," October 11, 2014, https://web.archive.org/web/20200921075830/https://www
    .performancegenetics.com/post/2014/10/11/the-lasix-debate-the-scientists-muddy-the
    -waters.

26 Natalie Voss, "Lasix Mythbusters: Drug Masking, TCO2, and Impact on Racehorse Break-
    downs," Paulick Report, October 21, 2022, https://paulickreport.com/horse-care-category/
    lasix-mythbusters-drug-masking-tco2-and-impact-on-racehorse-breakdowns.

27 Toby, *Unnatural Ability*, 194.

28 X. A. Zawadzkas, R. H. Sides, and W. M. Bayly, "Is Improved High Speed Performance Fol-
    lowing Frusemide Administration Due to Diuresis-Induced Weight Loss or Reduced Severity
    of Exercise-Induced Pulmonary Haemorrhage?" *Equine Veterinary Journal* 38, no. S36 (August
    2006): 291–93, https://doi.org/10.1111/j.2042-3306.2006.tb05555.x.

29 Natalie Voss, "New Furosemide Research Reveals Unexpected Impacts of the Medication,"
    Paulick Report, June 29, 2015, https://paulickreport.com/horse-care-category/vet-topics/
    new-furosemide-research-reveals-unexpected-impacts-of-the-medication.

30 K. W. Hinchcliff, K. H. McKeever, W. W. Muir, and R. A. Sams, "Furosemide Reduces
    Accumulated Oxygen Deficit in Horses during Brief Intense Exertion," *Journal of Applied
    Physiology* 81, no. 4 (October 1, 1996): 1550–54, https://doi.org/10.1152/jappl.1996.81.4.1550.

31 Ryan, "Lasix-Free Stakes."

32 Bob Baffert, January 4, 2023.

33 William C. Rhoden, "Wondering If Steroids Fueled a Run at Glory," *New York Times*, June
    8, 2008, https://www.nytimes.com/2008/06/08/sports/othersports/08rhoden.html.

34 Jack Shinar, "California Joins Growing List of States to Ban EPO," *BloodHorse*, August 22,
    2002, accessed September 10, 2024, https://www.bloodhorse.com/horse-racing/articles/186574
    /california-joins-growing-list-of-states-to-ban-epo.

35 "A Winner . . . but Not at All Costs," Paulick Report, November 16, 2010, https://paulickreport
    .com/news/a-winner-but-not-at-all-costs.

36 Toby, *Unnatural Ability*, 47.

37 "Racing: Dubai World Cup; Silver Charm Bleeds and Finishes Sixth," *New York Times*, March
    29, 1999, https://www.nytimes.com/1999/03/29/sports/racing-dubai-world-cup-silver-charm
    -bleeds-and-finishes-sixth.html.

38 Tim Wickes, "Letter to the Editor: Where's the Swamp?" *Thoroughbred Daily News*, July 26,
    2017, https://www.thoroughbreddailynews.com/letter-to-the-editor-wheres-the-swamp/.

39 Baffert and Haskin, *Baffert*, 137.

40 Bob Baffert, January 2, 2023.

CHAPTER 6 IT WAS THE POPPIES!

1 "Pick a Storyline to Follow," ESPN, November 5, 1999, https://www.espn.com.sg/sports/horse/news/story?id=152888.
2 Tim Yakteen, January 17, 2023.
3 Bob Baffert, January 2, 2023.
4 William Nack, "The Almighty Bob Baffert," Stacks Reader, accessed September 10, 2024, http://www.thestacksreader.com/the-almighty-bob-baffert/.
5 Nack.
6 Toby, *Unnatural Ability*, 185.
7 "Queen's Horse Estimate Tests Positive for Morphine," Reuters, July 22, 2014, https://www.reuters.com/article/sports/queens-horse-estimate-tests-positive-for-morphine-idUSKBN0FR29M/.
8 "Morphine Charges a Deja Vu for Frankel," *BloodHorse*, accessed September 10, 2024, https://www.bloodhorse.com/horse-racing/articles/196041/morphine-charges-a-deja-vu-for-frankel.
9 Steven Crist, "Lashkari Found Free of Drugs," *New York Times*, August 13, 1986, https://www.nytimes.com/1986/08/13/sports/lashkari-found-free-of-drugs.html.
10 Bob Baffert, January 4, 2023.
11 Bob Baffert, January 2, 2023.
12 Rob Fernas, "Dose of Reality," *Los Angeles Times*, July 4, 2001, https://www.latimes.com/archives/la-xpm-2001-jul-04-sp-18644-story.html.
13 "Morphine Charges a Deja Vu for Frankel," *BloodHorse*, accessed September 10, 2024, https://www.bloodhorse.com/horse-racing/articles/196041/morphine-charges-a-deja-vu-for-frankel.
14 Fernas, "Dose of Reality."
15 Bob Baffert, May 25, 2023.
16 Bob Baffert, January 4, 2023.
17 Joe Drape, "On Horse Racing; Baffert Seeking Redemption in a Summer That Has Gone Sour," *New York Times*, June 29, 2001, https://www.nytimes.com/2001/06/29/sports/on-horse-racing-baffert-seeking-redemption-in-a-summer-that-has-gone-sour.html.
18 Ingrid Fermin, June 12, 2023.
19 "Biancone Granted Conditional License in Kentucky," *BloodHorse*, accessed September 10, 2024, https://www.bloodhorse.com/horse-racing/articles/223125/biancone-granted-conditional-license-in-kentucky.
20 Walt Bogdanich and Rebecca R. Ruiz, "Turning to Frogs for Illegal Aid in Horse Races," *New York Times*, June 19, 2012, https://www.nytimes.com/2012/06/20/sports/horse-racing-discovers-new-drug-problem-one-linked-to-frogs.html.
21 https://ker.com/equinews/illegal-frog-juice-detected-racehorses/.
22 Clara Fenger, Maria Catignani, Jake Machin, and Thomas Tobin, "An In-Depth Look at Stall Contamination: A Total of 28 Substances Were Identified in Charles Town Ship-In Stalls as a Mix of Human Medications and Recreational Substances with Some Actual Equine Medications," University of Kentucky Maxwell H. Gluck Equine Research Center, 2017.
23 Rick Sams, June 28, 2024.
24 Toby, *Unnatural Ability*, 153.
25 Fernas, "Dose of Reality."
26 Rick Sams, June 28, 2024.
27 "Seinfeld: Poppy Seeds (Clip). TBS, 2014," YouTube, https://www.youtube.com/watch?v=mYzuQr7YVYg.
28 Rick Sams, June 28, 2024.
29 Baffert v. California Horse Racing Bd., 332 F.3d 613, accessed September 17, 2024, https://casetext.com/case/baffert-v-california-horse-racing-bd.

30 Baffert v. California Horse Racing Bd., Order, US District Court of the Central District of Calfornia, November 19, 2001.

31 Baffert v. California Horse Racing Bd., Order, US District Court of the Central District of Calfornia, November 19, 2001.

32 "Complete Text of CHRB's Baffert Ruling," ESPN, June 21, 2001, accessed September 10, 2024, http://a.espncdn.com/horse/news/2001/0621/1216845.html.

33 "CHRB Dismisses Baffert Morphine Case," *BloodHorse*, accessed November 4, 2024, https://www.bloodhorse.com/horse-racing/articles/171229/chrb-dismisses-baffert-morphine-case.

34 "CHRB Dismisses Baffert Morphine Case."

35 "CHRB Dismisses Baffert Morphine Case."

36 https://www.thoroughbreddailynews.com/pletcher-wins-round-in-supreme-court-over-forte -dq/; https://www.nytimes.com/2023/05/09/sports/horse-racing/forte-kentucky-derby-doping .html.

37 Joe Drape, "On Horse Racing; Baffert Seeking Redemption in a Summer That Has Gone Sour," *New York Times*, June 29, 2001, https://www.nytimes.com/2001/06/29/sports/on-horse -racing-baffert-seeking-redemption-in-a-summer-that-has-gone-sour.html.

38 Bob Baffert, January 2, 2023.

CHAPTER 7 **SUDDEN DEATH**

1 Ray Paulick, "Updated: Cardiac Failure Fatalities Spike in California, Baffert Barn," Paulick Report, April 10, 2013, https://paulickreport.com/news/ray-s-paddock/sudden-equine-fatalities -spike-in-california-baffert-barn.

2 Bob Baffert, January 2, 2023.

3 Rick Arthur, "Report on the Investigation and Review of the Seven Sudden Deaths on the Hollywood Park Main Track of Horses Trained by Bob Baffert and Stabled in Barn 61," California Horse Racing Board, 2013, https://www.chrb.ca.gov/veterinary_reports/baffert_sudden _death_report_final_1121.pdf.

4 Paulick, "Updated: Cardiac Failure Fatalities Spike in California, Baffert Barn."

5 William Nack, "Blood Money," *Sports Illustrated*, November 16, 1992, accessed September 10, 2024, https://vault.si.com/vault/1992/11/16/blood-money-in-the-rich-clubby-world-of -horsemen-some-greedy-owners-have-hired-killers-to-murder-their-animals-for-the-insurance -payoffs.

6 Tom Dixon, "Alydar's Final Hours," *BloodHorse*, accessed September 10, 2024, https://www .bloodhorse.com/horse-racing/features/alydars-final-hours-21207.

7 Arthur, "Report on the Investigation and Review."

8 Rick Arthur, January 4, 2023.

9 Rick Arthur, January 4, 2023.

10 Mike Marlow, January 2, 2023.

11 Mike Marlow, January 2, 2023.

12 Mike Marlow, January 2, 2023.

13 Baffert and Haskin, *Baffert*, 97.

14 Arthur, "Report on the Investigation and Review."

15 Arthur.

16 Arthur.

17 Arthur.

18 Bob Baffert, January 2, 2023.

19 Rick Arthur, email, June 28, 2024.

20 Arthur, "Report on the Investigation and Review."

21 Bob Baffert, January 2, 2023.

22 Arthur, "Report on the Investigation and Review."

23 Bob Baffert, January 2, 2023.

24 Joe Drape, "PETA Videos Prompt New York and Kentucky to Investigate Horse Trainers," *New York Times*, March 21, 2014, https://www.nytimes.com/2014/03/21/sports/peta-videos -prompt-new-york-and-kentucky-to-investigate-horse-trainers.html; New York Gaming Commission, "Staff Report in Regard to Allegations Advanced by the People for the Ethical Treatment of Animals in Regard to the Practices of KDE Equine, LLC et Al.," November 23, 2015, https://www.gaming.ny.gov/pdf/11.23.15.AsmussenReport.pdf.

00 Arthur, "Report on the Investigation and Review."

00 Bob Baffert, January 2, 2023.

26 Arthur, "Report on the Investigation and Review."

27 Bob Baffert, January 2, 2023.

28 Laura Nath, Andrew Stent, Adrian Elliott, Andre La Gerche, and Samantha Franklin, "Risk Factors for Exercise-Associated Sudden Cardiac Death in Thoroughbred Racehorses," *Animals: An Open Access Journal from MDPI* 12, no. 10 (May 18, 2022): 1297, https://doi.org/10.3390 /ani12101297.

29 Helena Carstensen et al., "Long-Term Training Increases Atrial Fibrillation Sustainability in Standardbred Racehorses," *Journal of Cardiovascular Translational Research* 16, no. 5 (2023): 1205–19, https://doi.org/10.1007/s12265-023-10378-6.

30 Janice Kritchevsky et al., "A Randomised, Controlled Trial to Determine the Effect of Levothy- roxine on Standardbred Racehorses," *Equine Veterinary Journal* 54, no. 3 (May 2022): 584–91, https://doi.org/10.1111/evj.13480.

31 Rick Arthur, email, September 18, 2024.

CHAPTER 8 **SOCIAL LICENSE TO OPERATE**

1   William Nack, "The Breaking Point," *Sports Illustrated*, November 1, 1993, accessed September 10, 2024, https://vault.si.com/vault/1993/11/01/the-breaking-point-a-rising-toll-of-racetrack -breakdowns-has-shaken-public-confidence-and-put-the-thoroughbred-industry-at-a-crossroads.

2   "Horsepower in the Bluegrass: The Economic Impact of Horse Racing," Kentucky Derby, accessed September 10, 2024, https://www.kentuckyderby.com/horses/news/horsepower-in -the-bluegrass-the-economic-impact-of-horse-racing/.

3   "Eight Belles' Death Sparks Controversy," CBS News, May 5, 2008, https://www.cbsnews .com/news/eight-belles-death-sparks-controversy/.

4   "PETA Wants Eight Belles' Jockey Suspended After Filly's Death," Associated Press, March 25, 2015, https://www.foxnews.com/story/peta-wants-eight-belles-jockey-suspended-after -fillys-death.

5   William Nack, "The DNA of Eight Belles' Tragic Breakdown," ESPN, May 16, 2008, https://www.espn.com/sports/horse/triplecrown08/columns/story?columnist=nack_ bill&id=3399004.

6   Nack, "The DNA of Eight Belles' Tragic Breakdown."

7   "Size of Field and Starts per Horse," Jockey Club, accessed September 20, 2024, https://www .jockeyclub.com/default.asp?section=FB&area=10.

8   "The Thoroughbred Safety Committee Soundness Issues: Dr. Larry Bramlage," Jockey Club, accessed September 20, 2024, https://www.jockeyclub.com/default.asp?section=RT& year=2008&area=11.

9   Natalie Voss, "Despite HISA Oversight, Parx Turf Course's Seasonal Bow Had a Bobble," Paulick Report, September 23, 2024, https://paulickreport.com/news/thoroughbred-racing/ despite-hisa-oversight-parx-turf-courses-seasonal-bow-had-a-bobble.

10 "Sale Companies Ban Off-Label Use of Bisphosphonates," *BloodHorse*, accessed September 10, 2024, https://www.bloodhorse.com/horse-racing/articles/232688/sale-companies-ban-off -label-use-of-bisphosphonates.

11 Dan Ross, "Joint Injections: 'Litmus Test' for HISA," *Thoroughbred Daily News*, August 16, 2023, https://www.thoroughbreddailynews.com/intra-articular-joint-injections-litmus-test -for-hisa/.

12 Ross.

13 Natalie Voss, "Lasix Mythbusters: Drug Masking, TCO2, and Impact on Racehorse Break-downs," Paulick Report, October 21, 2022, https://paulickreport.com/horse-care-category/ lasix-mythbusters-drug-masking-tco2-and-impact-on-racehorse-breakdowns.

14 Mary Scollay, October 31, 2022.

15 "Breeding, Drugs, and Breakdowns: The State of Thoroughbred Horseracing and the Welfare of the Thoroughbred Racehorse," US House of Representatives, June 19, 2008, https://www .congress.gov/event/110th-congress/house-event/LC7764/text.

16 "Breeding, Drugs, and Breakdowns."

17 Jay Hovdey, "Call Him Doctor Derby: Harthill Remembers Bad Old Days," *Daily Racing Form*, April 28, 2002.

18 Randy Moss, "Ruffian Remembered," ESPN, June 4, 2007, https://www.espn.co.uk/sports/ horse/columns/story?columnist=moss_randy&id=2892898.

19 Bill Finley, "New York Unveils Steroid-Free Racing," *New York Times*, January 1, 2009, https:// www.nytimes.com/2009/01/02/sports/othersports/02racing.html.

20 Lev Akabas, "Kentucky Derby Horses Aren't Getting Any Faster," *Sportico* (blog), May 1, 2024, https://www.sportico.com/leagues/other-sports/2024/kentucky-derby-horses-winners -record-secretariat-1234777428/.

21 "Hancock's Call for a Commissioner," Paulick Report, November 16, 2010, https://paulick report.com/news/the-biz/hancock-s-call-for-a-commissioner.

22 "Group Wants Racing Act to Regulate Medication," *BloodHorse*, accessed September 10, 2024, https://www.bloodhorse.com/horse-racing/articles/127617/group-wants-racing-act-to-regulate -medication.

23 Andrew Beyer, "After All These Years, Lasix Is 'a Polarizing Topic' in Horse Racing Again," *Washington Post*, August 31, 2011, https://www.washingtonpost.com/sports/horse-racing/after -all-these-years-lasix-is-a-polarizing-topic-in-horse-racing-again/2011/08/30/gIQAzPAsrJ_story .html.

24 Natalie Voss, "'Bring Rick Back'? Years Later, Dutrow's Ban Still Divides," Paulick Report, January 29, 2019, https://paulickreport.com/nl-art-1/bring-rick-back-years-later-dutrows-ban -still-divides.

25 Voss, "'Bring Rick Back'?"

26 John Pricci, "Whistleblower: State Actor Framed Trainer Rick Dutrow," *Horse Race Insider* (blog), February 16, 2020, https://www.horseraceinsider.com/kentucky-derby-winning-trainer -was-framed-by-new-york-state-actor/.

CHAPTER 9 THE RACING BUSINESS

1 "22nd Horse since December Dies at California's Santa Anita Park after Race Track Declared Safe," Fox 5 Atlanta, March 14, 2019, https://www.fox5atlanta.com/news/22nd-horse-since -december-dies-at-californias-santa-anita-park-after-race-track-declared-safe.

2 Mike Kane, "Antonucci: 'It Just Brings You Back to It,'" *Thoroughbred Daily News*, August 6, 2023, https://www.thoroughbreddailynews.com/antonucci-it-just-brings-you-back-to-it/.

3 Kane.

4 Tony Cobitz, "Re: How to Define a 'Super Trainer'?" X, March 22, 2024, https://x.com/ Tinky47flat/status/1771142845006520796.

5 Andrew Beyer, "Lukas's Derby Strategy Quantifiable," *Washington Post*, May 2, 1996, https:// www.washingtonpost.com/archive/sports/1996/05/02/lukass-derby-strategy-quantifiable /785d2d36-d013-4229-9733-fbff723395e4/.

6 Ray Paulick, "Pletcher Juveniles No One-Hit Wonders," Paulick Report, September 5, 2012, https://paulickreport.com/news/ray-s-paddock/pletcher-juveniles-no-one-hit-wonders.

7 Rick Arthur, "Report on the Investigation and Review of the Seven Sudden Deaths on the Hollywood Park Main Track of Horses Trained by Bob Baffert and Stabled in Barn 61," California Horse Racing Board, 2013, https://www.chrb.ca.gov/veterinary_reports/baffert _sudden_death_report_final_1121.pdf.

8 "Report Finds No Evidence That Illegal Drugs Contributed to 23 Horse Deaths at Santa Anita," CBS Los Angeles, March 10, 2020, https://www.cbsnews.com/losangeles/news/report -finds-no-evidence-that-illegal-drugs-contributed-to-23-horse-deaths-at-santa-anita/.

9 Mick Peterson, July 10, 2023.

10 Bill Finley, "Are Horses More Likely to Break Down on Wet Tracks? The Stats Say No," *Thoroughbred Daily News*, September 19, 2023, https://www.thoroughbreddailynews.com/ are-horses-more-likely-to-break-down-on-wet-tracks-the-stats-say-no/.

11 Rick Arthur, January 4, 2023.

12 https://www.washingtonpost.com/politics/the-president-in-the-room/2016/07/13/99228738 -4926-11e6-acbc-4d4870a079da_story.html.

13 Associated Press, "Austrian-Canadian Billionaire Frank Stronach Charged with Sexual Assault," *Guardian*, June 9, 2024, https://www.theguardian.com/world/article/2024/jun/09/billionaire -frank-stronach-charged-sexual-assault-canada.

14 "Frank Stronach Says His Accusers Are Motivated by Money," CBC News, YouTube, accessed September 20, 2024, https://www.youtube.com/watch?v=zB_80-PiMcI.

15 John Cherwa, "As Santa Anita Opens, Fix-It Man Tim Ritvo Ponders 'Problems Bigger than I Thought,'" *Los Angeles Times*, September 29, 2017, https://www.latimes.com/sports/more/ la-sp-santa-anita-ritvo-20170928-story.html.

16 Joanna Bliss, email, September 20, 2024.

17 T. D. Thornton, *Not by a Long Shot* (New York: PublicAffairs, 2007), 158.

18 "Shelbe Ruis, Santa Anita at Odds Over Wet-Track Scratch," *BloodHorse*, accessed September 10, 2024, https://www.bloodhorse.com/horse-racing/articles/231918/shelbe-ruis-santa-anita -at-odds-over-wet-track-scratch.

19 "Shelbe Ruis, Santa Anita at Odds Over Wet-Track Scratch."

20 New York Task Force on Racehorse Health and Safety, "Investigation of Equine Fatalities at Aqueduct 2011–2012 Fall/Winter Meet," September 2012, https://www.gaming.ny.gov/pdf/ NY%20Task%20Force%20on%20Racehorse%20Health%20and%20Safety.pdf.

21 "Investigation of Equine Fatalities at Aqueduct 2011–2012 Fall/Winter Meet."

22 "Open Letter from the Stronach Group," California Thoroughbred Breeders Association, accessed September 10, 2024, https://ctba.com/open-letter-from-the-stronach-group/.

23 California Horse Racing Board, "Report on Fatalities at Santa Anita Park from 12/30/18 through 3/31/19," March 10, 2020, https://www.chrb.ca.gov/veterinary_reports/CHRB-Santa -Anita-Fatalities-Report-3-10-20.pdf.

24 Dan Ross, "Joint Injections: 'Litmus Test' for HISA," *Thoroughbred Daily News*, August 16, 2023, https://www.thoroughbreddailynews.com/intra-articular-joint-injections-litmus-test-for-hisa/.

25 Bill Finley, "With No Main Track Musculoskeletal Racing Fatalities in '22, Santa Anita Continues to Make Strides on Safety," *Thoroughbred Daily News*, January 17, 2023, https://www .thoroughbreddailynews.com/with-no-main-track-racing-fatalities-in-22-santa-anita -continues-to-make-strides-on-saftey/.

26 John Cherwa, "Investigation into Horse Deaths at Santa Anita Finds No Unlawful Conduct," *Los Angeles Times*, December 19, 2019, https://www.latimes.com/sports/story/2019-12-19/ horse-racing-investigation.

27 Dan Ross, "Computer Assisted Wagering: Anatomy of a Deal," *Thoroughbred Daily News*, March 20, 2024, https://www.thoroughbreddailynews.com/computer-assisted-wagering-anatomy -of-a-deal/.

28 "Churchill Downs Incorporated Reports 2023 Fourth Quarter and Full Year Results," Churchill Downs Inc., February 21, 2024, https://ir.churchilldownsincorporated.com/news-releases/news-release-details/churchill-downs-incorporated-reports-2023-fourth-quarter-and.

29 Joe Drape, "Death of Another Horse at Santa Anita Rocks the Racing Industry," *New York Times*, April 1, 2019, https://www.nytimes.com/2019/04/01/sports/santa-anita-horse-deaths.html.

CHAPTER 10 **"EYES AND GUT"**

1 Joe Drape, "Justify Failed a Drug Test Before Winning the Triple Crown," *New York Times*, September 11, 2019, https://www.nytimes.com/2019/09/11/sports/horse-racing/justify-drug-test-triple-crown-kentucky-derby.html.

2 Bob Baffert, January 2, 2024.

3 Data provided by the Association of Racing Commissioners International.

4 Drape, "Justify Failed a Drug Test."

5 Bob Baffert, January 2, 2024.

6 Mike Marten, California Horse Racing Board, June 26, 2024.

7 "Agreement: CHRB to Order Justify DQ, Pay Ruis $300,000," *BloodHorse*, accessed September 10, 2024, https://www.bloodhorse.com/horse-racing/articles/275497/agreement-chrb-to-order-justify-dq-pay-ruis-300-000.

8 Rick Sams, June 28, 2024.

9 Rick Arthur, email, June 21, 2024.

10 Rick Arthur, email, June 20, 2024.

11 T. D. Thornton, "CHRB Settles with Ruis in '18 Santa Anita Derby Dispute Involving Justify DQ," *Thoroughbred Daily News*, March 8, 2024, https://www.thoroughbreddailynews.com/chrb-settles-with-ruis-in-18-santa-anita-derby-dispute-involving-justify-dq/.

12 Rick Arthur, January 4, 2023.

13 "Report of the Board of Stewards to the California Horse Racing Board: Week of Monday, May 11, 2020 through Sunday, May 17, 2020."

14 Drape, "Justify Failed a Drug Test."

15 Bob Baffert, January 2, 2023.

16 Mike Marlow, January 2, 2023.

17 "Drug Violations, Mislabeling in NYRA's Baffert Charges," *BloodHorse*, accessed September 10, 2024, https://www.bloodhorse.com/horse-racing/articles/255917/drug-violations-mislabeling-in-nyras-baffert-charges.

18 "NYRA Amends Baffert Complaint to Include Two Bute Positives from 2019," *DRF*, accessed September 10, 2024, https://www.drf.com/news/nyra-amends-baffert-complaint-include-two-bute-positives-2019.

19 Dan Ross, "CHRB Investigative Reports Add Details to NYRA's Amended Charges Against Baffert," *Thoroughbred Daily News*, January 5, 2022, https://www.thoroughbreddailynews.com/chrb-investigative-reports-add-details-to-nyras-amended-charges-against-baffert/.

20 "NYRA Adds to Baffert Files: Trainer Said 'Someone' Gave Bute to His Horses, Would Offer Reward to Solve Case," Paulick Report, January 4, 2022, https://paulickreport.com/news/the-biz/nyra-adds-to-baffert-files-trainer-said-someone-gave-bute-to-his-horses-would-offer-reward-to-solve-case.

21 Bob Baffert, January 2, 2024.

22 Rick Arthur, January 4, 2023.

23 Rick Sams, June 28, 2024.

24 New York Racing Association in the Matter of Robert A. Baffert, New York, January 24, 2022.

25 "KHRC, Baffert's Legal Team Present Arguments at Appeal," *BloodHorse*, accessed September 10, 2024, https://www.bloodhorse.com/horse-racing/articles/262498/khrc-bafferts-legal-team-present-arguments-at-appeal.

26 "CHRB Issues Complaint against Trainer Richard Baltas for 47 Horse Racing Violations," Yahoo Sports, June 22, 2022, https://sports.yahoo.com/chrb-issues-complaint-against-trainer-010230785.html.

27 Arkansas Racing Commission in the Matter of Bob Baffert, April 19 and 20, 2021.

28 "Arkansas State Racing Commission Meeting: Meeting Minutes," April 19, 2021, https://ssl-dfa-site.ark.org/images/uploads/racingCommissionOffice/RAC_4-19-2021__4-20-2021.pdf.

29 Beth Harris, "Arkansas Racing Officials Vote Not to Suspend Bob Baffert," Associated Press, n.d, https://www.kxan.com/sports-general/arkansas-racing-officials-vote-not-to-suspend-bob-baffert/; "Baffert's Oaklawn Winners Reinstated," *Arkansas Democrat Gazette*, April 21, 2021, https://www.arkansasonline.com/news/2021/apr/21/bafferts-oaklawn-winners-reinstated/.

30 Bob Baffert, January 4, 2023.

31 Bob Baffert, January 4, 2023.

32 Bob Baffert, January 4, 2023.

33 Natalie Voss, "Dead Horse's Medical Records Cast Light on Baffert's Evolving Relationship with Betamethasone," Paulick Report, September 5, 2023, https://paulickreport.com/news/the-biz/dead-horses-medical-records-cast-light-on-bafferts-evolving-relationship-with-betamethasone.

34 Associated Press, "Bob Baffert Hires Oversight after Multiple Horses Test Positive for Medical Violations," *Los Angeles Times*, November 4, 2020, https://www.latimes.com/sports/story/2020-11-04/baffert-hires-oversight-after-stables-drug-positives.

35 Bob Baffert, January 4, 2023.

CHAPTER 11 STUART JANNEY'S QUEST

1 "Stuart S. Janney III," Breeders' Cup, Equibase, n.d., https://www.equibase.com/breederscup/2016/owners/StuartJanney.pdf.

2 "Stuart S. Janney, III," Bessemer Trust, accessed September 15, 2024, https://www.bessemertrust.com/people/stuart-s-janney-iii.

3 "Ogden Phipps, Racing Titan, Dead," *DFR*, April 22, 2002, accessed November 20, 2024. https://www.drf.com/news/ogden-phipps-racing-titan-dead.

4 Max Hodge, "Letter to the Editor: 'Give the Jockey Club to the Industry,'" *Thoroughbred Daily News*, November 14, 2023, https://www.thoroughbreddailynews.com/letter-to-the-editor-give-the-jockey-club-to-the-industry/.

5 "Janney Elected Chairman of Jockey Club," *BloodHorse*, accessed September 21, 2024, https://www.bloodhorse.com/horse-racing/articles/105841/janney-elected-chairman-of-jockey-club.

6 Mark Johnson, *Spitting in the Soup: Inside the Dirty Game of Doping in Sports* (Boulder, CO: VeloPress, 2016), 14.

7 "'Dope' an American Term," *New York Times*, April 7, 1901, https://timesmachine.nytimes.com/timesmachine/1901/04/07/101186374.pdf?pdf_redirect=true&ip=0.

8 Johnson, *Spitting in the Soup*, 15; "Doping a Race," *Morning Call* (San Francisco), November 26, 1894, https://www.loc.gov/resource/sn94052989/1894-11-26/ed-1/?sp=5&st=image&r=-0.116,-0.066,0.746,0.289,0.

9 Toby, *Unnatural Ability*, 11.

10 Rick Sams, email, September 22, 2024.

11 Johnson, *Spitting in the Soup*, 122.

12 Johnson, 36.

13 Johnson, 36.

14 Johnson, 39.

15 Rebecca R. Ruiz, Juliet Macur, and Ian Austen, "Even with Confession of Cheating, World's Doping Watchdog Did Nothing," *New York Times*, June 15, 2016, https://www.nytimes.com/2016/06/16/sports/olympics/world-anti-doping-agency-russia-cheating.html.

16 "Interview with John Penza," Jockey Club, accessed September 21, 2024, https://jockeyclub .com/default.asp?section=RT&year=2022&area=7.

17 "Judge Orders Reinstatement of Fired DEA Agent," *Sarasota Herald-Tribune*, June 5, 2004, accessed September 21, 2024, https://www.heraldtribune.com/story/news/2004/06/05/judge -orders-reinstatement-of-fired-dea-agent/28809248007/.

18 "Judge Orders Reinstatement of Fired DEA Agent."

19 "Judge Orders Reinstatement of Fired DEA Agent."

20 "Timothy P. Harrington," 50-a.org, accessed September 18, 2024, https://www.50-a.org/ officer/MFK3.

CHAPTER 12 **THE COPS**

1 "Equestology: The Science of Performance Horses," Equestology, March 9, 2016, https://web .archive.org/web/20160309093644/http://equestology.com/.

2 Terry Wan, email, January 21, 2024.

3 A. G. Sulzberger, "At Military Contractor's Trial, a $100,000 Buckle," *New York Times*, July 27, 2010, https://www.nytimes.com/2010/07/27/nyregion/27fraud.html.

4 United States v. Seth Fishman, Southern District of New York, trial testimony of Angela Jett, January 21, 2022.

5 Bill Finley, "Navarro Cleared to Race at Stronach Tracks," *Thoroughbred Daily News*, September 27, 2017, https://www.thoroughbreddailynews.com/navarro-cleared-to-race-at-stronach -tracks/.

6 "Russian Mafia Boss Still at Large after FBI Wiretap at Trump Tower," ABC News, March 21, 2017, accessed September 21, 2024, https://abcnews.go.com/US/story-fbi-wiretap-russians -trump-tower/story?id=46266198.

7 "Two More Defendants Plead Guilty in Manhattan Federal Court in Connection with Russian-American Organized Crime Gambling Enterprise," press release, US Department of Justice, Southern District of New York, May 13, 2015, https://www.justice.gov/usao-sdny/pr /two-more-defendants-plead-guilty-manhattan-federal-court-connection-russian-american.

8 Randal Gindi, telephone interview, September 9, 2024.

CHAPTER 13 **"NOBODY GOES TO JAIL FOR AN EPOGEN POSITIVE"**

1 Shaun Richards, January 27, 2024.

2 Timmy L. S. Choi et al., "Identification of the Dermorphin Tetrapeptide [Dmt 1]-DALDA in a Seized Unlabelled Vial and Its First Detection in Horse Urine: A Case Report," *Drug Testing and Analysis* 16, no. 3 (March 2024): 268–76, https://doi.org/10.1002/dta.3536.

3 P. Teale, J. Scarth, and S. Hudson, "Impact of the Emergence of Designer Drugs upon Sports Doping Testing," *Bioanalysis* 4, no. 1 (January 2012): 71–88, https://doi.org/10.4155/bio.11.291.

4 Lawrence Ostlere, "Lance Armstrong Reveals How He Passed Drugs Tests to Win Tour de France," *Independent*, December 14, 2023, https://www.independent.co.uk/sport/cycling/ lance-armstrong-doping-drugs-tests-b2464036.html.

5 "'Thief-In-Law' Razhden Shulaya Sentenced in Manhattan Federal Court to 45 Years in Prison," press release, US Department of Justice, Southern District of New York, December 19, 2018, https://www.justice.gov/usao-sdny/pr/thief-law-razhden-shulaya-sentenced-manhattan-federal -court-45-years-prison.

6 Bailee Woolstenhulme, "Horses Officially Categorized as Livestock, Thanks to 2018 Farm Bill," Utah Farm Bureau Federation, February 26, 2019, https://www.utahfarmbureau.org/ Article/Horses-officially-categorized-as-livestock-thanks-to-2018-Farm-Bill.

7 United States v. Navarro et al., indictment, US Department of Justice, Southern District of New York, March 9, 2020.

CHAPTER 14 **THE BACKSIDE**

1 "Wage Judgment Against Asmussen Stable Totals Over $486K," *BloodHorse*, accessed September 21, 2024, https://www.bloodhorse.com/horse-racing/articles/275446/wage-judgment-against -asmussen-stable-totals-over-486k; T. D. Thornton, "Chad Brown Must Pay $1.6M for Federal Labor Violations," *Thoroughbred Daily News*, May 22, 2019, https://www.thoroughbreddaily news.com/chad-brown-must-pay-1-6m-for-federal-labor-violations/.

2 Frank Luengo, Sentencing Letter on Behalf of Jorge Navarro, United States v. Navarro, US Department of Justice, Southern District of New York, December 3, 2021.

3 Cristobal Morales, Sentencing Letter on Behalf of Jorge Navarro, United States v. Navarro, US Department of Justice, Southern District of New York, December 3, 2021.

4 Orietta Canet, Sentencing Letter on Behalf of Jorge Navarro, United States v. Navarro, US Department of Justice, Southern District of New York, December 3, 2021.

5 Canet.

6 John Koenig, Sentencing Letter on Behalf of Jorge Navarro, United States v. Navarro, US Department of Justice, Southern District of New York, December 3, 2021.

7 Gary F. Maluski, Sentencing Letter on Behalf of Jorge Navarro, United States v. Jorge Navarro, US Department of Justice, Southern District of New York, December 3, 2021.

8 James E. Harries, Sentencing Letter on Behalf of Jorge Navarro, United States v. Navarro, US Department of Justice, Southern District of New York, December 3, 2021.

9 "'Goodbye to a Friend': Elite Sprinter X Y Jet Dies of Apparent Cardiac Event," Paulick Report, January 8, 2020, https://paulickreport.com/news/thoroughbred-racing/goodbye-to-a-friend -elite-sprinter-x-y-jet-dies-of-heart-attack.

10 Bruce A. Turpin, "Line Sheet, Tannuzzo Sessions 2.0," United States v. Navarro et al., Exhibit C-1, US Department of Justice, Southern District of New York, November 21, 2022.

11 "Two Trainers Acknowledge Using Fishman's Drugs," *BloodHorse*, accessed September 21, 2024, https://www.bloodhorse.com/horse-racing/articles/256397/two-trainers-acknowledge -using-fishmans-drugs.

12 United States v. Seth Fishman, US Department of Justice, Southern District of New York, trial testimony of Special Agent Aaron Otterson, January 27, 2022.

13 United States v. Seth Fishman.

14 United States v. Seth Fishman.

15 Trial Exhibit GX-2014-Q, United States v. Seth Fishman, US Department of Justice, Southern District of New York, n.d.

16 Trial Exhibit GX-2018-B, United States v. Seth Fishman, US Department of Justice, Southern District of New York, n.d.

17 Trial Exhibit GX-2014-Q, United States v. Seth Fishman, US Department of Justice, Southern District of New York, n.d.

18 United States v. Seth Fishman, Southern District of New York, trial testimony, Special Agent Aaron Otterson, January 27, 2022.

19 United States v. Seth Fishman, trial testimony of Special Agent Aaron Otterson, January 27, 2022.

20 Trial Exhibit GX-191A-T, United States v. Seth Fishman, US Department of Justice, Southern District of New York, n.d.

21 Damian Williams, "Re: United States v. Jorge Navarro," US Department of Justice, December 10, 2021.

22 Bruce A. Turpin, "Line Sheet, Tannuzzo Sessions 2.0," United States v. Navarro et al., Exhibit C-1, US Department of Justice, Southern District of New York, November 21, 2022.

23 Williams, "Re: United States v. Jorge Navarro."

24 Williams.

25 Williams.

26 Williams.

27 Natalie Voss, "'Animal Abuse in the Service of Greed': Prosecutors Reveal More About Navarro's Doping Program, Boastful Text Messages," Paulick Report, December 11, 2021, https://paulickreport.com/news/the-biz/animal-abuse-in-the-service-of-greed-prosecutors-reveal-more-about-navarros-doping-program-boastful-text-messages.

28 Voss.

29 Bill Finley, "Navarro Cleared to Race at Stronach Tracks," *Thoroughbred Daily News*, September 27, 2017, https://www.thoroughbreddailynews.com/navarro-cleared-to-race-at-stronach-tracks/.

30 Voss, "'Animal Abuse in the Service of Greed.'"

31 "Monmouth Stewards Urge Large Fines for Gindi, Navarro," *BloodHorse*, accessed September 21, 2024, https://www.bloodhorse.com/horse-racing/articles/223520/monmouth-stewards-urge-large-fines-for-gindi-navarro.

32 "Monmouth Stewards Urge Large Fines for Gindi, Navarro."

33 Finley, "Navarro Cleared to Race at Stronach Tracks."

34 Bruce A. Turpin, Line Sheet, Tannuzzo Sessions 2.0, United States v. Navarro et al., Exhibit C-1, US Department of Justice, Southern District of New York, November 21, 2022.

35 Turpin.

36 Isaac Jimenez, Sentencing Letter on Behalf of Jorge Navarro, United States v. Navarro, US Department of Justice, Southern District of New York, December 3, 2021.

37 Frederick Delbrey Cruz, Sentencing Letter on Behalf of Jorge Navarro, United States v. Navarro, Southern District of New York, December 3, 2021.

38 Turpin, Line Sheet, Tannuzzo Sessions 2.0.

39 Turpin.

40 Frank Vespe, "X Y Jet and the Horses of the Navarro-Servis," Racing Biz, March 10, 2020, https://www.theracingbiz.com/2020/03/10/x-y-jet-and-the-horses-of-the-navarro-servis-indictment/.

CHAPTER 15 **BELONGING**

1 "Feb. 14, 2019," United States v. Garcia, 20-cr-160 (MKV), 11 (S.D.N.Y. Dec. 8, 2021).

2 Audrey Strauss, "The Government's Omnibus Brief in Opposition to the Defendants' Pretrial Motions to Suppress Certain Intercepted Communications and Evidence Obtained from Premises Searches, Cellphone Searches, and Searches of Electronically Stored Information," United States v. Garcia et al., US Department of Justice, Southern District of New York, September 2, 2021.

3 United States v. Seth Fishman, US Department of Justice, Southern District of New York, trial testimony of Adrienne Hall, January 27, 2022.

4 Trial testimony of Adrienne Hall.

5 Trial testimony of Adrienne Hall.

6 Trial testimony of Adrienne Hall.

7 Rick Sams, June 28, 2024.

8 Trial Exhibit GX-101A, United States v. Seth Fishman, US Department of Justice, Southern District of New York, n.d.

9 Bill Finley, "Caught Up in Fishman Scandal, Hall Tells Her Story," *Thoroughbred Daily News*, February 10, 2022, https://www.thoroughbreddailynews.com/caught-up-in-fishman-scandal-hall-tells-her-story/.

10 Rick Sams, June 28, 2024.

11 Trial Exhibit GX-107A, United States v. Seth Fishman, US Department of Justice, Southern District of New York, n.d.

12 Trial Exhibit GX-106A.

13 Trial Exhibit GX-105F.

14 "About Godolphin," Godolphin, accessed September 21, 2024, https://www.godolphin.com/about-us.

15 Trial Exhibit GX-105B, United States v. Seth Fishman, US Department of Justice, Southern District of New York, n.d.

16 United States v. Seth Fishman, US Department of Justice, Southern District of New York, trial testimony of Adrienne Hall, January 27, 2022.

17 Trial Exhibit GX-105C, United States v. Seth Fishman, US Department of Justice, Southern District of New York, n.d.

18 Finley, "Caught Up in Fishman Scandal, Hall Tells Her Story."

19 United States v. Seth Fishman, US Department of Justice, Southern District of New York, trial testimony of Adrienne Hall, January 27, 2022.

20 "Know the Risks Before You Inject," Chronicle of the Horse, accessed September 21, 2024, https://www.chronofhorse.com/article/know-risks-you-inject/.

21 Trial Exhibit GX-501D-501A, United States v. Seth Fishman, US Department of Justice, Southern District of New York, n.d.

22 Damian Williams, "Re: United States v. Lisa Giannelli," US Department of Justice, Southern District of New York, September 1, 2022.

23 United States v. Seth Fishman, US Department of Justice, Southern District of New York, trial testimony of Jamen Davidovich, January 27, 2022.

24 Williams, "Re: United States v. Lisa Giannelli."

25 United States v. Seth Fishman, US Department of Justice, Southern District of New York, trial testimony of Ross Cohen, January 26, 2022.

26 United States v. Seth Fishman, US Department of Justice, Southern District of New York, trial testimony of Ross Cohen. January 26, 2022.

27 Trial Exhibit GX-2006-W, United States v. Seth Fishman, US Department of Justice, Southern District of New York, n.d.

28 United States v. Seth Fishman, US Department of Justice, Southern District of New York, trial testimony of Ross Cohen, January 26, 2022.

CHAPTER 16 THE GHOST OF ALEX HARTHILL

1 Bill Heller, "Trainer of the Quarter—Jason Servis," *Trainer*, February 1, 2018, https://trainermagazine.com/north-american-trainer-articles/60uj45kkjv5qm7n8s95vnzesb244qh/2018/2/6.

2 David Grening, "Jason Servis Cuts His Own Path to the Kentucky Derby," Saratoga Living, May 3, 2019, https://saratogaliving.com/daily-racing-form-jason-servis-cuts-his-own-path-to-the-kentucky-derby/.

3 Garrett Servis, Sentencing Letter on Behalf of Jason Servis, July 13, 2023.

4 "Recommendation: Clenbuterol," Jockey Club Safety Committee, May 12, 2020.

5 "NY Commission Passes Clenbuterol, NSAIDs Restrictions," *BloodHorse*, accessed September 21, 2024, https://www.bloodhorse.com/horse-racing/articles/245018/ny-commission-passes-clenbuterol-nsaids-restrictions.

6 Damian Williams, "Re: United States v. Jason Servis," US Department of Justice, Southern District of New York, July 20, 2023.

7 Jonathan Lintner, "On Roll of a Lifetime, Servis Says Chatter Is 'Embarrassing,'" Horse Racing Nation, July 8, 2018, https://www.horseracingnation.com/news/On_roll_of_a_lifetime_Servis_says_chatter_is_embarrassing_123.

8 Williams, "Re: United States v. Jason Servis."

9 Williams.

10 Rita Glavin, Sentencing Memorandum on Behalf of Jason Servis, US Department of Justice, Southern District of New York, July 13, 2023.

11 Sid Fernando, "Taking Stock: Is SGF-1000 a PED?" *Thoroughbred Daily News*, February 28, 2023, https://www.thoroughbreddailynews.com/taking-stock-is-sgf-1000-a-ped/.

12 "HIWU Calls Attention to Dietary Supplement Regulations," *BloodHorse*, accessed September 21, 2024, https://www.bloodhorse.com/horse-racing/articles/267571/hiwu-calls-attention-to-dietary-supplement-regulations.

13 Fernando, "Taking Stock."

14 Fernando.

15 Fernando.

16 Dionne Benson, Letter to Matt Iuliano, "Re: SGF 1000 Analysis—UC Davis—CONFIDENTIAL—INTERNAL USE ONLY," February 5, 2014.

CHAPTER 17 THROUGH THE LOOKING GLASS

1 Robert Gearty, "Seth Fishman Sentenced to 11 Years in Prison," *Thoroughbred Daily News*, July 11, 2022, https://www.thoroughbreddailynews.com/seth-fishman-sentenced-to-11-years-in-prison/.

2 Gus Garcia-Roberts, "As His Doping Case Goes to Trial, a Veterinarian Says It's Horse Racing That's Corrupt," *Washington Post*, January 19, 2022, https://www.washingtonpost.com/sports/2022/01/19/seth-fishman-horse-racing-doping/.

3 Andrew Adams, March 14, 2024.

4 Gentry Estes, "Undefeated Maximum Security Is a Puzzling Kentucky Derby Contender," *Courier-Journal*, May 1, 2019, accessed September 15, 2024, https://www.courier-journal.com/story/sports/horses/kentucky-derby/2019/05/01/kentucky-derby-horses-2019-maximum-security-puzzling-contender/3640887002/.

5 Andrew Adams, March 14, 2024.

6 "Lawsuit Filed Against Trainer Chad Brown Over Alleged Domestic Violence Incident," Paulick Report, May 11, 2023, https://paulickreport.com/news/lawsuit-filed-against-trainer-chad-brown-over-alleged-domestic-violence-incident.

7 T. D. Thornton, "Chad Brown Must Pay $1.6M for Federal Labor Violations," *Thoroughbred Daily News*, May 22, 2019, https://www.thoroughbreddailynews.com/chad-brown-must-pay-1-6m-for-federal-labor-violations/.

8 Data from the Association for Racing Commissioners International.

9 Damian Williams, "Re: United States v. Kristian Rhein," US Department of Justice, Southern District of New York, November 24, 2021.

10 Williams.

11 Williams.

12 Williams.

13 Transcript, police interview with Jason Servis, August 14, 2019.

14 Williams, "Re: United States v. Jason Servis."

15 Rita Glavin, "Sentencing Memorandum on Behalf of Jason Servis," US Department of Justice, Southern District of New York, July 13, 2023.

16 Glavin.

17 Transcript, police interview with Jason Servis, August 14, 2019.

18 T. D. Thornton, "The Week in Review: Feds: Even Those Sold It Did Not Know Contents of SGF-1000," *Thoroughbred Daily News*, November 21, 2021, https://www.thoroughbreddailynews.com/the-week-in-review-feds-even-those-sold-it-did-not-know-contents-of-sgf-1000/.

19 Mary Scollay, email, June 5, 2024; "Drs. Scollay, Arthur, Hovda Voice Support of RCI's Proposed Regulation of Compounded Drugs," Paulick Report, January 12, 2015, https://paulickreport.com/news/the-biz/drs-scollay-arthur-hovda-voice-support-of-rcis-proposed-regulation-of-compounded-drugs.

20 Kristian Rhein, September 7, 2024.

21 "Top Sprinter X Y Jet Dies from Heart Attack," *BloodHorse*, accessed September 15, 2024, https://www.bloodhorse.com/horse-racing/articles/237813/top-sprinter-x-y-jet-dies-from -heart-attack.

22 "X Y Jet, Imperial Hint Fine after Grueling Efforts in Mr. Prospector," *DRF*, December 23, 2019, accessed September 21, 2024, https://www.drf.com/news/x-y-jet-imperial-hint-fine -after-grueling-efforts-mr-prospector.

23 Mikhael Rolffs, Sentencing Letter on Behalf of Jorge Navarro, United States v. Navarro, December 23, 2021.

CHAPTER 18 **THE RAID**

1 Calvin H. Scholar, "Defendant Sentencing Memorandum on Behalf of Rick Dane, Jr.," US Department of Justice, Southern District of New York, August 26, 2022.

2 "Former Harness Trainer Rick Dane Sentenced to 30 Months in Prison," Paulick Report, September 12, 2022, https://paulickreport.com/news/the-biz/former-harness-trainer-rick -dane-sentenced-to-30-months-in-prison.

3 Gary F. Maluski, Sentencing Letter on Behalf of Jorge Navarro, United States v. Jorge Navarro, December 3, 2021.

4 Cindy Harries, Sentencing Letter on Behalf of Jorge Navarro, United States v. Jorge Navarro, December 3, 2021.

5 Damian Williams, "Re: United States v. Seth Fishman," US Department of Justice, July 5, 2022.

6 Natalie Voss, "Fishman Case: Prosecutors Request 10 to 20 Years in Prison, Point to Emirati Involvement in Case," Paulick Report, July 7, 2022, https://paulickreport.com/news/the-biz /fishman-case-prosecutors-request-10-to-20-years-in-prison-point-to-emirati-involvement-in-case.

7 "Godolphin Horses in Training," Godolphin, accessed September 21, 2024, https://www. godolphin.com/horses/in-training.

8 "Fishman Sentenced to 11 Years in Prison," *BloodHorse*, accessed September 21, 2024, https:// www.bloodhorse.com/horse-racing/articles/261263/fishman-sentenced-to-11-years-in-prison.

9 Bill Finley, "The Week in Review: With Forte Non-DQ, New York Stewards Owe Public an Explanation," *Thoroughbred Daily News*, July 30, 2023, https://www.thoroughbreddailynews .com/the-week-in-review-with-forte-non-dq-nyra-stewards-owe-public-an-explanation/.

10 "Buy SGF-5000 Online (Super Growth Factor)," Best Equine Meds, accessed September 21, 2024, https://bestequinemeds.com/shop/other/buy-sgf-5000-online-super-growth-factor/.

11 Shaun Richards, September 20, 2024.

CHAPTER 19 **ALL HEART**

1 "Breeder Rice Elated Over First Grade 1 Winner Speech," *BloodHorse*, accessed September 9, 2024, https://www.bloodhorse.com/horse-racing/articles/242374/breeder-rice-elated-over -first-grade-1-winner-speech.

2 "Breeder Rice Elated Over First Grade 1 Winner Speech."

3 "Preakness Stakes 2021: Medina Spirit Takes Breeder Gail Rice from Backyard to Big Stage," NBC Sports, YouTube, accessed September 9, 2024, https://www.youtube.com/watch?v=D5T KZyQJux0.

4 Gail Rice, telephone interview, September 24, 2023.

5 William Nack, *Secretariat: The Making of a Champion* (New York: Hyperion, 2010), 14.

6 Amr Zedan, telephone interview, June 26, 2024.

7 Mike Marlow, January 2, 2023.

8 Mike Marlow, January 2, 2023.

9   "Life Is Good to Have Surgery for Ankle Chip," *BloodHorse*, accessed September 23, 2024, https://www.bloodhorse.com/horse-racing/articles/246780/life-is-good-to-have-surgery-for-ankle-chip.

10   Bob Baffert, January 4, 2023.

11   Bob Baffert, January 4, 2023.

12   Bob Baffert, January 4, 2023.

13   Amr Zedan, telephone interview, June 26, 2024.

14   Gail Rice, telephone interview, September 24, 2023.

15   Joe Drape, "Medina Spirit Wins the 147th Kentucky Derby," *New York Times*, May 1, 2021, https://www.nytimes.com/2021/05/01/sports/horse-racing/medina-spirit-wins-kentucky-derby.html.

CHAPTER 20 **THE POSITIVE**

1   "Audio: Baffert Angry, Defiant in Recorded Calls after Banned Drug Found in Medina Spirit's System," WVLT, May 5, 2022, https://www.wvlt.tv/video/2022/05/05/audio-baffert-angry-defiant-recorded-calls-after-banned-drug-found-medina-spirits-system/.

2   John Cherwa, "Kentucky Regulators Taped Calls without Consent with Baffert after Medina Spirit Test," *Los Angeles Times*, April 3, 2022, https://www.latimes.com/sports/story/2022-04-03/kentucky-regulators-calls-bob-baffert-medina-spirit.

3   Natalie Voss, "Hair Testing—What It's Good For, What It's Not Good For," Paulick Report, May 11, 2021, https://paulickreport.com/horse-care-category/hair-testing-what-its-good-for-what-its-not-good-for.

4   Toby, *Unnatural Ability*, 191.

5   Toby, 190.

6   Toby, 191.

7   Toby, 190.

8   Toby, 348.

9   Bob Baffert, January 4, 2023.

10   Bob Baffert, January 4, 2023.

11   "Bob Baffert's Full Response on Failed Drug Test by Kentucky Derby 147 Winner Medina Spirit," YouTube, 2021, https://www.youtube.com/watch?v=IFleIm0oGTg.

12   Michael Anderson, "Declaration of Michael Anderson," US District Court, Western District of Kentucky, January 17, 2023, 31.

13   Anderson, 30.

14   Gary B. Graves, "Churchill Downs Suspends Trainer Bob Baffert," Louisville Public Media, May 9, 2021, https://www.lpm.org/news/2021-05-09/churchill-downs-suspends-trainer-bob-baffert.

15   "Bob Baffert Defends His Reputation after Medina Spirit's Drug Test," *Dan Patrick Show*, YouTube, accessed September 9, 2024, https://www.youtube.com/watch?v=Akhz1CUy-HY.

16   Bob Baffert, September 16, 2024.

17   Bob Baffert, January 4, 2022.

18   "Baffert: Meds Applied to Derby Winner Had Steroid," ESPN, May 11, 2021, https://www.espn.com/horse-racing/story/_/id/31426817/bob-baffert-says-medina-spirit-was-treated-ointment-contained-steroid.

19   Kristian Rhein, September 7, 2024.

CHAPTER 21 **THE *SATURDAY NIGHT LIVE* EFFECT**

1   Mike Marten, email, June 26, 2024.

2   Bill Finley, "Medina Spirit Cleared to Run in Preakness," *Thoroughbred Daily News*, May 11, 2021, https://www.thoroughbreddailynews.com/baffert-attorney-says-agreement-reached-for-preakness-runners/.

3 Finley.

4 Amr Zedan, June 26, 2024.

5 "Spendthrift Farm 'to Hit the Pause Button' on Relationship with Bob Baffert, MyRacehorse Pulls Horses," Paulick Report, May 11, 2021, https://paulickreport.com/nl-art-1/spendthrift -farm-to-hit-the-pause-button-on-relationship-with-bob-baffert.

6 "Spendthrift Moving Some of Its Horses from Baffert's Barn," *DRF*, May 11, 2021, accessed September 23, 2024, https://www.drf.com/news/spendthrift-moving-some-its-horses-bafferts -barn.

7 "Medina Spirit Passes All Tests to Run in Preakness," *Thoroughbred Daily News*, May 14, 2021, https://www.thoroughbreddailynews.com/medina-spirit-passes-all-tests-to-run-in -preakness/.

8 "Bob Baffert Releases Statement," *Thoroughbred Daily News*, May 16, 2021, https://www .thoroughbreddailynews.com/bob-baffert-releases-statement/.

9 "NYRA Suspends Bob Baffert," New York Racing Association, accessed September 9, 2024, https://www.nyra.com/belmont/news/nyra-suspends-bob-baffert.

10 "NYRA Suspends Bob Baffert."

11 "Churchill Bans Baffert After Split Sample Confirmation," TrueNicks, accessed September 9, 2024, https://truenicks.com/articles/250573/churchill-bans-baffert-after-split-sample-confir mation.

CHAPTER 22 **21 PICOGRAMS**

1 Stuart Janney, June 26, 2024.

2 Eric Hamelback, August 23, 2023.

3 Bob Baffert, March 15, 2024.

4 Natalie Voss, "New York's Drug Testing Program Has Its Own 'Style,'" Paulick Report, March 12, 2015, https://paulickreport.com/news/ray-s-paddock/new-yorks-drug-testing-program -has-its-own-style; Emilie Munson and Matt Rocheleau, "N.Y. Issues Horse Racing Drug Violations at Lower Rate than Other States," *Times Union*, March 18, 2022, https://www .timesunion.com/news/article/new-york-horse-racing-drug-violations-16994784.php.

5 Chelsea Hackbarth, "Kentucky Judge Anxious to Remand Medina Spirit Case to Board of Stewards," Paulick Report, August 9, 2021, https://paulickreport.com/nl-art-1/kentucky-judge -anxious-to-remand-medina-spirit-case-to-board-of-stewards.

6 "KHRC Alleges Depletion of Medina Spirit Urine by Lab," *BloodHorse*, accessed September 9, 2024, https://www.bloodhorse.com/horse-racing/articles/251706/khrc-alleges-depletion- of-medina-spirit-urine-by-lab.

7 "Experts Blast Maylin Study of Medina Spirit Positive," *BloodHorse*, accessed September 9, 2024, https://www.bloodhorse.com/horse-racing/articles/259778/experts-blast-maylin-study -of-medina-spirit-positive.

8 Axel Gerdau, "Video: Surveillance at the Derby," *New York Times*, May 3, 2013, https://www .nytimes.com/video/sports/100000002203126/surveillance-at-the-derby.html.

9 Natalie Voss, "I Read Several Hundred Pages of Emails and Transcripts from the Medina Spirit Case So You Don't Have To," Paulick Report, July 20, 2022, https://paulickreport.com/news /the-biz/i-read-several-hundred-pages-of-emails-and-transcripts-from-the-medina-spirit-case -so-you-dont-have-to.

10 Natalie Voss, "Four Racetrack Veterinarians on Probation as Part of Agreement with California Board; Violations Could Include Medications Dispensed to Medina Spirit," Paulick Report, September 8, 2023, https://paulickreport.com/horse-care-category /four-racetrack-veterinarians-on-probation-as-part-of-agreement-with-california-board -violations-could-include-medications-dispensed-to-medina-spirit.

11 Clark Brewster, September 22, 2022.

12　Clark Brewster, September 3, 2024.

13　"Auction Buy Leads to Shake Up in Medina Spirit Appeal," *BloodHorse*, accessed September 9, 2024, https://www.bloodhorse.com/horse-racing/articles/263379/auction-buy-leads-to-shake-up-in-medina-spirit-appeal.

14　"With Conditions, Baffert Cleared to Participate in 2021 Breeders' Cup," Paulick Report, October 17, 2021, https://paulickreport.com/nl-art-1/with-conditions-baffert-cleared-to-participate-in-2021-breeders-cup.

15　John Cherwa, "New Syndicate Model of Horse Racing Ownership Is Proving to Be a Winner," *Los Angeles Times*, May 16, 2024, https://www.latimes.com/sports/story/2024-05-16/new-syndicate-model-of-horse-racing-ownership-is-proving-to-be-a-winner.

CHAPTER 23　THE BOTTOM LINE

1　T. D. Thornton, "Credibility Challenged, Former NY Steward Erupts at Baffert Hearing," *Thoroughbred Daily News*, January 27, 2022, https://www.thoroughbreddailynews.com/credibility-challenged-former-ny-steward-erupts-at-baffert-hearing/.

2　New York Racing Association in the Matter of Robert A. Baffert, New York, January 24, 2022.

3　New York Racing Association in the Matter of Robert A. Baffert.

4　"Bettors Lose Case Against Baffert, CDI in Appeals Court," *BloodHorse*, accessed September 18, 2024, https://www.bloodhorse.com/horse-racing/articles/276640/bettors-lose-case-against-baffert-cdi-in-appeals-court.

5　"Bettors Lose Case Against Baffert, CDI in Appeals Court."

6　New York Racing Association in the Matter of Robert A. Baffert.

7　New York Racing Association in the Matter of Robert A. Baffert.

8　New York Racing Association in the Matter of Robert A. Baffert.

9　O. Peter Sherwood, Hearing Report, New York Racing Association in the Matter of Robert A. Baffert, New York, April 27, 2022.

10　John Cherwa, "Bob Baffert Returns to Santa Anita Park after Suspension Expires," *Los Angeles Times*, July 4, 2022, https://www.latimes.com/sports/story/2022-07-03/bob-baffert-returns-to-santa-anita-park-after-suspension.

CHAPTER 24　HATE THE GAME, NOT THE PLAYER

1　New York Task Force on Racehorse Health and Safety, "Investigation of Equine Fatalities at Aqueduct 2011-2012 Fall/Winter Meet," September 2012, https://www.gaming.ny.gov/pdf/NY%20Task%20Force%20on%20Racehorse%20Health%20and%20Safety.pdf.

2　Natalie Voss, "Will Todd Get 'The Baffert Treatment'?" Paulick Report, June 15, 2023, https://paulickreport.com/news/ray-s-paddock/will-todd-get-the-baffert-treatment.

3　Todd Pletcher, September 18, 2024.

4　"NY Court to Weigh Due Process Rights in Pletcher Case," *BloodHorse*, accessed September 9, 2024, https://www.bloodhorse.com/horse-racing/articles/275920/ny-court-to-weigh-due-process-rights-in-pletcher-case.

5　New York State Gaming Commission license search, September 18, 2024, https://breakdown.gaming.ny.gov/index.php.

6　New York State Gaming Commission license search.

7　Bob Baffert, January 4, 2023.

8　Bob Baffert, January 2, 2023.

9　Rick Arthur, January 4, 2024.

10　Joe Drape, "Horse Racing; Lukas Makes Himself Seen and Heard Once Again," *New York Times*, May 30, 1999, https://www.nytimes.com/1999/05/30/sports/horse-racing-lukas-makes-himself-seen-and-heard-once-again.html.

11 Bob Baffert, January 4, 2023.

12 Eoin Harty, January 16, 2023.

13 Steve Lewandowski, June 26, 2024.

14 Bob Baffert, March 15, 2024.

15 Ogden Mills Phipps, "Phipps: When It Comes to Drug-Testing Reform, Transparency a Good Place to Start," Paulick Report, April 14, 2014, https://paulickreport.com/news/phipps-to -asmussen-stay-hom.

16 Bob Baffert, January 4, 2023.

17 "Baffert, Zedan Dropping Appeal of Medina Spirit Case," *BloodHorse*, accessed September 9, 2024, https://www.bloodhorse.com/horse-racing/articles/274605/baffert-zedan-dropping -appeal-of-medina-spirit-case.

18 "Churchill Downs Extends Ban of Baffert Through 2024," *BloodHorse*, accessed September 9, 2024, https://www.bloodhorse.com/horse-racing/articles/269893/churchill-downs-extends -ban-of-baffert-through-2024.

19 Bob Baffert, March 15, 2024.

20 Bob Baffert, January 4, 2023.

21 Cecilia Vega, "Horse Racing Cleaning Up Its Act under New Anti-Doping Rules," *60 Minutes*, CBS News, November 12, 2023, https://www.cbsnews.com/news/horse-racing-anti-doping -racetrack-safety-60-minutes-transcript/.

22 Bill Finley, "Addressing the 60 Minutes Piece, a Q&A with Stuart Janney III," *Thoroughbred Daily News*, November 28, 2023, https://www.thoroughbreddailynews.com/addressing-the -60-minutes-piece-a-q-a-with-stuart-janney-iii/.

23 Max Hodge, "Letter to the Editor: 'Give the Jockey Club to the Industry,'" *Thoroughbred Daily News*, November 14, 2023, https://www.thoroughbreddailynews.com/letter-to-the -editor-give-the-jockey-club-to-the-industry/.

24 *The Nick Luck Daily Podcast*, January 6, 2024.

25 Chad Brown, June 28, 2024.

CHAPTER 25 "WE'RE ALL JUST WHORES"?

1 "Horse Racing Anti-Doping Program," C-SPAN, accessed September 23, 2024, https:// www.c-span.org/video/?447431-1/horse-racing-anti-doping-program.

2 Karen Murphy, March 22, 2024.

3 Joe Drape, "Despite the Evidence, Trainers Deny a Doping Problem," *New York Times*, November 23, 2013, https://www.nytimes.com/2013/11/23/sports/despite-the-evidence-trainers-deny -a-doping-problem.html.

4 Matt Miller, "Trainer Pleads Guilty in Penn National Horse Doping Case," PennLive, December 17, 2014, https://www.pennlive.com/midstate/2014/12/horse_trainer_pleads_guilty _in.html.

5 "Horse Racing Anti-Doping Program."

6 "Horse Racing Anti-Doping Program."

7 Thomas M. Hunt, Scott R. Jedlicka, and Matthew T. Bowers, "Drugs, the Law, and the Downfall of Dancer's Image at the 1968 Kentucky Derby: A Case Study on Human Conceptions of Domesticated Animals," *International Journal of the History of Sport* 31, no. 8 (May 24, 2014): 902–13, https://doi.org/10.1080/09523367.2014.894024.

8 Toby, *Unnatural Ability*, 192.

9 Natalie Voss, "Veterinary Records Reveal Laoban's Last Season Punctuated by Difficulties in the Breeding Shed," Paulick Report, February 2, 2024, https://paulickreport.com/horse-care -category/veterinary-records-reveal-laobans-last-season-punctuated-by-difficulties-in-the -breeding-shed.

10 Seth Hancock, November 15, 2023.

11 "Jockey Club Asks US Judge to Dismiss Stallion Cap Lawsuit," *Thoroughbred Report*, April 1, 2021, https://www.ttrausnz.com.au/edition/2021-04-01/jockey-club-asks-us-judge-to-dismiss-stallion-cap-lawsuit.

12 22RS HB 496, Kentucky Legislature, accessed September 23, 2024, https://apps.legislature.ky.gov/record/22rs/hb496.html.

13 Dave Brynes, "Illinois Racetrack, State Racing Board Face RICO Claims over Dead Horses," Courthouse News Service, September 12, 2024, https://www.courthousenews.com/illinois-racetrack-state-racing-board-face-rico-claims-over-dead-horses/.

14 Natalie Voss, "Despite HISA Oversight, Parx Turf Course's Seasonal Bow Had a Bobble," Paulick Report, September 23, 2024, https://paulickreport.com/news/thoroughbred-racing/despite-hisa-oversight-parx-turf-courses-seasonal-bow-had-a-bobble.

15 Damian Williams, "Re: United States v. Jorge Navarro," US Department of Justice, December 10, 2021.

16 John Williams, October 27, 2023.

17 "HISA's First Quarter Metrics Show 38 Percent Decline in Racing Fatalities," Paulick Report, June 12, 2024, https://paulickreport.com/news/the-biz/hisas-first-quarter-metrics-show-38-percent-decline-in-racing-fatalities.

18 "Review of the 2023 Equine Fatalities at the Saratoga Race Course," New York State Gaming Commission, July 29, 2024.

19 "First Horse Racing Fatality of the 2024 Season in Saratoga Springs," WRGB, August 30, 2024, https://cbs6albany.com/news/local/first-horse-fatality-of-the-2024-season-in-saratoga-springs.

20 Scott Leeds, "Letter to the Editor: One Small Step for Horse Racing," *Thoroughbred Daily News*, August 29, 2024, https://www.thoroughbreddailynews.com/letter-to-the-editor-one-small-step-for-horse-racing/; "Letter to the Editor: When It Comes to Vet Scratches, 'An Abundance of Caution Is Never an Embarrassment,'" Paulick Report, September 12, 2024, https://paulickreport.com/news/ray-s-paddock/letter-to-the-editor-when-it-comes-to-vet-scratches-an-abundance-of-caution-is-never-an-embarrassment.

21 Horseracing Integrity and Welfare Unit, "HIWU'S Report on Its Investigation of the University of Kentucky Equine Analytical Chemistry Laboratory," September 17, 2024, https://assets.ctfassets.net/6mwruzwftvzd/Sj3O8SkfljUrd8wnYC9R3/a1e62deab146d80d8389ad839b4fab4b/HIWU_UK_INVESTIGATION_-_PUBLIC_REPORT_-_9.17.24_-FINAL.pdf.

22 "'Claims Are Made Without Evidence' As Dr. Scott Stanley's Attorney Responds to HIWU Accusations," *Thoroughbred Daily News*, October 4, 2024, https://www.thoroughbreddailynews.com/claims-are-made-without-evidence-as-dr-scott-stanleys-attorney-responds-to-hiwu-accusations/.

23 Bob Baffert, January 2, 2023.

24 Rick Sams, email, September 18, 2024; Natalie Voss, "What People Are Afraid of in the Wake of the UK Lab Story," Paulick Report, Patreon, n.d, https://www.patreon.com/posts/what-people-are-112366542.

25 Chelsea Hackbarth, "Welfare Summit: McKinsey Report Provides 'How To' Guide to Further Lower Fatalities," Paulick Report, June 25, 2024, https://paulickreport.com/horse-care-category/welfare-summit-mckinsey-report-provides-how-to-guide-to-further-lower-fatalities-.

26 Hackbarth, "Welfare Summit."

27 "What Is the Secret That Enables Germany to Punch so Far above Its Weight in Breeding; Topics: Deutsches Derby, Monsun, Germany, Direktorium," *Thoroughbred Racing*, accessed September 9, 2024, https://www.thoroughbredracing.com/articles/2147/country-where-stallions-who-have-ever-had-lasix-are-disqualified-breeding/.

28 Stuart Janney, June 26, 2024.

29 Fred Pope, "Racing's Upside Down Distribution Model," *Thoroughbred Daily News*, https://www.thoroughbreddailynews.com/pdf/oped/7-17i%20Op%20Ed.pdf.

30 Stuart Janney, June 26, 2024.

31 Kylie A. Legg et al., "A Bioeconomic Model for the Thoroughbred Racing Industry—Optimisation of the Production Cycle with a Horse Centric Welfare Perspective," *Animals: An Open Access Journal from MDPI* 13, no. 3 (January 30, 2023): 479, https://doi.org/10.3390/ani13030479.

32 Laura Hillenbrand, *Seabiscuit: An American Legend* (New York: Ballantine Books, 2003), 274.

33 Bob Baffert, March 15, 2024.

EPILOGUE

1 "Churchill Downs Suspends Saffie Joseph Jr. Indefinitely," NBC News, May 4, 2023, https://www.nbcsports.com/betting/horse-racing/news/churchill-downs-suspends-saffie-joseph-jr-indefinitely.

2 Natalie Voss, "Dead Horse's Medical Records Cast Light on Baffert's Evolving Relationship with Betamethasone," Paulick Report, September 5, 2023, https://paulickreport.com/news/the-biz/dead-horses-medical-records-cast-light-on-bafferts-evolving-relationship-with-betamethasone.

3 Shaun Richards, September 18, 2024.

4 Chelsea Hackbarth, "Dr. Scott Shell Suspended Two Years, Fined Total of $35,000 for 228 Hemo 15 Injections," Paulick Report, June 20, 2024, https://paulickreport.com/news/the-biz/dr-scott-shell-suspended-two-years-fined-total-of-35000-for-228-hemo-15-injections.

5 Todd Pletcher, September 18, 2024.

6 Natalie Voss, "Voss: Former UK Lab Director Equates SGF-1000 to Cold Water Therapy; Here's Why That's a Problem," Paulick Report, September 11, 2024, https://paulickreport.com/news/ray-s-paddock/voss-former-uk-lab-director-equates-sgf-1000-to-cold-water-therapy-heres-why-thats-a-problem.

7 "Jockey Club of Saudia Arabia and Jason Servis: Decision and Sanction," Jockey Club of Saudi Arabia, 2024.

8 Ray Paulick, "Will A New Chairman Shake Up The Jockey Club?," Paulick Report Patreon, November 19, 2024.

9 Ray Paulick, "Stuart Janney to Retire; Everett Dobson Chosen as Next Chair of the Jockey Club," Paulick Report, November 19, 2024, https://paulickreport.com/news/people/stuart-janney-to-retire-everett-dobson-chosen-as-next-chair-of-the-jockey-club.

10 Stuart Janney, June 26, 2024.

11 Wendell Berry, *Sex, Economy, Freedom, and Community* (New York: Pantheon, 1993).

12 Bob Baffert, text message, Juy 19, 2024.

ABOUT THE AUTHOR

Katie Bo Lillis is a senior reporter at CNN covering intelligence and national security. She previously worked for Defense One, where she traveled the Middle East covering America's wars. But she was raised in the saddle in rural Virginia, and her first love was Thoroughbred horse racing. She now lives on a farmette with a small barn in northern Virginia with her husband and son.